The Business of Private
Medical Practice

Critical Issues in Health and Medicine

Edited by Rima D. Apple, University of Wisconsin–Madison, and Janet Golden, Rutgers University, Camden

Growing criticism of the U.S. health care system is coming from consumers, politicians, the media, activists, and healthcare professionals. Critical Issues in Health and Medicine is a collection of books that explores these contemporary dilemmas from a variety of perspectives, among them political, legal, histori-cal, sociological, and comparative, and with attention to crucial dimensions such as race, gender, ethnicity, sexuality, and culture.

For a list of titles in the series, see the last page of the book.

The Business of Private Medical Practice

Doctors, Specialization, and Urban Change in Philadelphia, 1900–1940

James A. Schafer Jr.

Rutgers University Press

New Brunswick, New Jersey, and London

Library of Congress Cataloging-in-Publication Data

Schafer, James A., Jr., 1974– author.
   The business of private medical practice : doctors, specialization, and urban change in
Philadelphia, 1900–1940 / James A. Schafer Jr.
      p. ;   cm. — (Critical issues in health and medicine)
   Includes bibliographical references and index.
   ISBN 978–0–8135–6175–2 (hardcover : alk. paper) — ISBN 978–0–8135–6174–5 (pbk. :
alk. paper) — ISBN 978–0–8135–6176–9 (e-book)
   I. Title II. Series: Critical issues in health and medicine.
   [DNLM: 1. Private Practice—history—Philadelphia. 2. History, 20th Century—
Philadelphia. 3. Physicians—history—Philadelphia. 4. Urban Health Services—history—
Philadelphia. WZ 70 AP4]
   R728
   610.68—dc23   2013005962

A British Cataloging-in-Publication record for this book is available from the British Library.

Visit our website: http://rutgerspress.rutgers.edu

Manufactured in the United States of America

For my family, friends, mentors, students, and colleagues

Contents

Figures

Maps

Tables

Acknowledgments

As I near the end of this long journey, it is a great pleasure to reflect upon the many family, friends, mentors, students, and colleagues who have given me inspiration and encouragement over the years. Without them, this book would not have been possible. I first want to thank my parents, Jim and Margy, and my sister, Kirsti, for their unwavering love and support. I could not have asked for a more supportive and loving family. I attribute my love of knowledge and teaching to my parents, who have always served as my role models for the lifelong pursuit of education and intellectual exchange, both formal and informal.

When I began this research project back in 2002, as a doctoral candidate in the Program of the History of Science, Medicine, and Technology at Johns Hopkins University, many terrific professors helped me to formulate my ideas, long before I knew that my ideas would germinate and grow into a book. Mary E. Fissell spent countless hours helping me to develop my primary source research and interpretation skills. I apply everyday what I learned during my fieldwork with Mary. Graham Mooney provided timely suggestions on historical geography as my research headed in that direction. I am also indebted to Daniel P. Todes for his patient and careful advice. He saved me from many professional blunders and taught me about the practical challenges and rewards of the academic workplace. I also learned so much from my fellow students. Special thanks are due to the wonderful participants of the Dissertation Reading Group: Alexa Green, Andy Russell, Eric Nystrom, Hyungsub Choi, Allison Marsh, Massimo Petrozzi, and Melissa Grafe. Finally, I owe a huge debt of gratitude to my advisor, the late Professor Harry M. Marks. He welcomed a scientist-historian as his graduate student, and tailored my education to meet my needs and interests. Above all, he challenged me to become a well-rounded scholar, and I can only try to meet his high standards.

Since graduate school, I have been privileged to work with many energetic and generous colleagues and friends. Scott Knowles and Amy Slaton helped me to translate my research to a larger historical audience during my postdoctoral year at Drexel University. Martin Melosi, Jim Martin, and Eric Walther helped to bring me to the University of Houston in Fall 2008. Since arriving in Houston, Chairpersons Bob Buzzanco, John Hart, and Nancy Beck Young helped me to settle in and to make the most of intramural research support opportunities. As I began major revisions to my book manuscript, Todd Romero and Nancy Beck

Young took me under their wing with good humor, reading countless drafts and offering me encouragement to move forward when I needed it most. So many other colleagues have welcomed me to the University of Houston and have given me the gift of their time and wisdom, and I feel very lucky to have landed at such a fine institution. In particular, I'd like to thank Kairn Kleiman, Landon Storrs, Natalia Milanesio, Monica Perales, Raul Ramos, Philip Howard, Joseph Pratt, Mark Goldberg, Helen Valier, and Bill Monroe. Frank Holt also provided very timely and much needed editorial suggestions at an important moment in my revisions. Up the bayou at Rice University, I have also received critical feedback on my research from Cyrus Mody, Rebecca Goetz, Caleb McDaniel, and Wilson Will. Finally, from outside of Houston, Christopher Crenner helped me to rethink the central framework for the book by offering constructive criticism on full drafts of the manuscript at two very different phases of the revision process.

This book would not have been possible without generous funding from the following libraries, museums, and archives in Philadelphia: a Wood Resident Research Fellowship from the Library of the College of Physicians of Philadelphia (2002–2003); a Library Resident Research Fellowship from the American Philosophical Society (2002–2003); a Gloeckner Research Fellowship from the Archives and Special Collections on Women in Medicine and Homeopathy of the Drexel University College of Medicine (2003–2004); and a Mellon Visiting Research Fellowship from the Library Company of Philadelphia and the Historical Society of Pennsylvania (2003–2004). At the University of Houston, a New Faculty Research Grant (2010) also provided a vital boost to my follow up research and early manuscript revisions, along with a Junior Faculty Leave from my department during the Fall 2012 semester.

Without archivists, librarians, and other technical experts, historians would be lost in the tall grass. Christine Ruggere at the Rare Book Room of the Institute of the History of Medicine was my first port of call for many early research projects. I also had the great pleasure to work with Joanne Grossman and Barbara Williams at the Drexel University Archives and Special Collections. Joanne, in particular, helped me to identify many papers I might otherwise have overlooked. Special thanks are also due to Mike Angelo at Thomas Jefferson University Archive, to Max E. Moeller at the Historical Society of Pennsylvania, to Valerie Lutz at the American Philosophical Society, and to Ed Morman, all of whom made special efforts, despite being understaffed and overworked, to see that I had made full use of the rich archival resources in Philadelphia. Mary Alice Ernish also provided timely statistical advice during the early days of data collection and interpretation for this project. I also consulted at critical junctures with Amy Hillier at the Cartographic Modeling Lab of the University of Pennsylvania, who helped me determine the best use of technology for my historical needs. Bryce Schimanski and my brother-in-law, Tommaso Lesnick, also helped me to present my story in graphic form.

Finally, I would like to thank my best friend, domestic partner, and the love of my life, Jane, whom I cannot thank enough for all of her love and support. I could not have done this without you, Jane. You are my bedrock and the sweetness in my life. I look forward to our journey together, wherever it may lead. And to our son Julius—thank you for helping me to see the world in new ways, with love, patience, and wonder . . .

Abbreviations

AMA American Medical Association

AMD *American Medical Directory*

BHM *Bulletin of the History of Medicine*

CBD Central Business District

DUCOM Archives Archives and Special Collections on Women in Medicine and Homeopathy, Drexel University College of Medicine

HSP Historical Society of Pennsylvania

PCMS Philadelphia County Medical Society

PMJ *Pennsylvania Medical Journal*

JAMA *Journal of the American Medical Association* (issued 1883–1960; renamed *JAMA* in 1960)

LCPP Library of the College of Physicians of Philadelphia

TJU Archives Thomas Jefferson University Archives and Special Collections

UPA University of Pennsylvania Archives

WR *The Weekly Roster* (title varied, sometimes *The Weekly Roster and Medical Digest* or *The Weekly Roster of the Medical Organizations of Philadelphia*; issued 1905–1942; preceded by *Proceedings of the Philadelphia County Medical Society* and continued by *Philadelphia Medicine*)

The Business of Private
Medical Practice

Introduction

The health care "system" in the United States has many problems, with rising costs and declining access being the two most intractable. By any measure, we have the most expensive health care system in the world. As I write this introduction, the latest data on national health expenditure (NHE) show that the United States spent $2.6 trillion in 2010. This tally was equivalent to $8,402 per person and comprised 17.9 percent of the gross domestic product (GDP). To put these daunting figures in perspective, since 1960, when the United States spent $148 per person and 5.1 percent of GDP on health care, our NHE has been increasing faster than any other nation in the world: in 2010, the next most expensive health care systems spent $5,388 per person (Norway) and 12.0 percent of GDP (the Netherlands).[1] Unlike all other wealthy industrial nations, however, we lack universal health care, and many people in the United States have little or no access to basic health services.

Since the mid-twentieth century, our system has become a hybrid of private, employment-based health insurance and public health insurance for veterans, the elderly, poor children, and very poor non-elderly adults.[2] Because the majority of people in the United States receive health care benefits from their employers, this system is sensitive to economic downturns: during the aftermath of the latest recession, when average annual unemployment peaked at 9.6 percent of the workforce in 2010, the number of uninsured spiked to 49.9 million. This group of uninsured people comprised more than 1 in 5 American adults (aged 18 to 64 years).[3] To make matters worse, the size of our public insurance "safety net," already inadequate before the latest recession, has only been shrinking with state budgetary shortfalls, with political aversion to taxation to support social programs, and with growing cynicism about the value and necessity of the social welfare state. Even if the Patient Protection and Affordable Care Act of 2010 manages to survive ongoing legal and political challenges, an estimated 30 million people will remain uninsured, to say nothing of the millions of underinsured Americans who will remain but one major illness away from bankruptcy.[4]

Rising costs and declining access are more than esoteric policy concerns, as being uninsured (or underinsured) leads many Americans to forgo needed care, whether preventive, diagnostic, or curative: for example, nearly 1 in 14 Americans did not receive needed health care in 2010 because of cost.[5] Forgoing needed care leads to worse health care outcomes and higher costs for uninsured Americans. It means that progressive diseases, like cancer, are detected at later stages, with more dire prognoses.[6] Problems of health care access, in other words, cause suffering and preventable deaths. The Institute of Medicine estimated that in the year 2000, over 18,000 American adults (aged 25–64 years) died from causes attributable to lack of health insurance.[7] More recent analysis placed the number even higher, at more than 35,000 annually by 2005—equivalent to the tenth leading cause of death that year and greater than the number of deaths to due septicemia (34,136), suicide (32,637), chronic liver disease and cirrhosis (27,530), primary hypertension and hypertensive renal disease (24,902), Parkinson's disease (19,544), and homicide (18,124).[8]

Lack of access to affordable health care is not only linked to cost and insurance status, but to a variety of social and economic variables including age, race/ethnicity, income, employment status, size of employee group, and, of central importance for this book, place of residence. In a loosely regulated, free market economy supplied mostly by private producers and providers, health care goods and services are unevenly distributed, as producers and providers seek to maximize profit rather than to satisfy underlying needs. Where you live, in other words, largely determines what health care goods and services you can access, let alone afford. *The Business of Private Medical Practice* examines the origins of one of our health care access problems: the uneven distribution of doctor's offices, or private medical practices.

Even though private practice has consistently ranked as the first or second largest type of health expenditure over the last one hundred years, the structure and distribution of private practices have changed considerably.[9] In the early twentieth century, most doctors practiced out of their homes, with a shingle hung on the front stoop and patients recruited from the immediate neighborhood. As cities grew and mass transportation improved, doctors began to separate home and office, instead renting offices in central business districts in which they could treat patients recruited from an entire metropolitan area. Whether in the home or in the office, though, private practice remained an individual affair, as group practices were uncommon, especially large ones. As such, most doctors were solo practitioners who ran their private practices not unlike a small business, with the hopes of profit pinned to a large degree on office location.[10] With the rise of third-party payment, through private insurance companies by the 1950s and government agencies by the late 1960s, the administrative overhead for private practice began to grow considerably, and most doctors had to hire clerical staff to process the onerous paperwork generated in our inefficient system.[11] With mounting costs, solo private practice became less desirable, let alone feasible. Instead, especially with the rise of managed care and health maintenance organizations by the 1980s, more and more doctors began joining large, corporate-owned, group practices as salaried employees rather than opening individually owned or small group practices. Managed care practices have spared doctors from large start-up costs and some of the administrative hassles of billing; on the other hand, salary bonuses have incentivized short office visits and high patient throughput per diem, thereby reducing the job satisfaction of doctor-employees and compromising the quality and continuity of care for patient-customers.[12]

Alongside changes in the structure of private practice during the twentieth century, the distribution of doctors relative to the population also shifted radically. The 1920 federal census marked the first time in American history that the majority of Americans lived in communities larger than 2,500 people.[13] Despite the emergence of the United States as an urban nation, early health care economists and health policy reformers in the 1920s and 1930s noticed that doctors and hospitals were urbanizing more rapidly than the rest of the population. For the next several decades, most scholarly and policy discussion of access and distribution problems in American health care focused on these rural-urban divisions.[14] Such parochial concerns reflected the political climate during these years, when ambitious proposals to create universal access through national health insurance never gained enough support to reach the floor of the House of Representatives or the Senate. Instead, only incremental reforms that transcended political party and regional divisions could be legislated, such as the Hill-Burton Act of 1946, which provided grants and loans for hospital construction, especially in rural areas, or the Emergency Health Personnel Act of 1970, which created the National Health Service Corps to recruit young medical students and doctors to practice in "medically underserved" areas, especially rural counties, in exchange for medical school scholarships and student loan forgiveness.[15] Despite these and other initiatives, the problem of rural access to health care endures, though faster transportation and greater numbers of regional hospitals have provided some relief.[16]

The Business of Private Medical Practice focuses instead on the growing problem of access to doctor's offices *within* American cities, a topic neglected in early scholarly and political attention to rural-urban divisions at the county, state, or regional level. Health economists and social geographers only began to study intra-urban health care in the late 1960s, when the inner-city doctor shortage was first "discovered." Titles of provocative policy studies asked, "Where have the doctors gone?" or asserted that doctors were "misused" and "misplaced."[17] Much of the early literature focused narrowly on professional factors shaping the location of private practices, such as proximity to teaching hospitals.[18] But even the work that examined broader social and economic predictors of office location in cities, such as poverty and race, did not explore structural causes of maldistributed health care services, such as the profit motives of private doctors in a free market economy or the effects of urban change on resource distribution more generally.[19] Finally, most of the work in the 1960s and 1970s was ahistorical, only characterizing "the urban health crisis" rather than finding its first appearance. As a result, we still have almost no analysis of the origins, let alone the consequences, of unevenly distributed private medical practices in early twentieth-century American cities.[20]

In order to undertake more thorough examination of intra-urban doctor shortages and their relation to broader social inequality, this book relies upon a longitudinal case study of a single, informative, rapidly changing, industrial metropolis—Philadelphia, Pennsylvania—from 1900 to 1940. From the perspective of medical history, beginning this study in the year 1900 focuses analysis on the period of time after which the "medical marketplace" had acquired most of the regulatory and professional institutions we have today, from state licensing boards to more standardized medical schools and hospitals to a centralized and powerful American Medical Association.[21] Because these institutions severely restricted supply, they transformed the market for private medical practice, thereby making comparisons to earlier patterns of practice location more difficult, when doctors still competed with a diverse cast of healers for optimal locations and wealthy clientele. Ending the study in the year 1940 has the advantage of limiting analysis to the period of time before which third parties transformed payment in the medical marketplace. Because third parties imposed new billing practices that demanded ever more labor-intensive administration, they ushered in changes to the structure of private practices, as once small businesses gave way to larger firms and investor-owned corporations. However, the office location calculus for partners or corporate chief executive officers changed little from what had been established in the early twentieth century. Thus, this historical study of Philadelphia sheds light on the urban origins of some of our most fundamental health care access problems today.

From the perspective of both medical history and urban history, Philadelphia offers a good opportunity to study the geography of early twentieth-century private medical practice. Not only does Philadelphia have numerous rich repositories of archival material about doctors, but the city was well researched by scholars and public officials in this period. As such, there is no shortage of extant primary source material on the business of private practice in Philadelphia or on the broader social and economic forces that shaped the medical marketplace in the city. Furthermore, as the third largest city in this period, Philadelphia invites comparisons to other early industrial metropolises across the United States.

In order to identify proper cities for comparison, there are two primary considerations. First, what large cities had similar medical infrastructure, such as number of medical schools, annual production of medical graduates, doctor-to-population ratio, and hospital-bed-to-population ratio? Philadelphia was the leading medical center in the English colonies and Early Republic and its reputation was built largely on its precocious medical institutions. The city boasted the first public hospital (established in 1731), what became Philadelphia Almshouse Infirmary and later Philadelphia General Hospital; the first private hospital, Pennsylvania Hospital (established in 1751); and the first medical school, the University of Pennsylvania School of Medicine (established in 1765). The establishment of these early institutions reflected the peculiar social organization and health care needs of America's first metropolis, and these institutions in turn shaped the kinds of doctors who practiced in Philadelphia and the nature of the medical marketplace therein.[22] Even after New York City and Chicago overtook it in size, Philadelphia kept pace in the development of its medical infrastructure, remaining a top destination for medical students and doctors from around the United States (tables 1 and 2). For these reasons, New York and Chicago make obvious points of comparison, though a few smaller large cities, especially Boston, had similarly extensive medical infrastructure.[23] By contrast, rapidly emerging metropolises in the early- to mid-twentieth century,

Table 1. Medical Infrastructure, Ten Largest American Cities, c. 1910

City	Population		Medical Schools		Medical Graduates		Doctor Ratio		Hospital Bed Ratio		Specialization Rate (%)	
New York City	4,766,883	(1)	8	(2)	329	(3)	1:540	(9)	1:221	(4)	11.1	(6)
Chicago	2,185,283	(2)	12	(1)	599	(1)	1:479	(5)	1:305	(8)	13.1	(3)
Philadelphia	1,549,008	(3)	6	(5)	402	(2)	1:431	(3)	1:246	(7)	12.8	(4)
St. Louis	687,029	(4)	7	(3)	230	(5)	1:405	(2)	1:223	(5)	15.0	(2)
Boston	670,585	(5)	4	(6)	158	(6)	1:357	(1)	1:208	(3)	12.2	(5)
Cleveland	560,663	(6)	3	(7)	40	(9)	1:584	(10)	1:342	(10)	7.8	(9)
Baltimore	558,485	(7)	7	(3)	242	(4)	1:467	(4)	1:198	(2)	17.0	(1)
Pittsburgh	533,905	(8)	1	(9)	53	(7)	1:516	(7)	1:164	(1)	4.7	(10)
Detroit	465,766	(9)	2	(8)	45	(8)	1:492	(6)	1:327	(9)	10.8	(7)
Buffalo	423,715	(10)	1	(9)	34	(10)	1:526	(8)	1:232	(6)	8.5	(8)
United States	91,972,266		131		4,440		1:609		1:590		Not tabulated	

Notes: Rankings are listed in parentheses. Other than population, rankings are relative, not absolute. Doctor ratio is the number of residents per single doctor. Hospital bed ratio is the number of residents per single hospital and sanitarium bed. Specialization rate is the percentage of doctors in a city who have limited their private practices to a particular specialty, such as pediatrics or gynecology.

Sources: U.S. Bureau of the Census, *Historical Statistics of the United States: Colonial Times to 1970*, Bicentennial Edition, part 1 (Washington, DC: U.S. G.P.O., 1975), 8, 76; U.S. Bureau of Census, *Thirteenth Census of the United States: 1910*, vol. 4 (Washington, DC: U.S. G.P.O., 1910), 93, 164–65, 178, 192–93, 206; U.S. Bureau of Census, *Benevolent Institutions: 1910* (Washington, DC: U.S. G.P.O., 1913), 48, 272–75, 290–95, 300–301, 308–11, 320–31, 336–39, 346–49; *AMD* (1909). 32–41; and Campbell Gibson, "Population of the 100 Largest Cities and Other Urban Places in the United States: 1790–1990," Population Division Working Paper no. 27 (Washington, DC: 1998). Specialization rates calculated from skip-interval samples of doctors in each city as listed in the *AMD* (1909). Sample sizes were as follows: New York City (5%), Chicago (5%), Philadelphia (20%), St. Louis (10%), Boston (10%), Cleveland (20%), Baltimore (12.5%), Pittsburgh (12.5%), Detroit (20%), and Buffalo (20%).

Table 2. Medical Infrastructure, Ten Largest American Cities, 1940

City	Population		Medical Schools		Medical Graduates		Doctor Ratio		Hospital Bed Ratio		Specialization Rate (%)	
New York City	7,454,995	(1)	5	(1)	427	(3)	1:445	(1)	1:119	(7)	37.4	(5)
Chicago	3,396,808	(2)	5	(1)	574	(1)	1:558	(7)	1:144	(8)	37.1	(7)
Philadelphia	1,931,334	(3)	5	(1)	523	(2)	1:527	(5)	1:86	(3)	38.3	(4)
Detroit	1,623,452	(4)	1	(8)	60	(8)	1:700	(9)	1:187	(9)	44.5	(1)
Los Angeles	1,504,277	(5)	2	(5)	144	(7)	1:493	(4)	1:189	(10)	34.4	(9)
Cleveland	878,336	(6)	1	(8)	58	(9)	1:865	(10)	1:109	(5)	39.9	(3)
Baltimore	859,100	(7)	2	(5)	168	(6)	1:470	(2)	1:110	(6)	34.2	(10)
St. Louis	816,048	(8)	2	(5)	201	(5)	1:590	(8)	1:67	(2)	37.3	(6)
Boston	770,816	(9)	3	(4)	282	(4)	1:491	(3)	1:62	(1)	36.6	(8)
Pittsburgh	671,659	(10)	1	(8)	46	(10)	1:545	(6)	1:107	(4)	43.6	(2)
United States	131,669,275		77		5,097		1:800		1:107			

Notes: Rankings are listed in parentheses. Other than population, rankings are relative, not absolute. Doctor ratio is the number of residents per single doctor. Hospital bed ratio is the number of residents per single hospital bed (including bassinets). Specialization rate is the percentage of doctors in a city who have limited their private practices to a particular specialty, such as pediatrics or gynecology, though includes both partial and full specialists.

Sources: U.S. Bureau of the Census, *Historical Statistics of the United States: Colonial Times to 1970,* Bicentennial Edition, part 1 (Washington, DC: U.S. G.P.O., 1975), 8, 76 78; U.S. Bureau of Census, *Sixteenth Census of the United States: 1940,* vol. 3 (Washington, DC: U.S. G.P.O., 1940): part 1, 75; part 2, 222, 864; part 3, 367, 468, 599, 864; part 4, 363, 365; part 5, 48, 52, 54, 58; Campbell Gibson, "Population of the 100 Largest Cities and Other Urban Places in the United States: 1790–1990," Population Division Working Paper no. 27 (Washington, DC: 1998); "Description of Medical Schools," *JAMA* 115, no. 9 (1940): 701–8; and *AMD* (1940). Specialization rates calculated from skip interval samples of doctors in each city as listed in the *AMD* (1940). Sample sizes were as follows: New York City (5%), Chicago (5%), Philadelphia (20%), Detroit (10%), Los Angeles (10%), Cleveland (10%) Baltimore (10%), St. Louis (10%), Boston (10%), and Pittsburgh (10%).

such as Detroit and Los Angeles, tended to have underdeveloped medical infrastructure. As a result, their medical marketplaces were likely less diverse or competitive, and were primarily occupied by medical students and doctors of local origin.[24] Finally, smaller large cities, such as Pittsburgh or Cincinnati, tended to have a single medical school and just a handful of teaching hospitals that were controlled by a coterie of city doctors.[25] This state of affairs yielded very different market conditions, though much more work is needed to understand the relationship of medical schools and hospitals to the geography of private medical practice.[26]

Besides being compared to cities having similar medical infrastructure, Philadelphia must also be compared to cities undergoing similar social and spatial transformation in the early twentieth century. Again, New York City and Chicago comprise obvious peers, as these cities experienced analogous changes wrought by foreign and domestic immigration, by the early development of mass transportation, and by the growth and suburbanization of a white-collar middle class. In each instance, the emergence of the modern American metropolis came with greater social inequality, as high-paying jobs, good schools, and affordable, safe, quality homes were only available to certain social groups and in certain locations. In short, the organization of urban space became yet another manifestation of inequality in American society, whether in employment, education, or housing. Other large American cities decentralized in this period, such as St. Louis, Detroit, and Baltimore, though without preserving vital central business districts tied to vast transportation networks, such as those found in New York City, Chicago, Philadelphia, or even San Francisco. Furthermore, latecomer metropolises, like Los Angeles or Houston, never had a massive industrial urban core that left an imprint on labor, politics, and social life in the city.[27] For all of these reasons—both urban and medical—the particular patterns of private practice location in early twentieth-century Philadelphia are best generalized to New York City, Chicago, Boston, and perhaps San Francisco, though divergences from dissimilar large cities would be informative.

Using the example of Philadelphia, along with judicious reference to what scholarship is available for comparable cities, this book places private medical practice, and health care more generally, in the context of urban change and social inequality in American history. At the heart of the book are the following questions (chapters 3 and 5): Where were doctor's offices located? How and why did the geography of private practice change over time? What were the consequences of maldistributed doctor's offices in American cities like Philadelphia? What does the historical geography of private medical practice reveal about deeper structural causes of America's broken health care system? In order to answer these questions, we need a greater understanding of American doctors and the private practice of medicine in the early twentieth century (chapters 1, 2, and 4).

Most of what is known about the activities of American doctors during the early twentieth century is limited to the historical literature on medical "professionalization." This scholarly corpus explores the political and institutional reform of medical education, licensing laws, hospital administration, and food and drug safety at the national level, as well as how orthodox doctors established a self-regulating monopoly in the medical marketplace by wresting economic power from other healers.[28] More recent studies have revised the grand narrative of medical professionalization by identifying lingering sources of discord that undermined political and institutional reforms and by identifying a persistent ethos of individualism among orthodox doctors, which foiled some attempts at market regulation. It is now clear that the era of medical professionalization by no means produced a homogenous or unified corporation of American doctors.[29]

Revisions aside, two blind spots persist in the historical literature on American doctors in the early twentieth century. First, by focusing on professional reformers, historical studies have lavished attention on a small number of elite doctors who had the time, money, and power to lead political and institutional reform movements. Although the effects of these reforms rippled through the profession and the wider medical marketplace, one has to wonder what non-elite doctors were doing at this time. In an effort to shift the focus, many historians have explored the consequences of education and licensing reform for practitioners at the margins of the medical marketplace, such as "sectarian" healers like homeopaths and osteopaths, and for practitioners who were targets of outright persecution, such as midwives and chiropractors.[30] Unfortunately, non-elite doctors within the orthodox medical profession in the early twentieth century, especially rank-and-file general practitioners, have not received similar attention.[31]

The second blind spot arising from a focus on professionalization is that profession-building activities, such as attending medical society meetings or lobbying state legislatures, comprised only a very small part of what most doctors actually did. During this period, ordinary doctors spent most of their time *practicing medicine*—an activity that was as much a mundane occupation as it was an idealistic or nefarious profession. Frankly, not much is known about the activities of doctors in private practice, apart from a handful of studies, most of which examine the biographies of individual doctors rather than exploring the dynamics of private practice as a health care service in a larger medical market-place. What factors led doctors to select one career path over another in private practice, such as specialization over general practice (chapters 1, 2, and 4)? How did doctors make a living from private practice (chapters 2 and 4)? What factors influenced the selection of an office location and therefore the distribution of private medical care in American cities (chapters 3 and 5)? Such questions about the social and economic history of ordinary doctors have been missing from the history of American medical practice in the early twentieth century.[32]

A richer picture of urban medical practice at this time emerges from careful analysis of the working lives and private practices of doctors from a representa-tive cross-section of the medical community in Philadelphia. To uncover this detail, I use the collected papers of doctors, especially autobiographical memoirs that detail the career paths, business practices, and location decisions of doctors in private practice. As is so often the case in historical research, however, few papers of ordinary doctors have survived, either because these doctors regarded their lives as unremarkable or because collectors typically sought the papers of "great doctors."[33] Fortunately, a vast prescriptive literature written for a broad medical audience survives. This literature, which includes editorials published in medical student bulletins, alumni newsletters, and local and state medical journals, addresses a wide array of professional and pocketbook issues affecting the working lives of ordinary doctors at various stages of their careers. In addi-tion, a rich how-to literature, from advice manuals to published medical school commencement and graduation speeches, reveals what factors influenced criti-cal career and business decisions for ordinary doctors as well as elites.

The Business of Private Medical Practice also draws upon a core of quanti-tative material on doctors derived from statistical samples of the Philadelphia doctors listed in the 1909 and 1940 editions of the *American Medical Direc-tory*. The *AMD* included a wide range of valuable information, including not only biographical and career data for doctors, but also their office locations.[34] These samples have been combined with supplemental data from local medi-cal directories, local medical society membership lists, city directories, and ward-level federal census data in 1910 and 1940. Using these rich data, it is possible for the first time to track longitudinal changes in the careers of a com-munity of American doctors, including increasing inclination to limit private practice to particular specialties, such as obstetrics or otorhinolaryngology (chapters 1 and 4).[35] By mapping the office locations of Philadelphia doctors, it is also possible to identify and explain the specific market forces that shaped the geography of private medical practice (chapters 3 and 5). Whenever possible, quantitative trends in private practice are further illustrated by specific examples taken from the autobiographies of Philadelphia doctors, from local and national prescriptive literature, and even from classified advertisements for office space published in local medical journals. This new methodology reveals that immigration and suburbanization altered not only the social and spatial order of Philadelphia, but also the location decisions of doctors and the distribution of health care services in the city.

The longitudinal study of the changing careers and private practices of Philadelphia doctors is divided into two parts in this book—roughly 1900 to 1920 (chapters 1, 2, and 3) and 1920 to 1940 (chapters 4 and 5). There are two reasons for partitioning the analysis in this way. First, 1920 marked the beginning of significant social shifts in Philadelphia, from foreign to domestic immigration as the source of population growth and from a more centralized city to a sprawling suburban metropolis. These changes affected not only the social structure of the city but the market niches available for private medical care. Second, 1920 also marked the acceleration of changes in the careers of doctors and the business of private medical practice, as doctors increasingly specialized their practices and associated their businesses and careers with medical institutions, such as hospitals and medical schools.

Modern specialists first appeared in large European cities in the early nineteenth century and began to prosper in the large hospitals and medical schools of major cities by late century.[36] The United States trailed European specialization for most of the nineteenth century, largely because of the smaller size of its cities and the relatively few medical institutions that had been established. But by 1880, specialization rates reached 13 percent in booming American cities with well-developed medical institutions, like Philadelphia. As hospitals and medical schools became central to medical education and training, the specialists who flourished in these growing institutions became accepted members and later leaders of the American medical profession.[37] With the standardization of graduate medical education after World War I, American doctors specialized at ever greater rates: specialists tripled in representation between 1925 and 1962, from one-quarter to three-quarters of all American doctors.[38]

Until very recently, historical studies of specialization have tended to focus on specialty formation at the national level.[39] Two conditions favored the early growth of specialties: first, specialists needed a large urban population in order to have adequate demand for their services; second, specialists needed wealthy patients who could afford expert services.[40] As final ingredients, specialization required a regulatory framework and a professional ethos that supported, or at least did not retard, specialty formation. As historian and sociologist George Weisz has detailed, these conditions varied considerably at the national level: France and the United States favored specialty formation, whereas Britain did not.[41] Besides examining specialty formation in general, historians have also identified the social, intellectual, and institutional origins of individual specialties, such as pediatrics, or subspecialties, such as cardiology, but again the level of analysis has typically been national rather than local.[42]

The Business of Private Medical Practice instead focuses analysis of specialists at the city level, thereby placing medical specialization in the context of the changing social geography and expanding medical marketplace of an American city. What benefits did urban doctors derive from limiting their private practices to particular specialties in the early twentieth century (chapters 1, 2, and 4)? How did the business practices of specialists differ from those of general practitioners (GPs) in private practice (chapters 2 and 4)? Finally, to what degree did the location decisions and behaviors of specialists and GPs diverge, and what does this reveal about new niches in the changing urban market for private medical care (chapters 3 and 5)?

That economic self-interest and market forces shaped doctors' career and business decisions in cities like Philadelphia is the premise, not the conclusion, of *The Business of Private Medical Practice.* Instead, the fundamental contribution of the book is to map the consequences of economic self-interest and changing market forces for the distribution of doctors' offices and for the growth of medical specialization in early twentieth-century American cities: health care services were unevenly distributed across social and spatial boundaries, with poor and immigrant neighborhoods having ever fewer doctor's offices; similarly, specialization was fueled by broader market forces, such as metropolitan growth, the lucrative potential of specialty practice, and the pressure for doctors to differentiate services in a competitive marketplace. No other study of private practice at this time has linked these two processes. The central argument of this book is that the inequitable distribution of health care goods and services and the uncontrolled growth of expensive, specialty care were (as they remain) the inevitable, though deeply flawed, consequences of the informal organization of private medical care in a free market economy. In particular, the patterns of health care inequities that we have today were forged during the urban transformation of the United States in the early twentieth century.

Part I

1900–1920

Chapter 1

The Primacy of Private Practice

In a small, well-worn memorandum book, young Dr. DeForest Porter Willard Jr. (1884–1957), kept track of the highlights of his life and career in Philadelphia in the early twentieth century (table 3). His parents began the memo book to record childhood milestones, such as first words spoken, but Dr. Willard assumed authorship during adolescence. Apart from jotting down personal triumphs, such as winning golf championships in 1912 and 1913 and purchasing a Fiat roadster in 1916, Dr. Willard devoted most of his entries to career achievements, such as deployment dates for his medical service during World War I. Many of Dr. Willard's early career achievements had become typical by the early twentieth century and probably appeared in the personal papers of many of his peers. For example, after graduating from the University of Pennsylvania and earning his license in 1908, Dr. Willard undertook a voluntary hospital internship—in his case at the University of Pennsylvania Hospital. After completing his internship in 1910, Dr. Willard established his private medical practice. Dr. Willard's next career steps warrant closer inspection as they reflect some of the new opportunities available to young doctors in the early twentieth century. He quickly secured a number of institutional appointments, including staff positions at several Philadelphia hospitals and teaching positions at his alma mater. In addition, Dr. Willard limited his private practice to a single medical specialty— orthopaedic surgery—only a few years after graduating from medical school. The example of Dr. Willard begs the question: how common or accessible was his career path to specialism?

Table 3. Selected Events from the Memo Book of Dr. DeForest P. Willard Jr., 1908–1917

1908	May	Earned M.D. from the University of Pennsylvania (Univ. of Penn.), third in class.
	July	Began internship at University Hospital (in West Philadelphia).
1910	April	Finished internship.
	September	Did "some work" at St. Mary's Hospital (Kensington).
	October	Started private practice at 1901 Chestnut Street (Center City).
	November	Assistant Surgeon in Pathology, Univ. of Penn.
		Staff in Surgical Dispensary, University Hospital (West Philadelphia).
		Private assistant to Dr. Ed Martin (Clinical Professor of Surgery at Univ. of Penn.).
		Consulting Surgeon at the State Hospital for the Insane (West Philadelphia).
1911	February	Assistant Orthopaedic Surgeon at University Hospital (West Philadelphia).
	March	Consulting Surgeon at Haddock Memorial Home (a small hospital for infants in Center City).
	July	Bought a new automobile.
	October	Lecturer in Anatomy at University Hospital's School for Nurses (West Philadelphia).
		Gave two papers at the Clinical Congress of Surgeons of North America.
	November	Published first article, "Beck's Bismuth Paste Treatment" in the *Therapeutic Gazette*.
	December	Assistant Instructor in Orthopaedic Surgery, Univ. of Penn.
1912	January	Clinical Assistant at the Orthopaedic Hospital (Center City).
	April	Assistant Instructor in Surgery, Univ. of Penn.
	May	Consulting Surgeon for the Home for Consumptives (Chestnut Hill).
	July	Won golf championship. Took fishing trip.
	August	Moved private practice office to 1933 Chestnut (Center City).
	September	Gave paper at the Pennsylvania State Medical Society Meeting.
1913	March	Published article on "flat foot."
	April	Ordained elder in 2nd Presbyterian Church.
	May	Gave paper on "Splenic Anemia" at Academy of Surgery—later published.
	August	Won another golf championship.

(continued)

Table 3.   **Selected Events from the Memo Book of Dr. DeForest P. Willard Jr.,**
1908–1917 (*continued*)

	September	Gave paper with Dr. Dickson at the State Medical Society Meeting—later published.
	October	Assistant Surgeon, Home of the Merciful Savior for Crippled Children (West Philadelphia).
1914	June	Presented paper on "Results of Treatment of Scoliosis by Abbot Method" before the American Orthopaedic Association (AOA) Meeting in Philadelphia.
		Elected Fellow of the College of Physicians of Philadelphia.
	August	Vacation at the Lake Placid Club.
	September	Gave two papers at the Pennsylvania State Medical Society Meeting.
1915	January	Assistant Surgeon at Orthopaedic Hospital (Center City).
	May	Presented on "Association of Static Deformities in Children" at AOA meeting in Detroit.
	October	Assistant in Orthopaedic Hospital (Center City).
	November	Instructor in Orthopaedic Surgery, Univ. of Penn.
		Dispensary Chief for "Ward Z" at University Hospital (West Philadelphia).
1916	May	Elected to AOA membership.
	June	Appointed to AOA Scoliosis Committee.
	August	Bought a new Fiat Roadster.
	October	Attended Clinical Congress of North American Surgeons.
	December	Gave paper to the Chester County Medical Society.
1917	April	Received commission as 1st Lieutenant in the U.S. Army Medical Officers Reserve Corps.
	May	Ordered into active service and deployed.

Note: The terms of service were not indicated in the memo book.

Source: "Memorandum of Events in the Life of DeForest Porter Willard," DeForest Porter Willard Papers, 1884–1957, Unprocessed Collection, box 1, HSP.

This chapter examines the significance of private practice for the medical careers and livelihoods of Philadelphia doctors. As institutions played ever-larger roles in medical education and training during the professionalization of medicine in the early twentieth century, did private medical practice begin to decline in its importance to doctors? Had getting institutional appointments replaced setting up a private practice as the ultimate career objective? In order to ascertain the enduring significance of private practice, the chapter begins with an explanation of the growing role of medical institutions, especially medical schools, boards of medical examiners, and hospitals, in shaping the early careers of medical graduates. Despite the increasing standardization of medical education in this period, medical careers and incomes diverged considerably after graduation. General practice remained the default career path, but with every new class of medical graduates, larger numbers of young doctors aspired to specialize their private practices in the early twentieth century. As the following analysis of medical careers illustrates, stark differences emerged in the career paths of specialists and general practitioners (GPs), particularly the tendency to hold institutional positions. Finally, this chapter explores the extent to which growth of specialization stratified the medical profession, as only a few doctors, like Dr. Willard, could specialize in this period. Specialty careers often eluded other doctors, especially female, African American, and working-class medical graduates.

Becoming a Doctor in the Early Twentieth Century

Before the late nineteenth century in the United States, all it took for a person to become a doctor was the ability to attract clients who were willing to pay for one's medical services. Anyone could practice medicine, of any kind, with little to no formal education at a medical school and without any formal clinical training in a hospital. Although having a medical degree or hospital training might have given a doctor competitive advantage in certain market niches, these were by no means part of a legal barrier to practice. Some states had passed medical practice and licensing laws in the Early Republic, the strictest of which required an aspiring doctor to pass an examination administered by an authorized state or local medical society. It is doubtful that these laws achieved their regulatory objectives, and nearly all such laws were repealed by mid-century during the populist wave of disestablishmentarianism that characterized Jacksonian America. From a legal standpoint, then, there was almost "free entry into the professional practice of medicine" by the start of the Civil War.[1] Pennsylvania had the dubious distinction of having been one of the few states that *never* enacted medical practice and licensing laws in the Early Republic.[2]

By the late nineteenth century, however, the medical marketplace witnessed renewed and even strengthened regulation—a transformation that is now well understood by historians of American medicine. Beginning in mid-century, the profession began to unify around efforts to reform medical institutions from within, especially medical schools, and to wrest power from alternative healers in the marketplace such as homeopaths. These developments

rejuvenated medical societies at the local, state, and national levels and culmi-
nated in the 1901 reorganization of the American Medical Association into
a well-coordinated, three-tiered federation of constituent medical societies
wherein local society members automatically joined at the state and national
level. Growing unity and more effective organization enabled the medical profession to apply greater pressure upon state legislatures to strengthen medical
practice and licensing laws. These appeals gained traction during the Progressive Era, when grassroots organizations, journalist muckrakers, and political
activists throughout the United States pursued a legislative reform agenda
in the name of public interest and safety. The AMA and state medical societies argued that poorly trained doctors and quack alternative healers harmed
the public, whereas professional orthodox doctors, certified and protected by
licensing laws, could better guard the public health against the emerging hazards of modern, industrial life.[3] Determining the true motivation behind professional medical reforms—whether humanitarian benevolence or economic
self-interest—need not deter us here. Of more importance for our purposes is
that two reforms affected the career paths of would-be doctors by limiting entry
into medical practice: medical education reform and the passage of medical
practice and licensing laws.

The number of American medical schools expanded dramatically in the
nineteenth century, from 4 medical schools in 1800 to the zenith of 162 medical
schools in 1906. The entrance requirements and curricula varied considerably,
however, from rigorous institutions of higher learning to fraudulent diploma
mills.[4] By the 1880s, a few elite medical schools, including the University
of Pennsylvania, had begun to reform their curricula, raise entrance requirements, increase the time to degree, and add laboratory and clinical instruction.
In 1893, the Johns Hopkins University School of Medicine raised the bar for
medical school reform by requiring a bachelor's degree for admission and by
establishing a graded, four-year curriculum that began with laboratory-based
basic science courses and ended with hospital-based clinical instruction.
Many American medical schools either resisted or could not afford to implement these reforms, and many of these schools were later forced to close due to
declining enrollment or by the passage of new laws that established more strin-
gent requirements for medical degrees. Several Philadelphia medical schools,
however, kept pace with the reforms begun by their colleagues at the University of Pennsylvania. Jefferson Medical College and Woman's Medical College
of Pennsylvania, for example, had increased their entrance requirements and
updated their curricula by 1900.[5] The early support for education reform in

Philadelphia's medical schools reflected a desire on the part of the Philadelphia medical profession to preserve (what they perceived to be) its status as America's "City of Medicine."

With momentum building for medical school reform, the emboldened Pennsylvania Medical Society vigorously advocated for medical practice and licensing legislation. In 1875 and 1877, the Pennsylvania Medical Society introduced and successfully lobbied for the passage of the first state laws regulating the practice of medicine through licensure; future versions closed what loopholes existed in these initial laws. An 1881 revision, for example, increased the punishment for unlicensed practice from a $50 penalty fee to a misdemeanor with a $100 fine or a one-year jail sentence. The next revision, in 1893, required that all doctors entering medical practice apply for a state license, and further stipulated that applicants must have a medical degree and pass an examination by a board of medical examiners appointed by the governor from among the members of a state medical society. The most significant revision created a Bureau of Medical Education and Licensure in 1911, which was empowered not only to examine every medical-degree-holding applicant but to inspect the instruction and facilities of every medical school in Pennsylvania. The bureau reported its findings to medical schools and could refuse to examine graduates from any school not meeting the standards defined in the law—or four years of high school education and "a medical and surgical course of four years."[6] Thus, in Pennsylvania, as in many other states during this period, medical practice and licensing laws reinforced medical school reform.[7]

By the early twentieth century, this rising tide of reform and lawmaking had ushered in significant barriers for those wishing to become doctors and practice medicine. Not only were the professional and legal standards increasing but the efforts to enforce these standards and punish violators intensified as well, with licensed doctors assisting in the identification of scofflaws. For example, the Philadelphia County Medical Society encouraged its members to get to know "the medical newcomers in your neighborhood" and urged doctors to report those suspected of being unlicensed "quacks."[8] Although it is impossible to quantify the results of the campaign, the gradual disappearance of diatribes about unlicensed or fraudulent practitioners in the PCMS newsletter and journal—*The Weekly Roster*—suggests that, at the very least, such competitors posed an ever-dwindling market threat to licensed doctors. Having a state medical license, and therefore having a medical degree from a recognized medical school, had become prerequisites for becoming a doctor in Philadelphia by the first decade of the twentieth century.

In addition to medical schools and boards of medical examiners, hospitals comprised the other growing institutional influence upon the careers of young doctors, especially in mid-sized to large cities where hospitals had been established in record numbers in the decades between the Civil War and World War I. As with the establishment of boards of medical examiners, medical education reform contributed to the growth of hospitals.[9] As reformers such as Charles Elliot at Harvard University rejected didactic lectures in favor of hands-on learning, many medical schools sought opportunities for their students to gain clinical experience. To this end, reform-minded schools began to establish relationships with nearby hospitals or construct their own teaching hospitals as early as the 1870s.[10] In Philadelphia, for example, the University of Pennsylvania School of Medicine, Jefferson Medical College, and Hahnemann Medical College all established teaching hospitals in the 1870s, and Woman's Medical College cobbled together clinical instruction at various Philadelphia hospitals, clinics, and dispensaries from the 1880s until the establishment of its own teaching hospital in 1913.[11] In exchange for opening their wards to medical students, hospitals secured cheap labor. Because most hospitals continued to serve as charity institutions of last resort into the early twentieth century, inpatients had little power to object to serving as the "clinical material" for medical education in exchange for the free or nearly free inpatient care they received.[12]

The influence of late nineteenth- and early twentieth-century hospitals upon undergraduate medical education was unmistakable, but how did hospitals affect the careers of young doctors? After all, as eminent ophthalmologist Dr. George Norris recalled after he graduated from the University of Pennsylvania School of Medicine in 1899, "hospitals in my early days were still in bad repute" among patients and practitioners alike.[13] Despite their association with indigent patients and charity care, hospitals still attracted doctors after graduation. Indeed the first major career choice after getting a medical degree and a license was whether to begin private medical practice immediately or first pursue a hospital internship. Even though internships were not required for state licensure until 1914, when Pennsylvania became the first state to pass such an amendment to its licensing laws, growing numbers of young American doctors undertook a year or more of internship by the turn of the century.[14] Internships generally involved a yearlong engagement. The successful applicant would either volunteer or, at best, receive a small stipend plus room and board in the hospital. This arrangement enabled the intern to work in a number of hospital services and treat a wide range of patients, often under the supervision of a more senior staff member.[15]

For those who could afford to postpone setting up their first practice, the hospital internship could bestow many practical career benefits and greater prestige. Many reform-minded medical schools, such as Jefferson Medical College in Philadelphia, encouraged their senior students to apply for internships. The student-run journal *The Jeffersonian* even boasted that "practically all of the members of the class [of 1911] intend on becoming hospital residents."[16] The editorialist explained, "An internship in a good hospital is probably worth as much to a physician as his four years in medical school, while it is certain that in experience one year in a hospital is equal to a much longer time spent in private practice." The editorialist recommended internships in "the best hospitals," wherein an intern was "instructed at the bedside in the practical part of the healing art by the ablest men."[17]

Despite the potential benefits heralded by some, internships did not have universal appeal. For starters, many young doctors objected to the poor supervision and meager facilities at many of the hospitals that offered internships, as the Council on Medical Education (CME) of the AMA noted in its first national study of internships in 1904. According to the CME, it was "impossible to say" what proportion of students took "a year or more of hospital work after graduation," but estimated that proportion was likely less than half of all students. A later CME study estimated that there were three available hospital internships for every four medical school graduates in 1912.[18] Common reasons given for forgoing an internship were that graduates "did not want them," that they were going "directly into practice," or that "they were married" (and therefore could not tolerate the monastic boarding arrangements that typically accompanied a hospital internship).[19] Although no Philadelphia-based studies of internships were conducted at the time, analysis of area doctors in the *American Medical Directory* indicate that only 46 percent of 1908 graduates occupied internships in 1909.[20] Until 1914, when a year of hospital internship became a requirement for licensure in Pennsylvania, most Philadelphia doctors went directly into private practice after medical school (figure 1).

During this period, the private practice of medicine combined two methods of attending patients. The first, best understood as "family practice," was older, more familiar, and based on house calls. The doctor, having being summoned by a relative or friend of the patient, traveled to the patient's home to offer treatment. By the turn of the century, however, "office practice" had emerged as a second method of private medical practice, especially in American cities.

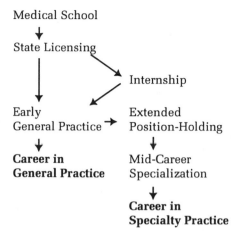

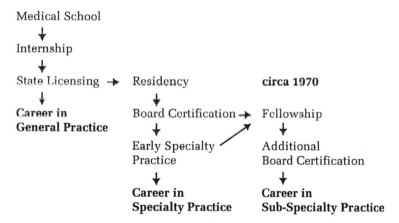

Figure 1. The Changing Career Paths of American Doctors

Working out of either a home office or a rented office in a central location, the doctor would assign certain hours of the day to treat ambulatory patients who came to the office. By the turn of the century, office practice outpaced family practice, especially in cities.[21]

In addition to private medical practice, the other mode of practice at the turn of the century could be described as "institutional medical practice," wherein a doctor practiced or taught medicine in a medical institution—such as a hospital, dispensary, medical school, public health department, military base, or even in a public school—typically part time and in exchange for a salary or small stipend, but occasionally on a volunteer basis. Medical schools and hospitals (or dispensaries) comprised the largest sources of institutional positions, and their faculty and staff were expanding dramatically at the turn of the century as medical schools and hospitals became essential steps in medical education and postgraduate career formation. In Philadelphia, between 1880 and 1910, the number of faculty in the city's six major medical schools expanded from 78 to 569. The diversification and expansion of medical school curricula and the growing enthusiasm for pedagogical specialization no doubt accounted for most of this increase.[22] Hospitals provided a similar burst of staff positions that was due in part to the hospital construction boom but also to the metamorphosis of these charity institutions into more widely used, fee-charging medical centers with educational and career opportunities valued by doctors.[23] By 1910, the number of medical and surgical staff positions in Philadelphia hospitals numbered 2,586 in one local medical directory—or roughly 1 position for every 1.28 doctors.[24]

Despite this rapid growth in institutional positions, though, very few of these positions were full-time, which meant that nearly every doctor in institutional practice also had a private practice.[25] In 1909, 95 percent of Philadelphia doctors had at least one private practice; of the remaining 5 percent, roughly half had internships and were therefore on a career path that, more often than not, led to private practice.[26] Even when combining private practice with a hospital position, most doctors viewed the latter as a career springboard for the former. Thus the establishment of a private practice was not only the first step in the careers of most young doctors (at least in the era before mandatory internships), it was also the primary interest of interns and doctors holding faculty and staff positions. As such, private practice must be viewed as the ultimate career objective in early twentieth-century medical careers, despite the growth of institutional practice. Since private practitioners represented nearly all (95 percent) Philadelphia doctors in 1909–1910, we should examine their careers more closely.

Career Differentiation and Professional Stratification

By the early twentieth century, medical careers more or less began the same way—by earning a medical degree, passing the state board examination for licensure, and establishing a private medical practice (see figure 1). The only optional step was the hospital internship, which nevertheless led to private practice in the long run. The uniformity of first career steps might lead one to assume that doctors had standard and therefore homogenous careers once in private practice. Nothing could be further from the truth, however. Once in private practice, medical careers diverged to such a degree that the medical profession was divided into distinct strata. Building on historical studies that have identified disparities in practice income and institutional tenure as signs of the "uneven rewards" of professional labor, I argue that the income and position holding were features, rather than causes, of stratification.[27] Instead, specialization was the most fundamental cause of career differentiation, as doctors who chose to limit their practices to particular specialties had markedly different personal and professional characteristics from general practitioners (GPs), including average income and institutional tenure. By identifying the role of specialization in career differentiation and professional stratification, we can better understand the complex and poorly organized system of private practice that arose in an era otherwise associated with growing standardization.

After graduation, licensure, and the optional hospital internship, young doctors overwhelmingly began their private practices as GPs. In part, general practice remained the default first career step because of the anemic growth of medical and surgical specialties until the early to mid-twentieth century. Even in large cities with expanding medical marketplaces and diverse market niches for private practice, specialization rates did not exceed 10 to 15 percent of the medical profession; in Philadelphia, for example, just 13 percent of doctors had specialized their practices in 1909–1910.[28] For young doctors fresh out of medical school, it was even more uncommon to specialize without first spending many years in general practice: only about 1 percent of Philadelphia doctors less than five years and 8 percent of Philadelphia doctors less than ten years out of medical school had specialized (figure 2).[29] In this regard, the young Dr. DeForest Porter Willard Jr. was unusual in that he began to limit his practice to orthopedic surgery within six years of his graduation in 1908.[30]

Why did so few young doctors specialize their practices? Although specialization had gained prestige and respectability by the early twentieth century, many older doctors who occupied positions as medical school professors and hospital department chiefs counseled young doctors against specializing too early. As Dr. Elizabeth L. Peck remarked in her presidential address to the annual meeting of the Alumnae Association of Woman's Medical College in 1901, "specialization is a necessity and a forced step in medical practice; but its premature development may be a drawback to the performance of the highest type of work. I trust the time will never come when the specialist springs forth from college full-fledged upon the world. An apprenticeship in general practice, and a reasonably long one, is of incalculable value."[31] Philadelphia

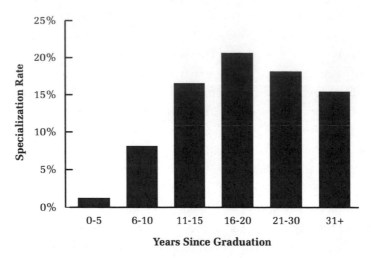

Figure 2. The Specialization Rate of Philadelphia Doctors by Experience, 1909

Source: AMD (1909) sample. Doctors not in private practice (32 of 664 in the sample) were excluded. Partial specialists were not listed in the AMD (1909). See appendix for details.

medical students received similar advice to that given to medical graduates. For example, Dr. Edwin B. Cragin acknowledged to a student audience at Jefferson Medical College in 1911 that "specialism in medicine is characteristic of the times, and specialism has come to stay." But he sternly warned his audience: "do not specialize too early." Instead, he suggested that "if you were to ask the best preparation for a good specialist I should say, develop yourself first as a man, second as a doctor, and third as a specialist."[32] The advice given to Philadelphia medical students and young doctors was consistent with that given to broader audiences.[33] The low specialization rate of young doctors indicates that they heeded such advice by busting their chops in general practice (see figure 2).

Even if some young medical graduates dismissed the alleged value of early general practice, they faced nearly insurmountable hurdles to immediate specialization. To begin with, there was no standard graduate medical education for pre-specialists to undertake in the early twentieth century, let alone legal or professional regulation of specialization.[34] Before the first world war, only a handful of universities and independent "polyclinic" medical schools offered graduate medical education of any kind, and these tended to be short six-week courses rather than the several-year course of residency later implemented in the largest surgical specialties by 1930s. A couple of early graduate medical institutions existed in Philadelphia, most notably the Philadelphia Polyclinic (established in 1883).[35] Given the limited domestic opportunities for formal, let alone standardized, graduate education in medical and surgical specialties, young pre-specialists could only gain clinical experience in their chosen specialty by undertaking a general internship and then slowly working their way up the institutional ladder at hospitals and dispensaries.[36]

To be sure, young pre-specialists might have had the opportunity in private practice to treat cases in their specialty of interest, but these cases would have been few and far between in general practice. Limiting a private practice to a particular specialty required a professional network to supply a steady stream of patient referrals and consultations. In order to establish such a network, the young doctor first needed recognized expertise in the chosen specialty and a good reputation among GPs in the area. These networks took time to establish, and involved years of clinical work in hospitals and dispensaries, tutelage in the private practices of recognized specialists, and even teaching work in medical schools.[37] Only by these means and through these institutions could young aspiring specialists acquire adequate caseloads in their chosen specialties.

Patterns of institutional tenure attest to the importance of position holding for the careers and private practices of specialists and pre-specialists. As medical schools expanded their faculty and as hospitals solicited the labor of doctors and interns, institutional positions became more prevalent than ever before from the late nineteenth to the early twentieth century. But these positions were not evenly distributed across the medical profession. Among Philadelphia doctors in 1909–1910, only 41 percent held any positions, and an even more select few (25 percent) held more than one position (table 4).[38] These position holders were far more likely to have specialized their practices than non–position holders (28 percent to 4 percent, respectively), and specialists held far more positions, on average, than GPs (2.78 positions to 0.67 positions, respectively).[39] Moreover, specialists continued to hold clinical and teaching positions throughout their careers, whereas GPs gradually left institutions after a few years in private practice (figure 3).

In such patterns of position holding, we can begin to see the ways in which specialization stratified the medical profession at this time. In order to specialize in private practice, a doctor required early and sustained access to institutional positions. For young doctors, landing an entry-level position was relatively easy because positions such as "assistant demonstrator" in a medical school or "assistant medical staff" in a hospital outpatient department or dispensary were abundant by comparison to the number of professorships and

Table 4.   **Differences in Experience, Specialization, and Institutional Tenure of Philadelphia Doctors, 1909–1910**

	All Doctors		Men		Women	
	N	%	N	%	N	%
Private Medical Practitioners in Sample	632	100	571	100	45	100
1. Experience (years since graduation)						
Practitioners with 0–10 years	207	32	182	32	19	42
Practitioners with 11–20 years	224	35	168	29	12	27
Practitioners with 21–30 years	127	20	115	20	9	20
Practitioners with 31 years or more	104	16	99	17	3	7
Practitioners with graduation data missing	12	2	7	1	2	4
2. Specialization (if any)						
No specialty listed (general practitioners)	547	87	490	86	42	93
Full specialists	85	13	81	14	3	7
3. Position holding (medical school faculty & hospital staff)						
Practitioners holding 0 positions	375	59	340	60	24	53
Practitioners holding 1 position	100	16	88	15	9	20
Practitioners holding 2 positions	70	11	65	11	4	9
Practitioners holding 3 or more positions	87	14	78	14	8	18
Practitioners holding any positions	257	41	231	41	21	47

Sources: AMD (1909) sample. Of 632 sample doctors in active practice, 616 had first names of discernable gender and 45 were women (7.3 percent). This gender ratio was slightly lower than that measured from federal census data (table 5). Partial specialists were not listed in the *AMD* (1909). Data on positions held by sample doctors were obtained from *The Professional Directory* (1910). See appendix for details.

hospital chiefships. Moving up the ranks, however, proved more difficult. As young doctors gained experience, they either climbed the institutional ladder or left institutional practice rather than suffer the indignity of competing for entry-level positions with the next cohort of doctors fresh out of medical school or internship, especially as these entry-level positions came with little to no salary. For young doctors who had no specialty aspirations, leaving institutional practice was likely the plan from the start. After gaining additional clinical experience, earning a reputation in a neighborhood, making professional

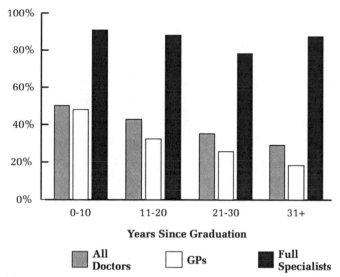

Figure 3. Differences in Institutional Tenure of Philadelphia Doctors, by Specialization and Experience, 1909–1910

Sources: AMD (1909) sample. Doctors not in private practice (32 of 664 in the sample) were excluded. Partial specialists were not listed in the AMD (1909). Data on positions held by sample doctors were obtained from *The Professional Directory* (1910). See appendix for details.

contacts, and having time to establish a private practice, the young GP left institutional practice altogether in order to focus on the ultimate career goal: running a lucrative private practice.[40]

Besides differing in their connection to institutions, specialists and GPs differed in the income they earned from private practice. Although the status and wealth of all doctors rose considerably with professionalization, private practice still had "uneven rewards," as there were wide ranging incomes across the medical profession.[41] In one of the earliest systematic studies of doctors' incomes, Harvard graduating classes from 1901 to 1910 had average incomes ranging from $362 to $1,237 one year after graduation.[42] To a large degree, income was determined by experience. Older doctors had more established and lucrative private practices than younger doctors who were just starting out.[43] Financial hardship also forced some young doctors to abandon the profession in their first few years. Even among graduates of Johns Hopkins, arguably the top medical school at the turn of the century, attrition rates reached 20 percent in the first five to ten years of practice as late as the graduating classes of 1897–1901.[44] Attrition thus winnowed the least successful doctors from the

profession and resulted in older cohorts that were comprised of more successful (and wealthier) doctors. However, for doctors of the same age, specialists
earned more than GPs on average.[45]

In summary, GPs and specialists had very different personal and professional characteristics. Although doctors in both strata had similar beginnings—
graduation, licensure, optional internship, establishment of general practice—GPs
and pre-specialists diverged considerably thereafter. Unlike GPs, specialists held onto institutional positions throughout their careers, as clinical and
teaching positions were central to their work. Specialists also tended to earn
more than GPs. But who were these early specialists? As we shall see, specialty
careers were not equally accessible to all medical graduates.

A Typology of General Practitioners

After Dr. DeForest Porter Willard Jr. completed his internship in 1910 and
began private medical practice, he was already well on his way to becoming
an orthopaedic surgeon. But as the son of the preeminent orthopaedic surgeon
in Philadelphia, Dr. DeForest Porter Willard Sr., the young Dr. Willard's path
to early specialization was shorter than most. It would be unfair to suggest that
young Dr. Willard lacked talent or did not deserve the success he achieved
so early in his career. From all available evidence, he became an outstanding
academic surgeon in his own right.[46] He did join his father's practice at 1901
Chestnut Street, a prime location, but he also had to take over when his father
died two weeks later. Nevertheless, the fact that his father had been a professor of orthopaedic surgery at the University of Pennsylvania and medical staff
at the Hospital of the University of Pennsylvania could only have helped the
young Dr. Willard in landing his first clinical appointments at Philadelphia
area hospitals (1910), in being elected to the exclusive College of Physicians
of Philadelphia (1914) and American Orthopaedic Association (1916), and in
establishing the professional networks necessary to specialize his private practice within a few years after internship (see table 3).

For the vast majority of doctors who were not like Dr. Willard Jr., the first
few years were comprised of general practice and entry-level institutional work
(see figures 2 and 3). Pre-specialists moved up the ranks and eventually specialized their private practices. But who were the rest of the GPs who comprised the
vast majority (86 percent) of doctors in cities like Philadelphia (see table 4)? To
answer this question, it is useful to distinguish two categories of GPs: first were
GPs who intended to remain GPs for their whole career, regardless of opportunities to specialize; second were GPs whose only career option was general

practice because they were unable to attain the institutional access and graduate medical education increasingly needed in order to specialize. Although it is
not possible to quantify the relative size of these two categories, this typology
highlights the importance of early twentieth-century medical institutions to
specialization, career differentiation, and professional stratification.

For those doctors who actively wanted to become GPs, general medical
practice was not just a default step; rather, it was the noblest career ambition in
medicine—to treat disease in all its forms. As one career advice author, Joseph M.
Matthews, put it in his *How to Succeed in the Practice of Medicine* (1905): "We
must admit that the one great 'specialty' is the general practice of medicine,
and the nearest approach to perfection is to be found in the person of the hon-
est, capable, and well-prepared 'country doctor.' From the drawing of a tooth
to the cutting off a leg; from prescribing for a simple 'belly-ache' to treating a
long-continued case of typhoid fever; from extracting an ingrown toe-nail to
saving life in a case of postpartum hemorrhage . . . He combines all specialties in his work. His responsibility is tenfold, or in proportion to the number of specialties, and his knowledge should be in the same positive ratio."[47]
This often-cited figure of the "country doctor" encapsulated arguments in early
twentieth-century medical rhetoric about the unappreciated value of the GP,
whether urban or rural. In this nostalgic trope, whatever the "country doctor"
lacked in scientific medical education and flashy laboratory knowledge, he or
she more than compensated for with a "take-action style" of medical practice
at the bedside. Nostalgic rhetoric about the "country doctor" or the old-time GP
glorified the "therapeutic imperative" assumed by these heroic figures.[48]

The foil for the country doctor was the "city doctor," who had more formal
education, institutional positions, and a greater likelihood to specialize as a result.
This trend did not escape the attention of career advice authors, many of who
were concerned about the growth of specialization in cities. As one satirical poem
published in the advice manual *How to Be Successful as a Physician* (1902) put it,

Of the genus "City Doctor" are species not a few;
There are many arrant humbugs, there are others learn'd and true.
The over-weening egotist will test you all he knows,
Some flourish on society, and some depend on clothes.
One city man's an oculist, a second treats the ear;
A third devotes himself to the lungs, and curious sounds doth hear.
A fourth, with his laryngoscope, will see your glottis quiver,
While many men the kidneys love, and many more the liver.

Some specialists prefer the joints, a few the brain and nerves;

Some spray away at old catarrhs, with hope that never swerves.

Some think a man in buttons, a coach and pair to drive,

May serve in lieu of wisdom and thus expect to thrive.

But 'mid these varied callings all, the man who heads the list

Is that gentle fingered ge-ni-us, the gy-ne-col-o-gist!

He's such a charming fellow, so clever in his way;

He always thrives in cities—I meet him everyday.

His rooms are overcrowded with ladies quite a host,

And if he has a wife, they trust she'll soon give up the ghost.

God bless these noble specialists in all they have to do;

And God have mercy on the souls of all the patients, too.[49]

Many doctors not only viewed general practice as the proper goal of a medical career but looked upon specialization with outright suspicion.

In the urban medical marketplace, nostalgia for the country doctor simply translated into nostalgia for the GP, at least in the early days of specialization. For example, in the early twentieth century, new or reform-minded institutions prioritized hiring doctors who possessed the latest knowledge of scientific medicine—knowledge that recent graduates from reformed medical schools might have possessed but that an experienced, rank-and-file doctor, who had never set foot in a laboratory, might well have lacked. In 1910, editorials in local newspapers questioned the wisdom of hiring "full-time" professors at the University of Pennsylvania School of Medicine. According to critics, it was unwise to hire young laboratory-savvy hotshots over the traditional graybeard practitioner-professor who had earned a reputation through years spent at the bedside.[50]

To some degree, the low opinion of specialism voiced by advice book authors and in the kerfuffle over hiring priorities at the University of Pennsylvania School of Medicine were vestiges of older professional ideology, when embattled elite doctors asserted that healers who claimed to have special (often "hidden") knowledge of disease were nothing more than itinerant quacks.[51] As a case in point, Philadelphia ophthalmologist Dr. George W. Norris recalled a story told to him about his father's decision to specialize. According to the story, George's father had "made specialization in Philadelphia respectable," later becoming the first professor of ophthalmology at the University of Pennsylvania. Many of his father's colleagues, however, had initially discouraged his father from specializing. One pleaded, "Willie, you must reconsider. You must not disgrace your eminent father and your highly esteemed and distinguished family by becoming a Quack!"[52] Although specialization had become more respectable by the time George Norris graduated from medical school in 1899, some doctors still regarded specialism as a necessary evil at best. As one contemporary advice author asked rhetorically in 1905, "Is it necessary for the welfare of the people to have other specialties outside of the division of medicine and surgery?"[53] Sentiments like these suggest that both those who admired general practice and those who disdained specialization formed the ranks of doctors who expressly wished to become GPs.

Many doctors, however, were unable to specialize, regardless of their affinities. Some of these doctors no doubt lacked the ability or knowledge to specialize. In many cases, though, institutional discrimination on the bases of gender, race, or social class denied women, African American, and working-class doctors the opportunity to get the education and institutional positions needed to specialize (see figure 3). We cannot know what percentage of women, African American, and working-class doctors wanted to specialize but could not do so because of institutional discrimination. It is possible, however, to identify the challenges faced by this second category of GPs in the early twentieth century.

Even earning a medical degree was difficult for many aspiring doctors from underrepresented groups: very few medical schools admitted women, African Americans, or even working-class applicants, and the few that did were generally guilty of symbolic inclusion. By the end of the nineteenth century, a handful of American medical schools had been founded by or specifically for these marginalized medical students. Woman's Medical College of Pennsylvania (established in 1850), for example, was one of three U.S. medical schools that admitted only women. Many of these schools, however, became the unintended (or deliberate) victims of medical education reform because underfunding prevented these schools from making the expensive upgrades to laboratory and clinical facilities that influential education reformers, like Abraham Flexner, pressured medical schools to undertake. Flexner and his ilk, however, were indifferent to the possibility that medical education reform would force many medical colleges for women, African Americans, and working-class medical students to close their doors.[54] A few medical schools like these did survive, but often suffered scathing evaluations even as they made good-faith efforts to meet the new standards. Flexner, for example, singled out for criticism schools like Temple University School of Medicine in Philadelphia (established in 1901), which offered night classes in order to accommodate working-class students. In his condescending opinion, part-time medical education in "night schools" that catered to "poor boys" undermined the goal of elevating and standardizing medical curricula.[55] In addition to discriminatory admission policies, the new admission requirement of college education further prevented many marginalized and low-income students from attending medical school and becoming doctors.

Because of discrimination, women, African Americans, and the working class were underrepresented as doctors. Although the social class background of doctors could not be measured in 1909–1910, there is unmistakable underrepresentation of women and African Americans in private practice relative to other occupations (table 5).[56] Even when doctors from underrepresented groups managed to matriculate to and graduate from medical school, their career paths were often restricted to general practice. In some cases, members of these three groups of doctors fell under the influence of essentialist logic about what sorts of careers best suited them. This logic, at times voiced by inculcated peers, limited the definition or expectation of career success for women, African American, and working-class doctors to general practice. In most cases, though, these underrepresented doctors were simply excluded from specialty career paths by old-boy networks that controlled access to the graduate medical education and institutional positions that were becoming necessary to specialize.[57]

Women doctors, in particular, often wrestled with the essentialist logic of mentors and colleagues, both male and female, that held that general medical work, especially among the poor and in free dispensaries, was not only a moral and charitable imperative, but one for which women were ideally suited by virtue of their gender.[58] Dr. Elizabeth Peck, an alumna of the Women's Medical College, advanced the two main reasons why women doctors might have

Table 5. **The Gender, Race, and Nativity of Doctors versus All Occupied Persons in Philadelphia, 1910**

Category	Percent of Physicians & Surgeons	Percent of Occupied Persons
White men, native-born	77.0	43.8
White men, foreign-born	11.7	23.7
African American men	2.2	4.2
Other men	0.1	0.2
Women	9.1	28.2

Source: U.S. Bureau of the Census, *Thirteenth Census of the United States, 1910* (Washington, DC: U.S. G.P.O., 1914), vol. 4, *Population*, 181, 193, 428–29, 588–89. The 1910 census did not subdivide women physicians and surgeons by race and nativity. Percentages are rounded to the nearest tenth of a percent, and therefore do not necessarily total 100 percent. See appendix for details.

felt "called" into general and not specialty medical practice: "there are many influences that tend to make woman the general practitioner: her interest in the family life, the care of children, the fact that most women who have thus far studied medicine have done so with a serious mind, desiring not only to gain a livelihood, but to work for the best good of the community, and seeing their fullest opportunity in this field. This motive actuates, as I believe, the majority of physicians, but seems to be earlier developed in the medical woman than in her brother practitioner."[59] In Peck's logic, women more often became GPs because this career path fulfilled the prescribed roles of womanhood. This kind of assumption about the proper role of women doctors was common in medicine but also reflected broader Progressive Era reform ideology, which had at its core what historians have labeled a "maternalist" form of essentialism.[60] Women doctors who did manage to specialize, though, continued to face stereotypes that limited the specialties that they sought, or that were prescribed for them, to a handful of fields for which women were thought to have been ideally suited, such as pediatrics, obstetrics, gynecology, psychiatry, and public health.[61]

But what larger effects did essentialist stereotypes or lived gender roles have for women in private practice? Evidence from the *American Medical Directory* (1909) indicates that in Philadelphia, women doctors had half the rate of specialization of their medical brethren—or 6.7 percent versus 14.2 percent (see table 4). Conformity to gender expectations can explain some of this difference. It is also clear that many women GPs expressly wished to become specialists but could not because they were excluded from graduate medical education and institutional positions. In a 1900 letter to her fellow alumnae, in which she reviewed the prospects for women to practice medicine in Philadelphia, Dr. Helen Murphy complained, "In no other city has the woman doctor had as bitter and as slowly yielding a prejudice to overcome." What women needed most, in her estimation, was "a wider open door to hospitals."[62] Although analysis of medical directories indicates that women doctors had statistically indistinguishable rates of position holding from men in 1910, most of these opportunities came from medical institutions founded by or dedicated to women medical staff and faculty.[63] But even women who had the access and opportunities to specialize faced a final gender-specific hurdle—the possibility of having their careers sidetracked by family demands. For women who wanted to mix private practice, motherhood, and marriage, the flexible hours and residential offices common to general practice were more appealing than the downtown office buildings and long hours of institutional positions common to specialty medical practice.[64]

Like women doctors, African American doctors were sorely underrepresented by comparison to other occupations. Despite the growing African American population in Philadelphia, there were very few African American doctors in the city (see table 5). In part, this reflected the broader underrepresentation of African American doctors in the United States, which resulted from structural racism and discriminatory admissions practices of undergraduate colleges and medical schools. African American doctors who managed to matriculate to and graduate from medical school faced further institutional discrimination and stereotypes that limited their career options to general practice or, at best, a handful of specialties. Until the 1930s, formal discrimination limited the number of Philadelphia hospitals in which African American doctors could get internships and staff positions to two, both of which had only recently been founded by or for African American doctors: Frederick Douglass Memorial Hospital (established in 1895) and Mercy Hospital (established in 1907). For the handful of African American women doctors at this time, the double bind of sexism and racism even further limited their ability to specialize, especially with the advent of mandatory hospital internships in 1914. The addition of this requirement ignored the effects of sexual or racial discrimination in hiring practices for hospital internships.[65]

Although it is not possible to determine the specialization rate of Philadelphia's few African American doctors, it is likely that most practiced general medicine in order to address the health care needs of their primary clientele— African American residents.[66] At this time in Philadelphia, African Americans suffered disproportionately from basic health care problems rooted in poverty and thus could not afford specialist care, except in free dispensaries and hospitals.[67] Some African American doctors no doubt practiced specialty medicine at Frederick Douglass or Mercy, but their private practices were almost certainly not limited to specialties. What specialty work African American doctors did outside of hospitals mostly came in the form of public health work in tuberculosis clinics. In part, African American doctors engaged in this field of specialty work because of a desire to address the immediate health needs of their community.[68] In addition, though, public health was one of the few specialty fields that African American doctors could enter at this time without much resistance from the white medical establishment. On top of the effects of embedded institutional racism, an essentialist logic, rooted in a paternalistic understanding of the proper professional interests and duties of African American doctors, limited the definition and expectation of success to general practice and public health work for African American doctors at this time.[69]

Working-class doctors also had difficulty specializing their private practices in the early twentieth century. Besides having to confront the expectation that they would naturally want to tend to the general medical needs of rural towns or impoverished urban neighborhoods, working-class doctors also had difficulty affording graduate education and gaining access to institutional positions, especially internships. It was common in this period before the standardization of graduate medical education, for example, for hospitals not only to make internship decisions on the basis of competitive examination but to consider the social background of the applicant. In a lecture given to the students of Jefferson Medical College in 1906, Dr. J. Torrance Rugh acknowledged that hospitals considered the "influence" of an internship applicant as much or more than his or her examination scores, personal qualifications, or class standing.[70] Limited access to institutional positions necessarily limited the specialization opportunities for working class doctors, as well as women and African American doctors.

As this chapter has shown, private medical practice remained the primary career objective despite the rise of institutions as centers of medical education and practice by the early twentieth century. That being said, doctors depended upon institutional positions in order pursue career objectives outside the walls of medical schools and hospitals. Doctors may have begun their careers more or less the same way, as GPs in private practice, and for many doctors, general practice was the ultimate objective. However, growing numbers of doctors desired to specialize, and access to institutions separated successful from unsuccessful aspirants. Pre-specialists secured institutional positions in hospitals, dispensaries, and medical schools, and leveraged these positions into referral and consultation networks that sustained the private specialty practices that orbited these institutions.[71] Access to these positions depended to a degree upon the intellectual affinities and aptitudes of applicants. However, institutional access also depended upon social background, as discrimination on the basis of gender, race, and social class severely limited the career options for women, African American, and working-class doctors.

In the case of Dr. DeForest Porter Willard Jr., his interest in specializing was not unique for his generation of medical graduates (see table 3). After licensure and hospital internship, he started a private practice and pursued appointments at various hospitals and medical schools in the city. The young

Dr. Willard distinguished himself from his peers, though, in the pace of his transition to specialty practice. Although not typical of pre-specialists, Dr. Willard did represent the growing divide between specialists and GPs in the early twentieth century. As specialization became more common and acceptable, the career paths of GPs and specialists diverged ever sooner after medical school. Although Dr. Willard boldly skipped the proving grounds of general practice, his career path would become common for pre-specialists by mid-century. The specialization of American medicine was well under way, and its monumental effects on the business of private medical practice and on the organization of health care in American cities were taking shape.

Chapter 2

The Doctor as Business Owner

As American doctors aspired to new professional status, an internal debate raged about the proper role of the commercialism in medicine, and Philadelphia doctors were no exception. For example, in a contentious paper read before the Philadelphia County Medical Society in 1901, Dr. John B. Roberts distinguished "proper and just enterprise and thrift in one's professional work and what is an improper commercial spirit." As a surgeon, Dr. Roberts had witnessed the most deplorable billing practices of his time: price gouging, upselling expensive prosthetics over affordable alternatives, referring patients to private hospitals in which one had part ownership, demanding payment from patients on the operating table, fee-splitting with GPs who referred patients, and taking kick-backs from pharmacists, medical supply companies, and life insurance companies in exchange for referrals, endorsements, and confidential patient records. According to Dr. Roberts, these practices should distress anyone "who believes that the medical man belongs to a liberal profession and not to that portion of the body economic, whose sole object is the accumulation of money."[1]

In stark contrast to loathsome figure of the avaricious specialist conjured up in debates about ethical standards stood the nostalgic figure of the self-sacrificing old-time doctor, who cared little about timely remittance or who knew nothing of efficient bookkeeping. The pages of medical journals were littered with tributes to the imaginary old-time doctor, who also made appearances in popular magazines such as the *Ladies' Home Journal* and *Harper's*.[2] For some, the old-time doctor aroused pity, and many county medical societies, including Philadelphia's, collected funds to support old-age homes for poor but pure old-time doctors lest they should have to see out their days in a poor-house. As the organizers of one such home in upstate New York explained, "It is a real home for physicians and surgeons who have been honorable in their conduct and yet have fallen victims to the common foes, poverty or broken health."[3] For others, though, the plight of the old-time doctor demonstrated the need to adopt modern accounting methods in private practice. As Dr. Daniel Cathell, author of the most popular advice book series, *The Physician Himself*, opined, "To fight the battles of life successfully it is as necessary for even the most scientific physician to possess a certain amount of professional tact and business sagacity as it is for a ship to have a rudder."[4] For Dr. Roberts and his ilk, the dilemma was how to reconcile the business of private practice and the emerging profession of medicine.

To assert that private practices functioned as small businesses at this time is hardly controversial. Historians of medicine have long used the metaphor of the "medical marketplace" to describe the economies of exchange between heal-ers and patients before the emergence of the modern regulatory state.[5] Market demand originated with patients, who bought medical goods and services; mar-ket supply came from healers, who sold their goods and services. In the relatively free market of early modern Europe and America, patient-buyer-consumers had innumerable options, and freely mixed and matched good and services based on their preferences and budgets. The openness of the early modern marketplace fostered competition and generated market niches that were filled by a vast array of healer-producer-providers. In mid-nineteenth-century America, for example, orthodox doctors competed with Thomsonians, homeopaths, hydropaths, sun-dry itinerant healers, and patent medicine vendors, to name just a few.[6]

Despite the explanatory power of the term "medical marketplace," more work is needed to identify local market variations and to explain the effects of regulation.[7] The conditions of the medical marketplace in the United States, for example, had changed dramatically by the early twentieth century as an emerg-ing orthodox medical profession gained legitimacy and status and acquired state-sanctioned power to regulate supply.[8] As has been well studied, orthodox doctors profited from new regulation.[9] Other changes to the business of private practice, however, remain poorly understood. For example, how did individual doctors integrate the financial goals of private practice with new career oppor-tunities in medical institutions, especially hospitals, which were expanding in American cities?[10]

Besides needing to account for the effects of regulatory and economic change, analysis of the urban medical marketplace in the early twentieth century must also account for the ways in which private practice differed from other kinds of businesses, such as groceries or laundries. Unlike product-based businesses, such as groceries, where the cost and quality of fresh produce, canned goods, pantry items, and even butchered meat were becoming standardized, service-based businesses, like private practice or laundries, were difficult to commoditize, as these services had no exchange value and necessarily differed from provider to provider. Although vendors benefited by establishing trust with clients, especially when selling products whose quality was not readily ascertained, service providers depended on establishing trust. The level of trust required for inexpensive or low-risk services like laundering, though, was much lower than for expensive and high-risk services, like the diagnosis and treatment of an illness.[11] But unlike buying produce or paying for laundry services, laypersons struggled to discern what was good health care with the growth of highly technical, scientific medicine in the early twentieth century; consumers did not require expert assistance in deciding whether to buy broccoli or launder a shirt, but this was not the case for a patient needing an X-ray or lab test.[12] The widening gap between lay and expert medical knowledge in part explains why the American public supported regulation, wherein state licensing laws guaranteed the basic qualifications of doctors. Because health or even life itself was on the line, doctors could not rely on their licenses alone to attract patients. Instead, success in private practice depended upon establishing trust, perhaps more than in any other small business.[13] In other words, contrary to the beliefs of today's advocates of health care privatization, buying broccoli and buying health care services were two radically different consumer experiences in the early twentieth century, as they remain today.[14]

But how did doctors establish trust in private practice? Were there different business models in private practice? Did private practice follow the trends toward corporatism and efficiency found in other businesses, including groceries, by the 1920s?[15] This chapter addresses these lingering questions about the business of private practice in the changing medical marketplace of early twentieth-century American cities. In order to address the larger tension between commercial and professional agendas, I examine the relationship between financial and career goals of individual doctors as revealed in memoirs and popular advice. Using specific examples of business pressures faced in practice, we can begin to understand the larger debate about business ethics portrayed in conflicting tropes of early twentieth-century doctors, from the greedy specialist criticized by the likes of Dr. Roberts, to the old-time doctor pitied by aid associations, to the naïve scientist-doctor counseled by advice authors such as Dr. Cathell.

Medical Careers and the Business of Private Practice

Many doctors embraced, even if only privately, the business side of private practice, and considered sound business practices and education in medical economics to be important tools for improving both their incomes and professional standing. For example, when surveyed about the subjects needing more instruction in medical school, Harvard medical graduates from 1901 to 1910 listed a "business course" near the top, with only "pharmacology and therapeutics" and "clinical instruction" ranking higher. Several respondents even suggested creating a chair in the "Conduct of Private Practice."[16] The perceived lack of practical business instruction explains why a vast advice literature for young doctors flourished in this period, particularly as career paths became more complex. Following graduation from medical school, young doctors faced an inevitable series of career choices, all of which affected the future of their businesses. These choices included whether or not to take a hospital internship, how to set up a private practice, how to build clientele, and how to make ends meet while waiting for patients. Even in mid-career, established doctors faced choices such as how to manage a growing practice and whether or not to limit a practice to a particular specialty. Upon closer examination, business concerns not only influenced but were often the primary factors directing the career decisions of young doctors in the early twentieth century.

The Uncertain Value of Internship

After passing state licensing examinations, the first career choice facing medical graduates was whether to undertake a hospital internship or to head directly into private practice (see figure 1). As noted previously, internships offered career benefits, particularly for pre-specialists who needed to build their clinical experience and professional networks.[17] But internships did not hold universal appeal, as evidenced by the fact that less than half of medical graduates undertook internship in 1910. This held true even in large cities like Philadelphia, where medical schools promoted graduate medical education earlier than most.[18] In part, many doctors chose immediate private practice because until 1924, the supply of internships did not match the annual production of medical graduates.[19] But demand also lagged because the internship required immediate financial sacrifices of doctors.

Of primary concern was that the internship provided austere room and board and very little, if any, stipend. For example, Dr. Edith Flower Wheeler, an 1897 graduate of Woman's Medical College of Pennsylvania, noted that her salary during her internship year at the West Philadelphia Hospital for Women was "board and lodging only"—the equivalent of about $5 dollars a week ($260 for the year).[20] By comparison, the nearby Philadelphia Orthopaedic Hospital paid its head housekeeper $300 and the ward maids $144 for the year 1900. Thus intern labor had little market value in terms of pay, or the equivalent of mid-level cleaning staff.[21] By contrast, Harvard medical graduates from 1901 to 1910 who went directly into private practice earned roughly $750 in their first year of practice.[22]

To add insult to injury, former interns in the Harvard study did not earn significantly more in their first year of practice than did graduates who had gone directly into practice.[23] Anecdotal evidence from Philadelphia confirms these findings: Drs. Catherine MacFarlane and Ellen Culver Potter, graduates of Woman's Medical College of Pennsylvania in 1898 and 1903, respectively, each undertook an internship at Woman's Hospital of Philadelphia, but each reported meager earnings from the first year in practice afterward—MacFarlane earned $206 and Potter just $188.[24] From a business perspective, the problem with an internship was that it postponed the establishment of a private practice in the short run and did not guarantee greater income until years later. When considering an internship, the graduate with loans to repay had to weigh possible career gains against certain financial hardship.[25]

Why did it ever make sense, from a business perspective, to subject oneself to the deprivations of internship? For starters, if a senior medical student did not have any promising leads for setting up a private practice, then internship was not much of a sacrifice, and perhaps even a welcome career waypoint. For young doctors in these circumstances, the internship provided modest income security and the chance to get his or her bearings before having to hang a shingle. For example, when describing his early career after graduating from the University of Pennsylvania School of Medicine in 1899, Dr. George W. Norris recalled that he was "fortunate in attaining an internship at Pennsylvania Hospital." Then, "slowly" he "accumulated a practice" while "connected with various hospitals—the Polyclinic, the Orthopedic, the Episcopal, the Philadelphia General, and the Phipps Institute and finally . . . a Chiefship at the Pennsylvania [Hospital]."[26]

Some Philadelphia medical faculty even counseled their students to use institutional positions as a strategy for building a private practice. Dr. Harriet L.

Hartley, clinical professor of surgery at Woman's Medical College, warned students and alumnae that "practice comes slowly; some days are very bright and others very dull." She then advised, "If hospital and dispensary practice are open to the physician, she derives much benefit from daily association with more experienced doctors—she keeps abreast of the new ideas in medicine. Her connection gives her prestige in the neighborhood [where she practices]. A good clinician is usually followed to her office by the best of her hospital patients. Thus the time of waiting for a practice is made much easier by keeping busy."[27] For Dr. Hartley, the career and financial benefits of internship were inseparable. Similarly, in a 1908 speech about the "practical points to be borne in mind by the young beginner," Dr. Philip H. Moore advised Jefferson students to plan their internships around their future goals for private practice: "To those who go into a hospital I would say that when possible select your hospital service in the place where you expect to practice medicine, for while you are serving as a resident you will become acquainted with a large number of people, who, with fair and right treatment, will become your friends and afterwards your patients."[28]

Some interns were "adopted" by an older doctor on staff at the hospital. Young doctors were even advised to "try to make the close personal acquaintance of one of the members of the visiting staff, as it will be many dollars in your pocket. He will probably be flattered by your attentions and will do all in his power to advance his protégé after you leave the institution."[29] Even if making such acquaintances did not lead to adoption, then at least they entitled one to "ask the opinion of all of the attending physicians and surgeons as to a suitable place for beginning practice." After all, they were "in a position to know of any good berths that may be open."[30] Thus, from a business perspective, the internship year bought time for a young doctor unready to open up a practice—time to make career decisions, time to build up clientele, and time to make contacts among the hospital staff that could lead to career advancement and to financial security in early private practice.

All of this suggests that internship might have had long-term financial benefits. Indeed, the Harvard study found that former interns earned more by their tenth year in practice than their classmates who had gone directly into private practice.[31] Internship yielded career and financial returns for Drs. MacFarlane and Potter in the long run as well: both became prominent Philadelphia doctors, with MacFarlane earning $2,200 and Potter $1,508 from private practice by the tenth year after graduation.[32] Their incomes were even higher if including earnings from part-time salaried positions in hospitals and medical schools, which both doctors had in abundance and which both doctors garnered through the institutional networks they had established during their internships. The potential for long-term career and financial gains explains why so many doctors were willing to risk short-term losses in internships. As one advice author jested, "If you can't afford it [the internship], borrow the money, if you cannot borrow it, steal it."[33]

Interns nevertheless kept an eye out for golden opportunities to start up their practices, even if that meant absconding from their internship. In a feeble attempt to "discourage these resignations," the Board of Managers at Saint Christopher's Hospital for Children (near Kensington in North Philadelphia) resolved in 1901 to require interns to pay a deposit at the beginning of their term, which they forfeited if they resigned "before they have completed full terms of service for which they are appointed."[34] Deposits became commonplace in the years before state-mandated internships, and amounted to significant sums for recent graduates: for example, Philadelphia General Hospital (in West Philadelphia) required $100 deposits of interns, to be returned "upon the completion of his full term of service in a satisfactory manner."[35] The fact that some interns forfeited their deposit suggests that young doctors jumped at good business opportunities to open a practice. If no opportunity came during the first year, then at least the doctor had received what long-term benefits—both career and financial—that the internship could provide.

For those doctors who did finish internships, formal graduate medical education did not have to end there. As one advice author put it, "After you have finished your hospital course and if you do not feel like beginning a practice, a year or two spent in post-graduate study in America or Europe is of great advantage."[36] Because only a handful of cities, such as New York, Philadelphia, and Chicago, had graduate medical instruction at the turn of the century, many American doctors journeyed to European institutes, hospitals, and universities, where rich clinical and research programs had been offered for decades.[37] Before the turn of the century, the American doctors who pursued formal graduate study generally did so in order to compensate for undergraduate medical education that had been lacking in practical laboratory or clinical instruction. As American medical schools reformed their curricula and facilities by the 1920s, graduate medical education in the United States shifted from remedial training for mid-career doctors to rigorous specialty training for young pre-specialists who had already received broad training as interns. Study abroad began to fade as a result.[38]

As with hospital internship, young doctors weighed the benefits against the costs of additional education. From a career perspective, graduate medical education promised many benefits, particularly for pre-specialists. First, additional education honed practical medical and surgical skills. Second, even though nearly all doctors started private practice as GPs (see figures 1 and 2), graduate education enabled a young doctor to cultivate specialty interests and could even lead to early specialization. Graduate education came with financial costs, though. For young doctors at the end of a long internship, additional education further delayed starting a private practice; for more established doctors, additional education took time away from building their practices. Other costs were more tangible, such as lecture fees and the expense of travel, lodging, and board if going abroad. Financial hardship alone limited the field of doctors who could consider graduate medical education. To some degree, these costs could be offset in the long run if additional education enabled the doctor to distinguish him or herself from the competition and to capitalize on this enhanced status by commanding higher fees or by attracting more patients. But, as one advice author cautioned, those who intended to "go to Europe for the prestige" needed to know that it "seldom counts for very much, unless one has been well established for some years in some locality before going abroad."[39]

Whether in a hospital internship, a short course in a "polyclinic" medical school, or in study abroad, young doctors weighed the costs and benefits of graduate medical education in very practical terms. In this decision process, the short-term demands of needing to make a living and build a business usually trumped whatever long-term career benefits that internship or graduate medical education might offer. For these reasons, the majority of Philadelphia doctors entered directly into private practice until 1914, when Pennsylvania became the first state to require a year of hospital internship before doctors could be licensed.[40]

Hanging a Shingle

Inevitably, whether directly out of medical school or after an internship or other graduate study, all young doctors turned their attention to the goal of setting up a practice. Dr. Martin E. Rehfuss, a Jefferson Medical College alumnus who set up his Philadelphia practice in 1914, remarked upon this awkward transition from student to business owner:

> Every one of us had some unusual experience in beginning a practice. . . .
> I remember so distinctly that after spending four years in the medical
> school and two years as an intern in a large hospital, I went to Europe
> and three years elapsed before I returned to my native Philadelphia. I
> had several offers to remain in Paris, another rather flattering one to join

an internist in New York and one in Washington, but Philadelphia was my home and I thought that I would rather begin at the bottom of the ladder in Philadelphia. Somehow I felt at home there, though I shall never forget the feeling of loneliness and strange uncertainty when I realized that I was to begin the practice of medicine.[41]

Prestigious graduate education did not spare Dr. Rehfuss from the arduous task of setting up his first private practice. In this regard, setting up a practice was a kind of professional equalizer. To be sure, some young doctors started their first enterprise with competitive advantages, whether in terms of greater financial resources or more extensive patronage networks than their peers. And yet, every doctor had to achieve three important business objectives in setting up a first practice: select a good location (in other words, profitable); rent or buy the best office space one could afford; and manage start-up costs for equipment and furnishings. Failure to achieve these three business objectives could lead to professional obscurity or worse—financial ruin.

Finding a good location had perhaps the most immediate and enduring influence upon the success of any small business, including a private medical practice. For obvious reasons, a young doctor needed to select a location in which he or she had a reasonable chance to attract clients before going broke from the fixed costs of overhead. Thus from the moment a new practice opened, a financial and career clock began to tick. Most contemporary advice authors, like Daniel Cathell, warned that "unless you gain popular favor by a display of ability, acquire a good and favorable reputation, and build up a fair practice in your first six or eight years, the probabilities are that you never will."[42]

Adding to the felt pressure of finding a good location were the prohibitive costs of leaving a poor location. Relocation cost money and it was difficult to retain clientele already cultivated. As Dr. C. R. Mabee, author of *The Physician's Business and Financial Adviser* (1900), put it, "If you remain in your first location or near by, you will be better off, as removals often cause the commencing of life all over again."[43] A fellow advice writer, Dr. Thomas F. Reilly, and author of *Building a Profitable Practice* (1912), used even plainer business metaphors: "once you locate don't move about to another section or even another street, if you can possibly help it, as every year in one house is in itself an increment in your capital stock, otherwise known as your reputation, and frequent moving much impairs the capital."[44] Perhaps it was for these reasons that the 1908 graduates of Jefferson Medical College were counseled to "consider whatever advantages any location has, your preference for it, or objection to it, then make your choice and go to it with the determination of staying there until you succeed."[45] For a young doctor with barely enough money to open a practice, the first location selected was likely the one and only shot at surviving, let alone thriving, in the marketplace. One had to get it right.

In selecting a location, the first consideration was the general locale, and both the city and the country were thought to have distinct prospects. Competition was generally lower in the country, but fees were smaller and there were fewer opportunities to supplement practice income with salaried work. On the other hand, cities were notoriously overcrowded with doctors, but they had "the most opportunities for study, advancement and eventual financial gain," provided one could endure the competition.[46] Familiarity and personal preference were perhaps the most important factors in choosing between city and countryside, for it was commonly advised that "a person brought up in the city generally does better in the city than in the country, and a man brought up in the country generally does better in the country than in the city."[47] The doctors at the center of this study had obviously chosen Philadelphia over country practice; perhaps it is not surprising that nearly all of them (90 percent) had graduated from Philadelphia medical schools and were therefore already familiar with the city.[48]

Once decided on an urban locale and a specific city, doctors next had to select a specific neighborhood. Chapter 3 considers in great detail the social, professional, and economic factors that directed the location decisions of urban doctors and the consequences of these decisions for the distribution of health care in large cities like Philadelphia in the early twentieth century. For our purposes here, it is only necessary to know that young doctors considered the relative merits of different market niches when selecting a specific neighborhood in which to locate their private practice.

After a good location, the next important business objective was to select the best office space one could afford without becoming burdened by the fixed cost of rent or mortgage. Although private practice continued to include home visits after the turn of the century, it had become customary for urban doctors to receive ambulatory cases in an office, whether in a home office or in a separate rented office.[49] In general, both doctors and patients benefited from this arrangement. The doctor could save on the expense and hassle of having to travel to every patient's home. The savings in transportation costs meant that doctors could charge less for an office visit than a home visit, which patients appreciated; the savings in time meant that doctors could see more patients in the office, thereby earning more per diem while charging less per patient. In other words, office practice had practical business appeal for urban doctors.[50]

The selection of the office space itself boiled down to basic microeconomics. The most limiting factor was the cost of rent or the added expense of buying a house with an extra room for an office. In general, young doctors were advised that "in commencing practice you ought to have at least a capital of about $500–$150 for equipment and $350 to supply your first year's deficiency. At the end of that time, in most instances, you can make your living expenses."[51] The fixed cost of office space, though, amounted to the greatest share of these living expenses and there were a number of business strategies for balancing quality and affordability, depending upon the means of the doctor and the neighborhood in which he or she planned to locate. Doctors lacking the capital to invest in real estate settled for renting office space. Single doctors, who had no spouse to help with the odds and ends of running a household and taking calls from patients, economized by renting an apartment or a room in a house and utilizing some living space therein for consultation, at least during daytime hours.[52] For example, Dr. Howard A. Kelley gave tips to Jefferson Medical College students on how to economize when setting up a first office practice:

> When I left the hospital, I was unwilling to lose the precious opportunities of following the traditional course of settling downtown, and waiting for some older doctor to adopt me, and to die and leave his practice, [so] I took up quarters in a weaver's family, in a little two-story house at 2316 N. Front Street, where I had a bed room (the family parlor), which was my consultation room by day, and the dining room which served as a waiting room, including board and all, for seven dollars a week. I slept on a sofa bed at night near the front window, and any one who knew where I was, could have thrown up the sash and caught me as I lay in bed by the foot.[53]

At seven dollars a week, Dr. Kelley still spent $364 a year for these two multipurpose rooms in the working-class neighborhood of Kensington. Only select Philadelphia doctors with great reserves of start-up money could afford to rent, let alone buy, a full house with an office.

Besides the weighing the costs of prospective offices, doctors also considered the business fortunes of other doctors in the area. In many cases, a young doctor even bought or rented the office of a previous doctor-owner. For example, a 1915 classified advertisement in *The Weekly Roster*, the main periodical of the Philadelphia County Medical Society, read, "Doctor's office for Rent. Room is 18x18 ft. Has 3 large windows from floor to ceiling. Reception Hall or Room. Has been the office of the late Dr. A. P. Good for 25 years. Built up practice to about $8,000.00 yearly. Dr. Good died last March. Office is furnished and is located at 622 N. 48th St. J. A. Nesbett, Bell-610, 622 N. 48th St."[54] The alleged success of this West Philadelphia office no doubt attracted some renters. But other advice warned against renting the office of a deceased doctor, "unless you can take it up within a week or two of the physician's demise."[55] If a practice had lain fallow for longer, then the patients of the previous renter/owner would have moved on to other doctors in the neighborhood.

Often the very practice itself was for sale with the office space—not just mortar and bricks, but the client list as well. This type of transaction was so common that the classified advertisements in *The Weekly Roster* usually included a section of "Practices for Sale." As one seller stated the terms of the sale in 1914, "Will sacrifice my $2,500.00 Practice in Kensington to Purchaser of my House and Stable at $5,900.00. All up to date. Owner going west. Answer to Dr. W. 20. Manhattan Advertising Service, 201 S. 4th St."[56] The few young doctors who might have been able to afford such a practice were advised to use caution. After all, there were no guarantees that the clientele of the previous doctor would remain loyal to a young new doctor at the same office address. In his *Building a Profitable Practice* (1912), Dr. Thomas Reilly listed what prospective buyers of private practices should expect and how they could negotiate more favorable terms: "You should have a few months' personal introduction by the retiring physician. It is only in case that there is absolutely no competition that you can expect to reap any sum approximating that received annually by the seller. In small towns, you need not expect to retain more than one-third of the former practice. In large cities it will not average more than one-fourth. [But] Even this introduction is a powerful lever in aiding your success. When buying a practice, make a hard and fast bargain that the seller must never again take up general practice in that city."[57] These business arrangements necessarily depended upon trust between the seller and the buyer, and did not always end satisfactorily.

For example, after Dr. Rita Finkler graduated from Woman's Medical College in 1915 and finished her internship at the Polyclinic Hospital, she decided to open a practice just up the road in Newark, New Jersey, so her husband could be closer to his job in New York City. By chance, Dr. Finkler learned that Dr. Lillian Shustman was selling her practice in Newark and moving to Hightstown. As Dr. Finkler put it, "We made a deal by which I would take over the lease on her apartment-office, she would introduce me to some of her patients and notify the others. I agreed to pay her $600.00 for this; $500.00 at once and $100.00 at the end of the year. We parted amicably and I never thought a written agreement was necessary." Unfortunately for Dr. Finkler, Dr. Shustman returned to Newark a short time later and began to contact her old patients. Dr. Finkler worried because many patients proved unwilling to go to a "new and unknown doctor" such as herself and went back to Dr. Shustman. Other patients, however, "were very unfavorably impressed by [Dr. Shustman's] proposed action and considered it dishonest and underhand. They decided that they would have nothing to do with her." Dr. Finkler recalled her first confrontation after Dr. Shustman returned: she "finally came in and told me how dissatisfied she and her husband were in Hightstown. She just had to come back, and besides, we did not have any written agreement! I was boiling mad, considered her unethical and dishonest. Written or not, I ordered her out of my house and vowed never to speak with her again." Dr. Finkler then resolved, as she put it, to "apply myself very diligently to hold the practice I had, and to develop a new following."[58]

After selecting office space, young doctors struggled to contain start-up costs without depriving the new practice of the vital equipment and furnishings needed to conduct business and to look the part of a respectable and trustworthy young doctor. Of the $500 recommended for setting up a practice, $150 was intended to cover equipment, but this large sum could be exhausted quickly even if young doctors purchased only the "practical instruments and necessary medicines." Recognizing the need for guidance, several Jefferson faculty members published a list for 1903 graduates intended to help "save the thoughtful from buying the whole store."[59] As Dr. Philip H. Moore later put it to the graduating class of 1908 at Jefferson, "Equip yourselves with such offices and apparatus as you really need, and as far as possible, as you are able to pay for." He further warned, "To cripple one's self on the installment plan for books, apparatus, and extravagant furnishings is poor policy, and a source of constant worriment. Save yourselves from it by the exercise of ordinary common sense."[60] Going into debt meant interest payments and thus higher fixed costs. This not only hurt the bottom line but inhibited reinvestment in the practice.

Waiting for Patients

After settling on a location, selecting office space, and purchasing equipment and furnishings, young doctors needed to attract patients while making ends meet. Practice income had to exceed fixed costs, and fast. Staying in business was such a common concern that it became good material for dark humor. For example, the editors of *The Jeffersonian*—a student-run newsletter of Jefferson Medical College—reprinted a mock dialogue cut from *Harper's Bazaar*, entitled

"Saving Doctors," which read, "Knicker—'There are plenty of books telling how to save life while waiting for the doctor.' Bocker—'Yes. What we need is one telling the young doctor how to save life while waiting for the patient.'"[61] This concern over "waiting for patients" surfaced in many commencement speeches and advice articles in Philadelphia medical publications. In 1911, for example, Dr. Harriet L. Hartley, a clinical professor of surgery, tried to dispel what she considered to be a common delusion among senior medical students at the Woman's Medical College of Pennsylvania (her alma mater):

> Surrounded as she is in her college days by only the successful of her calling, professors almost too busy to fill the scheduled hours, the student of medicine often looks forward to much more rapid returns in her medical life than usually fall to her lot. The blue moments, the periods of waiting, the poor pay for good work, bound to be part of her experience, are all unforeseen. Armed with a knowledge of disease and its treatment, made clearer and more comprehensive by a year's residence in a hospital, she feels she has only to establish an office, erect a nice brass sign on the window sill and the bell will merrily peal. Yes, it will peal, but the batteries are not apt to need replenishing the first few months. The public notices the advent of the sign, then it seems to forget.[62]

To some degree, women doctors in the early twentieth century still had difficulty earning patient trust outside of gynecological or obstetrical needs, which Dr. Hartley relayed as well.[63] The overall point of Hartley's advice, however, applied to all doctors: having a good education and a good location could confer competitive advantages, but they by no means guaranteed financial success. Getting even a well-planted first practice to germinate required close attention and care. By looking at a specific example of a young doctor in the first days of practice, we can see the business strategies used in order to survive while "waiting for patients."

In her unpublished autobiography, Dr. Catherine MacFarlane, who would become a renowned Philadelphia gynecologist and a distinguished faculty member at Woman's Medical College, described the financial pressures of her first days in practice. After graduating from Woman's Medical College in 1898, finishing a year of internship, and working for two years as an obstetrics instructor and a dispensary staff member, Dr. MacFarlane decided to set up her first practice. In 1901, she purchased a home and office in the suburb of Germantown that she hoped would be a good practice location, because "it had been occupied for many years by Dr. Charles Currie, a very successful physician."

In her estimation it was "an ideal Doctor's house."[64] But after she hung out her shingle, she confessed "most of my time was spent in the reception room looking out through the neat Swiss curtains and wondering how it happened that nobody rang the doorbell or needed the services of a young doctor like me."[65] As mentioned earlier, her first year's income amounted to $206.00—a paltry sum even for a rookie.

The first strategy for surviving the slow days was to keep up appearances by hiding any signs of financial desperation. In Dr. MacFarlane's case, she made every effort to keep her home and office presentable, including the white marble steps at the front of her house, which, she complained, "had to be scrubbed every day." She scrubbed them early in the morning, because "it would not have been professional for me to be seen doing this." Eventually, she was able to afford the cleaning services of a neighborhood girl from time to time.[66] Dr. MacFarlane used what little money she earned in her first year and reinvested it in her practice, especially in items that would preserve or enhance her image. In order to avoid the indignity and inefficiency of walking to house calls, Dr. MacFarlane made her first purchase a bicycle, which she rode with her black bag strapped to the handlebars. For some purchases, though, Dr. MacFarlane had to economize. For example, when she could finally afford her "great ambition"—a horse and buggy—she had to settle for a second-rate mare with weak ankles that caused the poor animal, from time to time, to fall down while pulling her buggy.[67] Throughout these lean early years of practice, Dr. MacFarlane scrimped and saved as best she could, but nevertheless depended upon her parents for support.[68] Despite pinching pennies, Dr. MacFarlane always tried to present a respectable, professional image in public even as she dealt with the mundane problems of running a small business out of her house.

One of the ironies in the business of private practice was that new professional norms discouraged doctors from advertising their services directly to patients. Both the 1903 and 1912 versions of the AMA's Code of Ethics criticized as "incompatible with honorable standing in the profession" those doctors who resorted "to public advertisement or private cards inviting the attention of persons affected with particular diseases; to promise radical cures; to publish cases or operations in the daily prints, or to suffer such publication to be made . . . to boast of cures and remedies; to adduce certificates of skill and success, or to employ any of the other methods of charlatans."[69] Violators risked expulsion from local, state, and national chapters of the AMA.

There were, however, surreptitious ways of advertising directly to patients, as Dr. Albert V. Harmon outlined in his cleverly titled how-to guide, *Large Fees and How to Get Them: A Book for the Private Use of Physicians* (1911). An adroit doctor could "get before the public" by joining a church and attending its social functions, by taking part in community events, by donating conspicuously to local charities, or by joining local fraternal orders.[70] Even though these activities cost money and time, they bought visibility and respect with influential neighbors. Eventually, participation in societies, clubs, and churches led to leadership positions—positions that might get the doctor's name in the paper, according to Dr. Harmon. "Of course he protests that others are better fitted, etc., but he doesn't mean it. He is elected and again there is legitimate excuse for getting more publicity."[71]

Contacting established doctors in the neighborhood also drew attention to a new practice. This strategy presumed that the newcomer had not already alienated colleagues by using sketchy advertising methods. Under normal circumstances, it was even considered disrespectful not to notify other doctors upon arriving in a new location. Besides reassuring established doctors about one's intentions, notification enabled a young doctor to solicit surplus clientele or to offer (paid) assistance for night calls or for laboratory analysis of urine or bacteriological cultures, if necessary.[72] When Dr. MacFarlane made her introductions, she reported mixed results. One local doctor offered her an assistantship, which she accepted gratefully, but another doctor merely patronized her with the obvious advice that "if you open your office on Main Street and do not drink, I am sure you will succeed." Dr. MacFarlane retorted that she had already opened her office on Main Street (Germantown Avenue), that she did not drink, and that she too hoped she would succeed.[73] Similarly, when Dr. Martin Rehfuss opened his first practice in Philadelphia in 1911, he sent four hundred business cards to his new colleagues, but he noted that it was "many months before [he] heard from anyone of them."[74] Although it did not always generate new clientele, contacting new colleagues at least started one off on the right foot.

Besides networking, young doctors often sought temporary salaried positions in order to earn much needed supplemental income, but also to expand their patronage network and perhaps draw new clients. In a chapter on "Extra-Practice Sources of Income," one advice book author noted that while "on the threshold of practice many of you will feel that you cannot afford to get along without some financial aid for the first year or so of waiting for practice. Some men borrow three or four hundred dollars for this purpose. Others seek extra-practice-means of keeping the wolf from the door."[75] The author detailed the benefits, in terms of salary and client-building opportunities, and costs, in terms of time away from building up a private practice, of half a dozen commonly available salaried positions, such as in the military, in public health, in state-run hospitals, in insurance companies, and in early laboratories.[76] These extra-practice sources of income were often combined with hospital and dispensary positions, which, although not typically remunerative, provided valuable experience and built a doctor's reputation in the neighborhood.[77] Thus, although doctors like MacFarlane took positions in order to advance their careers and to cultivate interests in medical specialties, paid positions also served as immediate sources of extra income to offset disappointing returns from early private practice, as important sites for networking with other doctors who might refer surplus clientele, or as opportunities to attract prospective clients.

To some extent, a young doctor simply had to wait for various business strategies to work while not committing any grave professional error in the meantime. In Dr. MacFarlane's case, she conceded that "the Germantown doctors were good to me" because she got many of her first clients by referral. In the end, though, she attributed her success to sheer patience: "eventually people began to see [my] sign and ring the doorbell."[78] After new patients began to trickle in, the key to building a practice was to satisfy these first patients and earn their trust. As with any new business, satisfied customers not only provided repeat business but free advertisement by word-of-mouth. As such, all the advice given to young doctors on setting up a practice stressed the need to provide the best possible care to a patient, because good care was the ultimate method of distinguishing oneself from the competition.[79]

Managing Growth and Career Transitions

After the early lean years, an established practice suffered the normal growing pains of any small business. Once doctors earned enough net income to repay any start-up loans, there were many ways to reinvest money in order to increase the profitability of a practice. From a business perspective, it made a good deal of sense to reinvest in better office furnishings, in new diagnostic equipment, and in an automobile. If it was true, as advice book authors claimed, that the public scrutinized every aspect of a doctor's office and image for signs of competence and trustworthiness, then reinvestment in office space, equipment, and transportation increased the efficiency and appeal of a private practice. Dr. MacFarlane, for example, reinvested profits by gradually upgrading her mode of transportation. At first she made house calls on foot, then on bicycle, and then by horse and buggy. By her tenth year in practice, by which time she held many hospital positions and had opened a second office in Center City,

Dr. MacFarlane decided to buy a car in order to cut her commute time between offices. At first, she could only afford a low-end model, which often broke down en route. Finally, after about fifteen years in practice, she could afford a reliable car—one with an electric "self-starter" rather than a hand crank (which she was not strong enough not operate).[80] Dr. MacFarlane's reinvestments increased her efficiency and burnished her public image—both of which increased the profitability of her practice. As with any business venture, one had to spend money in order to make more money.

Besides making regular decisions about reinvestment, an established doctor at some point considered how to maximize profits in a growing business. After tapping all of the available clientele in his or her neighborhood, an established doctor could increase profits by expanding to branch offices. For example, as Dr. MacFarlane developed interests in gynecology, she opened a second office in the Center City. By locating in a convenient and central location, she could draw gynecological patients from a wider radius than from her suburban Germantown office. Dr. MacFarlane nevertheless kept her first general practice, which had become the cornerstone of her income and reputation.[81] Although expanding to branch offices could increase profits, there were risks involved. For example, *The Physician's Business and Financial Adviser* (1900) claimed it was "seldom if ever that more than one office can be made to pay. People who know you have two offices often do not know at which office they will find you, and for this reason they send for some other doctor, especially in emergency cases. In addition there is the added work and worry to keeping up double offices in addition to the expense, and it is one case in one hundred where one office is not discontinued in a short time."[82] The development of telephony and faster transportation by the mid-1910s, however, mitigated many of these earlier inefficiencies of branch offices.

While expanding to branch offices could increase the radius of a practice otherwise limited by local demand in the original office location, some established doctors had the opposite problem—they had more patient demand in their neighborhood than they could handle. In this situation, a doctor could hire assistants to help with surplus cases, and plenty of young doctors in large cities were eager to earn extra income in this way. Hiring assistants, however, required additional management and ran the risk of breeding local competition. For this reason, doctors with the luxury of too many patients often used this opportunity to maximize their profits by raising fees—a strategy consistent with the principles of supply and demand. Although young doctors kept fees low in order to attract as many patients as possible, established doctors could raise fees to increase profit, and even to get rid of extra or unwanted clientele. As Dr. Hartley put it to alumnae of Woman's Medical College in 1911, "As her practice grows, the busy doctor can weed out and get rid of a great deal of hard and poorly paid work by increasing her fees."[83] Those who could not afford the higher fees would go elsewhere, and the established doctor could thereby earn more while working the same number of hours. This business strategy effectively limited clientele to the affluent while fobbing off charity cases to younger doctors in the neighborhood. In those local markets with a short supply of doctors, affluent patients paid more for the services of an established doctor, and younger doctors were certainly grateful for being referred charity and low-fee clients from their elders. Even in markets with balanced supply and demand, a more established or skilled doctor could raise fees and still remain competitive, provided that he or she offered medical services that were valued more than those offered by younger, less capable, or less trusted doctors.

Besides the decision of whether to use branch offices or higher fees to raise profits, an established doctor also faced the mid-career decision of whether or not to limit practice to a particular specialty of interest, such as obstetrics or pediatrics. In making this important decision, the feasibility of specializing often trumped whatever affinities, abilities, and career goals an established doctor with specialty aspirations might have had. For example, after discouraging a student audience at Jefferson Medical College from specializing too early, Dr. Edwin B. Cragin conceded that "the time may come in the life of any one of you when the limitation of your field of work is either necessary or distinctly desirable." He hastened to add, however, that the decision "should depend largely upon two conditions. 1. Your opportunities for work. 2. Your natural taste and fitness for work."[84] Market opportunity trumped a doctor's individual affinities and abilities when deciding whether to specialize.

Although specialty practice typically commanded higher fees and income, specialists first had to adapt to a different business model in order to succeed. In general practice, a doctor could depend on walk-by business in the neighborhood in which he or she located. To be sure, young doctors starting a first practice welcomed referrals of surplus clients from established doctors nearby, but such referrals were not the basis of general practice. Specialty practice, on the other hand, did not have walk-by or drop-in clients. Passersby of an obstetrician's office, for example, did not suddenly decide to go inside for treatment. Rather, specialists depended upon GPs for patient referrals and consultation requests.[85] It was therefore difficult to specialize before developing the institutional and collegial networks needed for referrals and consultations. These networks took years to build, and usually required the aspiring specialist first to pay his or her dues in general practice and then to develop recognized ability in his or her chosen specialty, typically through extensive work in hospitals and dispensaries and through teaching positions in medical schools. Although there were no legal barriers to specializing, limiting a practice to a single specialty simply was not feasible (from a business standpoint) without extensive preparation.

Practical business barriers further explain why so few doctors fully specialized within five or ten years after medical school (see figure 2). Not only was general practice viewed as the ideal first career step, even for those who hoped to specialize later on, but young doctors could succeed in general practice in ways that they could not in specialty practice until much later in their careers. Furthermore, even when deciding to specialize, many established doctors opted for *partial* specialization until they could depend upon income from referrals and consultations. For example, after ten years in practice and after having held many hospital and teaching positions, Dr. MacFarlane began to limit her practice to obstetrics and gynecology in 1908. At first, though, MacFarlane only spent two nights a week treating patients with specialty complaints in her Center City office; she spent the rest of her time in general practice treating the usual range of patients in her Germantown office.[86] Although aspiring specialists like Dr. MacFarlane might have preferred earlier specialization, the viability of specialty practice, from a business perspective, was the primary consideration in making this important mid-career decision.

Because of their career and financial dependence on private medical practice, doctors necessarily factored their goals for practice into their career choices. Given the nature of private practice, business considerations often directed career choices that might, at first glance, seem to have been matters solely of preference and aptitude. When considering an internship, for example, doctors not only considered possible career benefits of further clinical education, but also the financial impact of an internship on their future practices and incomes. Similarly, in order to achieve certain business objectives in practice, aspiring specialists adapted their career paths in order to cultivate the necessary institutional affiliations and collegial networks. In other words, medical careers and the business of private medical practice remained inextricably linked in the first two decades of the twentieth century.

Shared Business Problems and the Limits of Cooperation

Setting up a practice, waiting for patients, building clientele, and managing growth—these were ordinary small business problems that could be managed individually. Doctors may have received advice or assistance, but none of these problems threatened the place of solo private practice as the fundamental unit of the medical marketplace. Other business problems, however, either required or benefited from professional cooperation in order for the individual doctor to solve them effectively. The problems of excessive competition from oversupply and of fee collection from delinquent patients offer a window into the business othos of urban doctors at the turn of the century. By comparing the willingness of doctors to cooperate in solving these shared problems, we can see the tension between individualism and professional cooperation that shaped the business of private practice for much of the early twentieth century.

In the unregulated premodern medical marketplace, oversupply constituted the most common business problem in private practice. Without legal barriers to limit the supply of healers, average fees were low, as healers underbid one another to compete. Even though early regulation had increased significantly by the late nineteenth century, urban doctors still faced an oversupply of orthodox doctors. By raising admissions standards, overhauling curricula, and increasing graduation requirements, medical education reform raised the quality while lowering the production of medical graduates. After having peaked at 162 schools and 5,304 graduates in 1906, only 96 American medical schools remained in 1915 and these produced just 3,536 graduates.[87] As a result, the doctor-population ratio declined, even in the large cities to which doctors flocked. In Philadelphia, for example, the number of doctors dropped from 249 to 187 doctors per 100,000 residents between the years 1900 and 1920.[88] Thus medical education reform had the direct result of reducing competition by limiting supply of orthodox doctors. This reduction, it was hoped, would increase the market value of private medical care.

American doctors also rallied around professional efforts to reduce competition further by eliminating "sectarian" competitors, who had arisen in the nineteenth century due to populist rejection of elite orthodox medicine, to patient dissatisfaction with the perceived harshness of orthodox therapies, and to the repeal of nearly all legal barriers to medical practice.[89] Amid the felt chaos of urbanization and industrialization by the turn of the century, however, the American public appealed for state regulation of matters affecting health and safety, and orthodox doctors used this political opportunity to assert their legitimacy, grounded in scientific expertise, to lead the Progressive

Era charge to reform medical practice.[90] In the process, orthodox doctors waged war on sectarian "quackery" and succeeded in lobbying for stricter licensing laws granting orthodox doctors the exclusive rights to conduct state licensing examinations in states like Pennsylvania by the 1910s.[91] Despite facing hostile examiners on state boards, alternative healers did not vanish overnight, but the writing was on the wall. The more institutionalized medical sects, like homeopathy and osteopathy, conformed their medical school curricula and practices to those of orthodox medicine in order to survive.[92] Although medical heterodoxy persisted in various forms throughout the twentieth century, orthodox doctors had cornered the market for private practice in most states by World War I and used their new regulatory powers to persecute sectarian competitors to the fullest extent of the law.

In a marketplace ordinarily characterized by competition between small business owners, doctors nevertheless cooperated to limit supply for several reasons. Because oversupply within the orthodox profession lowered fees, it was in the economic self-interest of every practicing doctor to limit growth in their ranks—a monopolistic goal that harkened back to the earliest trade guilds in medieval Europe. Orthodox doctors could also agree on the supply-side threat posed by alternative healers. Although orthodox doctors provided some unique goods and services, alternative and orthodox market niches overlapped to a significant degree. It was therefore in the economic self-interest of every doctor to restrict if not eliminate sectarian competition. The lofty rhetoric of professional reform during the Progressive Era inspired collective action at the same time as it gave humanitarian cover to the financial advantages of reducing competition by limiting supply in the marketplace.

Fee collection comprised the other major business problem that tempted doctors to cooperate. Contemporary editorialists considered incomplete or delayed fee collection to be pervasive problems in private practice. To some degree, effective fee collection began with good accounting habits, and doctors had notoriously poor skills in such basics of running a business. For some doctors, such ineptitude connoted honesty and diligence.[93] Advice books devoted significant space to the basics of accounting and fee collection, because, as the author of *The Physician's Business and Financial Adviser* (1900) argued, "every doctor must live by his practice, and in order to do this, he must establish a regular business system."[94] Advice included tips on how to encourage patients to pay in cash, how to insist politely on payment up front, how best to account for unpaid fees, how frequently to settle accounts with patients, and what to do with delinquent patients. In general, doctors dared not be too pushy in demanding payment up front, because patients held the ultimate power—the option to see another doctor who was willing to wait for payment. Furthermore, in cases of medical urgency or emergency, many doctors either thought it was immoral to ask for money up front or felt that doing so would harm their public image (and thereby future business). Thus doctors often collected fees long after services had been rendered.[95] Here again, private practice differed from other small businesses, like groceries or laundries, in which payment was expected at the point of sale and in which there was no moral or professional expectation to provide free goods and services to those in need.

When collecting fees, doctors typically billed the patient. This interaction proved uncomfortable enough for some, but downright awkward when patients haggled with the doctor or simply did not reply. In these circumstances, advice books like *Building a Profitable Practice: Being a Text-Book on Medical Economics* (1912) recommended sending first a "suggestive letter," followed by an "argumentative," then an "urgent," and finally a "drastic letter."[96] We can see this epistolary strategy at work in the letters of Dr. Thomas R. Neilson, an 1880 graduate of the University of Pennsylvania who became a well-known Philadelphia surgeon. Dr. Neilson's first letters often began with a polite but pleading tone, one intended to invoke sympathy. For example, he asked of one patient who had proposed paying his bill in installments, "May I ask what intervals you intend to make these payments? Being myself practically a wage earner, too, I would like to have some idea of when my earnings will be available."[97] When diplomacy failed, Dr. Neilson became more insistent. He wrote to one unresponsive patient in November 1906, "I would esteem it a favor if you would kindly settle my bill for professional services rendered to you in May 1905. I have sent a bill to you several times, but have not as yet heard from you, although, in view of your promise on leaving the hospital to send me a check, I had expected a prompt settlement of the account. A remittance at an early date will be appreciated."[98] Dr. Neilson's position as a successful surgeon and professor at the University of Pennsylvania did not mean he was above haggling, either. To one patient who paid only $20 of his bill with the excuse "this is the best I could do at this time," Dr. Neilson replied that he was "much obliged . . . for the remittance," but then insisted on the remainder. He justified his position in his March 1912 reply: "As to the amount of my bill, I made my minimum charge of $10 per week for cases not requiring operative treatment. [Your wife] was under my care for 3 1/2 weeks—from March 15 till April 10 [1911], making the amount of the bill $35.00, which I felt to be a perfectly reasonable charge for the services rendered. I thank you for your check on that account, and am quite

willing to wait for the balance until the time you name."[99] As the letters of
Dr. Neilson indicate, success did not spare him one of the most common business tasks—having to collect fees.

At some point, every doctor encountered a patient who had no intention of
paying. Under these circumstances, doctors did have legal options. But in some
cities, like Philadelphia, doctors also banded together at the local level to help
identify and expose chronically delinquent patients in order to prevent such
patients scamming one doctor after another. A group of Philadelphia doctors
who practiced in the working-class neighborhoods of the Northern Liberties,
Kensington, and Fishtown formed the Northeast Medical Club in 1907, with
the stated purpose "to guard against loss from irresponsible and dishonest persons." Local doctors were invited to join for one dollar a year, which bought
them access to a list, printed yearly, of the names of allegedly delinquent
patients submitted by other club members. In a recruiting advertisement placed
in *The Weekly Roster*, entitled "Northeast Physicians Unite for Protection," the
club boasted that seventy-five members had already joined. According to the
advertisement, a similar business association had been operating in West Philadelphia for several years.[100] Because revenue lost to patient delinquency threatened the livelihoods of all, doctors proved willing to cooperate in order to solve
this shared business problem, at least in certain locations. Although it is not
possible to gauge the success of the Northeast Medical Club, its mission under-
scores the extent to which economic interests alone—that is to say, interests
without a lofty professional reform dimension—could also inspire cooperation
in the medical marketplace.

Besides exchanging lists of delinquent patients, urban doctors also hired
collection agencies to settle their largest outstanding accounts. Collection agencies eliminated the hassle of tracking down delinquent patients, but charged as
much as 20 percent of the fees collected. In a scheme inspired by the new ideals
of corporatism and efficiency during the "managerial revolution" in American
business, Chicago doctors banded together in 1907 to form their own collection
agency, to be run and operated by the Chicago Medical Society.[101] The agency
promised to protect the business interests of member doctors, save money by
cutting out private middlemen, and lower collection costs by providing the
economy of scale of a single, large business firm. Unfortunately for Chicago
doctors, they proved to be incompetent businesspeople, and the society's collection agency went bankrupt four years later, with the CMS having to write
off its initial investment. Even though it failed, historian Thomas Goebel has
argued that the CMS experiment using an "organizational and managerial

response to the problem of overdue accounts illustrates the extent to which business values had permeated American medicine."[102] If nothing else, the episode proves that pragmatic commercialism coexisted with professional idealism in medicine at this time.

When it came to other shared business problems, though, doctors proved unwilling to cooperate, particularly on measures that were perceived to restrict individual economic interests or impose corporate entities between doctors and patients in the marketplace. At times, this led to private practice being out of step with contemporary developments in American business.[103] For example, despite widespread agreement that the growth of medical specialties raised the cost and inefficiency of private medical care as patients were referred from one specialist's office to the next, county medical societies routinely criticized early proposals to organize and manage specialty care through private group practice. The most famous proponent of private group practice was Boston's Dr. Richard Cabot, who extolled the virtues of private group clinics like the innovative Mayo Clinic in Rochester, Minnesota, as managerial solutions to the problem of specialism.[104] In a contentious article published in the popular *American Magazine* in 1916, Cabot reasoned that group clinics could reduce the cost of private medical care by consolidating diagnostic facilities and equipment and could improve the quality and efficiency of medical care by centralizing case management and facilitating consultation between specialists.[105] Critics alleged that private group clinics demoted doctors to salaried employees and undercut fees of solo practitioners in the surrounding community. Medical societies in many states, including Pennsylvania, rebuked Cabot for his "unethical" public attack on his fellow practitioners and claimed group clinics violated the AMA's "Principles of Medical Ethics," which stipulated "it is unprofessional for a physician to dispose of his services under conditions that . . . interfere with reasonable competition among the physicians of a community."[106]

For ideological rather than practical reasons, large group practices remained extremely rare in the early twentieth century; instead, solo private practice endured as the business model and professional ideal in the marketplace.[107] Historian Donald Madison noted the irony of individualism crystallizing in private practice at the same time as bureaucracy and corporatism ruled in most other American enterprises. As he put it, "Physicians were the exception. Instead of joining other commercial and professional associations in heralding the advantages of consolidation and scientific management . . . organized medicine's leaders determined to end their sojourn with the organizational society. Forgoing the search for modernization, they preached instead a kind of antimodernism that would be protective of the dominant small-business and artisan values held by the majority of medical practitioners."[108] Although some county medical societies like Chicago (and later Philadelphia) experimented with corporatism in the form of society-run collection agencies, managed fee collection neither threatened the small business ethos of doctors nor altered their market access to patients, and doctors were only willing to cooperate or to adopt new business strategies under those limited conditions.

Economic Self-Interest and Professional Stratification

Individualism not only undermined cooperation but led each doctor to protect his or her own economic self-interest in private practice. The divergent business interests of GPs and specialists, and of young doctors and established doctors, reinforced professional stratification observed in the divergent career paths of these groups, and led to conflict and rivalry as doctors in each stratum defended their business interests. Young doctors at times resorted to "contract practice," much to the consternation of established doctors, and GPs and specialists locked horns over the issue of "dispensary abuse." In both disputes, doctors in different strata accused each other of using "unfair" business practices that placed commercial above professional goals.

In the mid-nineteenth century, when professional overcrowding became particularly pronounced, medical societies intervened in the marketplace by establishing "fee schedules" of the minimum charges for office and home visits and for routine procedures. Schedules were updated periodically to cover new procedures, adjust to the cost of living, and account for the increasing expense of medical treatment. Doctors, however, were not obliged to follow fee schedules, even though adopting minimum fees helped to prevent underbidding and to establish the fees a delinquent patient could be held legally accountable for not having paid.[109] Despite the price-fixing goals behind fee schedules, market forces ultimately determined the fees able to be charged in practice, and the oversupply of doctors and alternative healers devalued the price of private medical care into the early twentieth century. For example, even as late as 1917, the minimum fees of $2 for "treatment at the bedside" and $1 for office visits agreed upon by the newly formed Physicians' Business Association in Philadelphia were nearly unchanged from the fees adopted by the College of Physicians of Philadelphia in 1843.[110] Perhaps this was why the Physicians' Business Association hoped that "all will cooperate and restore the profession to its traditional high caste as well as to secure economic independence for each of its members."[111]

The problem with fee schedules was that price reduction was often the tool of last resort for a young doctor desperate to attract patients. The most common strategy for underbidding at the turn of the century was contract practice, wherein a doctor agreed to provide medical services for a company or organization for a flat rate, typically not more than two dollars per employee (or member) per annum. By this arrangement, a young doctor could secure a modest living if under contract with an organization having several hundred members. So-called lodge practice in a benevolent society or fraternal order were the most common forms of contract practice, especially in cities having large immigrant populations who were separated from their families and therefore from traditional domestic care networks. Lodge practices were not uncommon, and about 9 percent of adult males in Pennsylvania paid membership dues to an organization that entitled them to the contracted services of a doctor in 1907.[112]

In response to the rising tide of contract practice in industrial cities, the AMA branded all forms of contract practice as unethical and many county medical societies expelled members who violated these standards. Critics argued that contract practice cheapened the social status of the doctor to that of a wholesaler; "doctoring lodges and families by the head, like butchers kill hogs, or shearers shear sheep, should be below your dignity. No physician respects himself who does this."[113] Worse yet, lodge doctors were blamed for further lowering the market value of private medical care as organizations could get doctors to bid against one another for contracts. Finally, critics insisted that contract practice yielded inferior medical care, as lodge doctors were too busy to conduct thorough examinations and had little financial incentive to provide expensive treatment, even if indicated.[114] In an effort to drum up support for Philadelphia doctors to sign a 1905 pledge not to engage in contract practice, *The Weekly Roster* explained its hazards: "its very inexpensiveness must appeal to an ever-widening public that is incapable of judging as to cheapness and quality. The danger to physicians is certainly not a minor one. In such a manufacturing metropolis as Philadelphia the evil must constantly grow unless a firm stand is taken by the profession."[115]

Although no young doctor was foolish enough to praise lodge practice in print, the dire straits of the overcrowded marketplace drove some to risk professional ostracism by accepting contract practice. Editorialists cautioned that "the evil is very tempting to the beginner," because it could be used to build up clientele quickly and to reach an untapped class of patients often too poor to pay for medical care.[116] Sympathetic observers blamed market forces rather than young doctors for the growth of contract practice, urging prevention rather than punishment as a deterrent. As one Philadelphia editorialist appealed in 1913, "See to it that every young man not only is urged to join the society, but is given his share of work therein. No fear but you will see to it that he gets his share of the dead-head work in the community. Give these men work, and by attrition they will soon be assimilated and become proficient workers."[117] In other words, if older doctors expected younger doctors to adopt ethical business practices, then they needed to help younger doctors find work by referring surplus cases to them.

The dispute over contract practice reveals that divergent business interests in private practice led to conflict between young and established doctors. Similar disputes arose between GPs and specialists. Although they shared certain problems, like fee collection, GPs and specialists relied upon two fundamentally different business models in private practice: GPs relied upon walk-ins from in the neighborhoods around their offices whereas specialists relied upon the patient referrals and consultation fees from other doctors. As such, specialists spent years developing networks and gaining expertise through teaching positions in medical schools and staff positions in hospitals (see figure 3). It was therefore in the economic self-interest of specialists and pre-specialists to protect the supply of patients to hospitals and dispensaries, because these institutions provided, in the bodies of charity patients therein, the learning and teaching opportunities doctors needed in order to specialize in private practice. As these two institutions grew and became central to medical care in American cities, they also became sites for intra-professional conflict and rivalry. In particular, GPs and specialists fought bitterly over the proper role of dispensaries.

The first American dispensaries were established in the late eighteenth century, and were typically funded by private donations or by municipal taxes. These charitable outpatient institutions grew rapidly during the nineteenth century, as social reformers sought to control the poverty and poor health associated with urbanization and immigration. Philadelphia's first dispensary was founded in 1786; the number grew to thirty-three by 1877, and reached sixty-one in 1903.[118] Dispensary doctors typically handled minor ambulatory cases, provided vaccinations, performed minor surgeries, and wrote and filled prescriptions. These doctors volunteered their time, and dispensary patients paid little to nothing for services. In exchange, dispensaries provided valuable career opportunities for doctors and needed medical care for the working class in cities. With the arrival of the second wave of immigrants to already crowded slums at the turn of the century, the health conditions of the urban poor further deteriorated, which meant that dispensary patients often presented with more extreme and advanced illnesses due to their inability to afford regular medical care. As a result, specialists came to regard dispensaries as "feeders" for interesting "clinical material" not ordinarily encountered in office practice.[119]

As the role of dispensaries expanded, rank-and-file doctors became disillusioned with these medical charities in the early twentieth century. The still crowded medical marketplace in American cities generated intense competition, and many local doctors regarded neighboring dispensaries as nothing more than competitors for a finite supply of private patients. Dispensaries also served the narrow interests of elite doctors—namely those with specialty aspirations who were willing (and able) to volunteer their time. As the goodwill of ordinary doctors declined, dispensaries came under fire. Opponents charged that dispensaries failed to conduct proper means testing to weed out the presumed freeloaders from the truly needy, thereby robbing local doctors of clientele.[120] Many county medical societies investigated alleged "dispensary abuse" and recommended solutions. For example, the Philadelphia County Medical Society periodically appointed committees "for the purpose of looking into the methods and results of dispensary practice." In 1903, one such committee concluded from a survey of 481 Philadelphia doctors and 61 dispensaries that as many as 50 percent of dispensary patients received undeserved free care.[121] In 1914, another PCMS committee recommended that dispensaries hire social workers to determine the financial need of patients, and suggested raising the nominal fees charged.[122] In an era of heightened xenophobia and widespread public debate about the proper role of charity, it is perhaps no surprise that county medical societies uncovered widespread dispensary abuse.[123] But rank-and-file doctors, especially GPs, blamed perceived dispensary abuse as much on incompetent administrators and deceitful patients as on specialists, who were assumed to have turned a blind eye to the damage dispensaries inflicted on the private practices of nearby doctors.

This intra-professional rivalry became particularly heated after the turn of the century as GPs tried to explain perceived declines in their returns from private practice. Besides blaming the general oversupply of doctors, GPs found other culprits. Some even blamed the success of public health projects like water filtration plants, which lowered the chronic morbidity from infectious and contagious diseases like typhoid fever. As one Philadelphia doctor so frankly reasoned, "Every advance in sanitation, in providing better conditions for workmen and employees, serves to deplete his [the doctor's] income."[124] The declines in fees were thought to harm GPs more than specialists, as the fees of the specialists were "adjusted to the importance and difficulty of the work, his own reputation, and the means of the patient. The fees of the general practitioner, on the other hand, are fixed and small."[125]

Other GPs explained the income gap by accusing specialists of poaching patients with general complaints. One Philadelphia editorialist exclaimed in 1911, "Now Mr. Specialist, if you are a real specialist, who makes his living at the special work, and expect the profession to send you work, you will not do this, but will send them [patients] back to the old reliable family doctor, and the Lord knows he [the GP] is constantly having his income curtailed in enough ways without you aiding and abetting in the work."[126] To defend against poaching, GPs tried to learn the most common specialty procedures in order to avoid referring business elsewhere. As one advice author put it, "I do not mean that you should pose as a specialist, but that you should handle the ordinary cases that come to your office. . . . Every patient that you must turn over to another department of medicine spells failure for you, as far as that patient is concerned."[127] Specialists, in turn, tried to limit the scope of general practice by publishing advice in county and state medical journals on what the GP should know of certain specialties (very little) and when the GP should request consultation or refer patients to the specialist (immediately).[128]

In this climate of heated competition in private practice, GPs came to view dispensaries as symbols of their changing fortunes in the profession and in the marketplace. Not only did GPs view these institutions as the breeding grounds for specialist competitors, but the doctors who worked therein were either successful enough to donate their time or were willing enough to sacrifice their time in order to develop specialty skills. As such, one author blamed the persistence of dispensary abuse on "well-established physicians," like specialists, for whom "it is not a matter of direct interest whether patients are treated for free at the dispensaries or not."[129] The fear was that without the cooperation of dispensary staff, comprised mostly of specialists who had no interest in raising dispensary fees and thereby jeopardizing their supply of "clinical material," the pressure needed to eliminate dispensary abuse might never be brought to bear, thereby further endangering the survival of the GP. In the estimation of the editorial staff of the *Pennsylvania Medical Journal,*

> the general practitioner of today is ground between two rough surfaces—as it were—the consultant above and the dispensaries and hospitals below. In other words the consultant gets all the cream while the dispensaries cut very extensively into the lower class and very appreciably into the desirable middle class. . . . It is said the average consultant not only plainly seeks more purely consultation work in this class, but is ready

to act in the capacity of family physician when he gets the chance; and that he invariably does this among the rich. And then the dispensaries, on the other hand, relax quite all efforts at discrimination, treating every one that comes along, even throwing out strong inducements.[130]

Rural doctors in neighboring Montgomery County agreed that specialists were to blame for the inability of GPs to make a living in Philadelphia. One editorialist in the *Montgomery County Medical Bulletin* even linked the problem of dispensary abuse to that of the "lodge practice evil," by noting that specialism generated a class rift among Philadelphia doctors. First, there were "those connected with colleges or having political influence, or married to rich wives. Each morning they exchange patients from the country (sent by their former patients), so that each specialist gets a slice, each scratches each other's back; [and] in the afternoon they slave to keep their hospital clinics full." By providing each other with referrals and by giving free treatment to dispensary patients, the author charged that elite specialists created an underclass of Philadelphia doctors, or "those fighting for existence strapped to lodges, contracts, and individual insurances with no time for scientific work, [and] dying and leaving a family unprovided for."[131] Although this Montgomery County doctor indulged in hyperbole at times, his indictment of city specialists captured the sentiment of many Philadelphia-area GPs at this time.

Thus in the first two decades of the twentieth century, the individualism so valued by doctors, in general, led different strata to protect their respective business interests in private practice, even at the risk of intra-professional conflict and rivalry. These business interests were determined by age and specialization. Desperate to protect their economic self-interests, some young doctors defied prohibitions against contract practice enacted by their elder counterparts, who could afford the luxury of idealism from the offices of their established private practices. Contract practice eventually faded in the 1920s, but not because established doctors succeeded in shaming their younger colleagues. Instead, as regulation tamed oversupply, market conditions became more favorable for younger doctors to establish private practices without resorting to contract work.[132] Similarly, GPs and specialists butted heads over the proper role of dispensaries, as this institution had very different career and financial value to each group. This business conflict soured relations between GPs and specialists in other matters of professional concern in this period. For example, GPs found little reward in taking time from making a living to answer questionnaires received from academic specialists keen on publishing "collective investigations" into the epidemiology and treatment of various diseases using data gathered from the bedside experience of hard-working GPs.[133] Altogether, the disputes over contract practice and dispensary abuse reveal that different strata of the medical profession had different visions for the proper balance between commercial and professional interests in private practice.

After Dr. John Roberts finished his impassioned plea to his audience at the Philadelphia County Medical Society in the spring of 1911, a lively discussion followed in which his indictment of commercialism was met by skepticism and even scorn. Many doubted that the worst offenses, especially kickbacks, were common, and others defended many of the billing and fee practices that Dr. Roberts had criticized. As Dr. J. Madison Taylor, an eminent Philadelphia neurologist, replied, "The medical man having no salary, except the occasional and always small one for teaching, cannot act the good Samaritan in all particulars and indefinitely, and ought therefore to be recognized as worthy of richly-merited emoluments . . . his talent, labor, and maturity of judgment should be worth as much as the public is capable or willing to pay."[134] Many of his colleagues agreed. Dr. Louis J. Lautenbach, an established GP in the audience, even claimed that "in order to raise the standard of the medical profession as a whole[,] the profession should put a higher value on their services."[135] Commercial interests were complimentary, not inimical, to professional ideals.

As this ethical debate and my analysis of the business of private practice reveal, the fundamental nature of the medical marketplace remained unchanged in the early twentieth century, despite the rise of professional regulation. Private medical practices still functioned as small businesses, and old-fashioned individualism endured in the American medical profession. Even as new career paths emerged in specialty practice and in the medical institutions upon which specialists depended, doctors continued to base their career decisions upon economic self-interest in private practice. Doctors did follow some contemporary trends in American business by cooperating on occasion to solve shared business problems, but only so long as cooperation did not restrict the freedom of solo practitioners to compete for patients in the marketplace. Individualism yielded different strata of doctors who protected their respective business interests. Because of the divergent business interests of young and established doctors, of GPs and specialists, conflict and rivalry pervaded an age customarily assumed to have yielded a unified profession.[136]

Chapter 3

Downtown Specialists
and Neighborhood GPs

In her unpublished autobiography, Dr. Catherine MacFarlane recounted her medical career in Philadelphia, from studying as a medical student at Woman's Medical College (1895–1898), to training as an intern at Woman's Hospital (1898–1899), to working and teaching in an obstetrical clinic (1899–1901), to setting up her first private medical practice (1901), to specializing in gynecology (1908), to being appointed as professor of gynecology at her alma mater (1922), by which time she had earned a reputation as one of the city's top gynecologists.[1] As we have seen, the career moves of early twentieth-century American doctors were inseparable from the business considerations of private practice, and Dr. MacFarlane was no exception. Just like any small business, location mattered, and nearly every development in Dr. MacFarlane's career coincided with a change in her practice location. Thus her career path to urban specialty practice, like those of her peers, traversed the complex terrain of the industrial metropolis. From medical study and internship just north of Center City (1895–1899), to deliveries in the immigrant ghettoes of South Philadelphia (1899–1901), to house calls and office practice in suburban Germantown (1901–1908), to specialty office practice in Center City near the posh Rittenhouse Square (1908), Dr. MacFarlane's circuitous path raises interesting questions about niches in the urban medical marketplace (maps 1 and 2). This chapter examines the relationship between urban space, medical careers, and the business of private practice in the early twentieth century.

Career and business advice given to young doctors at the turn of the century emphasized the critical importance of finding a "good location." As Dr. Daniel

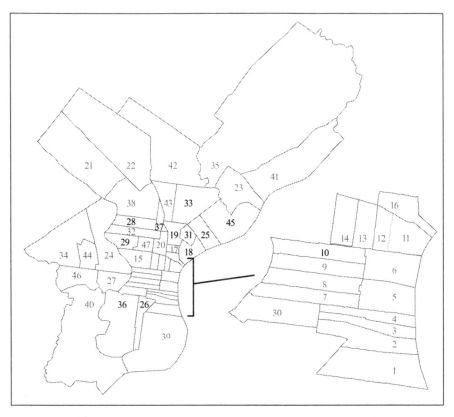

Map 1.   Ward Map of Philadelphia City and County

Note: Ward maps in this book use the forty-seven wards in 1909 for all analysis. The overall area of Philadelphia city and county remained fairly stable after 1848. The four wards (48–51) added from 1909–1940 did not change overall ward boundaries, but just subdivided wards 36, 42, and 46. See *Ward Genealogy of the City and County of Philadelphia*, comp. Allen Weinburg and Dale Fields, with Charles E. Hughes Jr. (Philadelphia: Dept. of Public Records, 1958).

Cathell explained in the opening pages of *The Physician Himself*, "Unless you have the locality and place of residence already selected, you may find it the most difficult problem of your life . . . to balance and weigh the advantages of this, that, or the other nook, crook, or corner."[2] Closer examination of popular advice literature reveals a detailed location calculus that urged doctors to consider regional, local and even street-level factors before deciding where to set up shop. Criteria included population density, accessibility, local demand, local competition from other health professionals, and the social background of prospective clientele. But did doctors heed the advice that they received? If so, what were the consequences of their collective "location behavior" for the geography of private practice and the availability of health care services more generally?[3]

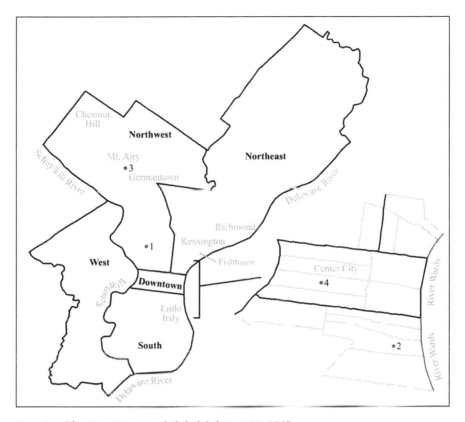

Map 2. The Five Districts of Philadelphia, 1900–1940

Note: The five districts (in dark lettering) used in my analysis of Philadelphia were first defined by Sam Bass Warner Jr. in *The Private City: Philadelphia in Three Periods of Its Growth*, 2nd ed. (Philadelphia: University of Pennsylvania Press, 1987), 160. Major neighborhoods discussed are also listed (in lighter lettering). Numbers (1–4) refer to the changing location of Dr. Catherine MacFarlane's medical practice, 1899–1908.

More and more medical graduates, like Dr. MacFarlane, followed advice to practice medicine in growing cities, like Philadelphia. Although this trend reflected the urbanization of Americans as a whole, doctors urbanized at a much faster rate (table 6) because cities offered benefits seldom found in rural practice. Cities had more doctors per capita than the countryside, but the population density and well-developed infrastructure of cities meant that doctors could cut the time and cost of house calls, thereby increasing profits. Patients could also easily access a doctor's office in the city, thereby offsetting the higher cost of overhead in cities by the greater fees earned from larger patient volume. Expanding metropolitan transportation networks stretched the effective radius of urban medical marketplaces into the countryside, thereby mitigating some of the deflationary effects of heightened competition in cities. Additionally,

Table 6.   **The Urbanization of Doctors in the United States in 1906 and 1923**

Community Size	Percent of Population		Percent of Doctors	
	1906	*1923*	*1906*	*1923*
Less than 25,000	69.1	62.6	59.8	50.6
25,000–100,000	8.9	10.5	10.5	12.0
More than 100,000	22.0	26.9	30.2	37.4

Source: Lewis Mayers and Leonard V. Harrison, *The Distribution of Physicians in the United States* (New York: General Education Board, 1924), 164–66.

urban doctors had more opportunities to gain experience (and enhance their income) through clinical appointments and part-time salaried work in medical institutions.[4] Large cities nurtured the careers and incomes of early specialists in particular. Vast patient populations promised full caseloads for specialists, and large cities had the medical institutions that specialists needed for training and for building networks for consultations and patient referrals—the bread and butter of any specialist's office practice.[5]

But even though cities attracted American doctors, finding a "good location" in a city proved difficult given the rate at which cities were changing. As industrial growth, foreign immigration, and domestic migration transformed the social and spatial order of cities in the early twentieth century, market demand and health care needs shifted within each urban medical marketplace. How did these seismic changes in cities like Philadelphia shape the location behavior of doctors, and therefore the geography of private practice? Curiously, Dr. MacFarlane changed locations many times, even though some advice of the time period suggested that relocations were to be avoided.[6] Was she making poor choices relative to contemporary advice, or was she deftly navigating the marketplace as her career progressed and as the city developed around her? These questions can only be answered by comparing advice and behavior in the broader context of urbanization.[7]

To date, historians know precious little about the distribution of private practices *within* early twentieth-century cities, let alone the market forces that caused doctors to select certain locations over others. A handful of intra-urban case studies suggest that doctors preferred affluent neighborhoods and central business districts.[8] This chapter builds on these studies by adding more individual variables (experience, specialization, and social background) to the analysis of doctors, by adding more ecological variables (race and nativity of residents) to the analysis of different locations in the city, and by using more

detailed mapping scale (ward level) to analyze location behavior and the result-
ing geography of private practice in the city. To this quantitative analysis I
have added extensive examination of advice literature and of doctors' papers in
order to identify group and individual rationales for location selection.

This approach yields a far more complex and nuanced picture of the
relationship between urban space, medical careers, and the business of private practice in the early twentieth century. Cities like Philadelphia had many
different niches in which to practice medicine. These niches were defined
by social, professional, and spatial boundaries and by the different kinds of
doctors who practiced medicine therein. For percipient young doctors like
MacFarlane, this dynamic medical marketplace offered new opportunities for
building their careers and businesses. As different neighborhoods developed
homogenous residential populations (by social class or race and nativity) or
specialized functions (residential, work, industrial, or commercial), doctors
specialized their private practices in order to adapt to and compete in different
corners of the emerging metropolis. Although some doctors no doubt chose
poor locations (relative to contemporary advice) or otherwise deviated from
being "rational maximizers" in classical economic terms, the location and specialization behaviors of doctors were attuned to, if not wholly determined by,
broader changes in American cities.

Doctors and the Social Geography of Philadelphia

Like other important American cities, Philadelphia grew rapidly during the first
two decades of the twentieth century. After New York and Chicago, Philadelphia
was the third largest American metropolis, with a population of 1.29 million in
1900 that swelled to 1.82 million by 1920.[9] Foreign immigration from Southern
and Eastern Europe, as well as domestic migration, especially of African Americans from the southern United States, fueled this population boom—the largest in the city's history. Even though relatively few immigrants disembarked in
Philadelphia by comparison to New York City, foreign-born immigrants grew to
roughly one-quarter of city residents by 1910. African Americans constituted
roughly 6 percent of Philadelphia residents by 1910.[10] Philadelphia's population
boom went hand in hand with growth in industry and manufacturing: new arrivals came in search of work, and firms were attracted to the supply of cheap labor
in the city.[11] As a result of these twin forces, Philadelphia also ranked as the third
largest manufacturing center in the United States in 1910.[12]

Job opportunities in industry and manufacturing, though, were not equally
accessible to all residents at this time. Foreign immigrants most often found

employment in low-wage, semiskilled and unskilled jobs in the city's bustling clothing manufacturing sector. Newcomers also found work in various shipping jobs on the docks and wharves along the Delaware River (see map 1), then the second largest American seaport. On occasion, immigrants were hired in the textile mills or machine-building industries, though native-born whites monopolized this skilled and semiskilled labor market. African Americans had fewer options than foreign immigrants, and found employment primarily in domestic service and manual labor. As W.E.B. Du Bois explained, "The causes of this peculiar restriction in employment of Negroes are twofold: first, the lack of training and experience among Negroes; second, the prejudice of the whites."[13]

Two features of Philadelphia's social geography affected doctors and the market for private medical practice: residential segregation and the differentiation of the city into distinct districts with specialized functions. Nineteenth-century Philadelphia had been a fairly compact city, with relatively heterogeneous neighborhoods that mixed housing and commerce and had diverse residential and occupational composition. To be sure, early forms of residential segregation and spatial differentiation existed: the wealthiest residents lived on the main streets, while the poorest residents lived on the overcrowded and unsanitary back alleys. And yet one could find a representative cross-section of social groups and occupations within any given neighborhood, at least in the densely populated and developed area of the central city.[14] This social and spatial heterogeneity, along with the absence of professional regulation of medical education or licensure, led to evenly distributed opportunities for healers in the early nineteenth-century medical marketplace. Although elite graduates of the University of Pennsylvania School of Medicine monopolized practice along the most affluent main streets, doctors with degrees in the rest of the city practiced next door to less credentialed healers, such as "cuppers, bleeders, dentists, surgeon-barbers, and apothecaries."[15] The heterogeneous nineteenth-century city yielded more evenly distributed private medical practice.

With immigration and industrial growth, however, the organization of the city changed dramatically by the end of the century, and with it the medical marketplace. First, neighborhoods became more socially homogeneous, with the newest arrivals living in just a handful of city blocks (maps 3 and 4). In part, the "opportunity structure" of the city caused this residential segregation.[16] Many of the industrial and manufacturing firms, especially the smaller to mid-sized firms, were interdependent and thus tended to cluster together.[17] But because clustered factories, mills, and workshops produced substantial noise and air pollution, few residents wanted to live in the industrial quarters, leaving these areas with the lowest rents. New arrivals to Philadelphia thus found employment and cheap housing only in particular neighborhoods. Foreign immigrants lived mostly in the "river wards," which contained readily available, semiskilled and unskilled jobs in the garment sweatshops (wards 4–5), in the wharves and docks of the seaport (wards 1–6, 11, 16, and 18), and in the factories, workshops, and mills of industrial neighborhoods in the Northern Liberties, Kensington, Fishtown, and Richmond (wards 11, 12,

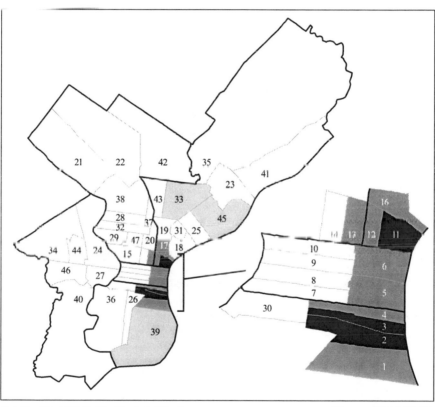

Foreign-Born White Residents in Ward   **Mean = 26.4 ± 12.6%**

| N | <26.4% | N | 26.4 - 39.0% | N | 39.0 - 51.6% | N | >51.6% |

Map 3. Residential Segregation by Nativity in Philadelphia, 1910

Source: U.S. Bureau of the Census, *Thirteenth Census of the United States, 1910* (Washington, DC: U.S. G.P.O., 1913), vol. 3, *Population*, table 5, 605–8. Map numbers indicate city wards. 24.7 percent of Philadelphia residents were immigrants in 1910. The map, however, compares immigrant residency rates in each ward to the mean of all city wards, which was 26.4 percent ± 12.6 percent. The city was then divided into four categories: wards below the mean rate, wards within one standard of deviation above the mean rate, wards one to two standards of deviation above the mean rate, and wards above two standards of deviation above the mean rate.

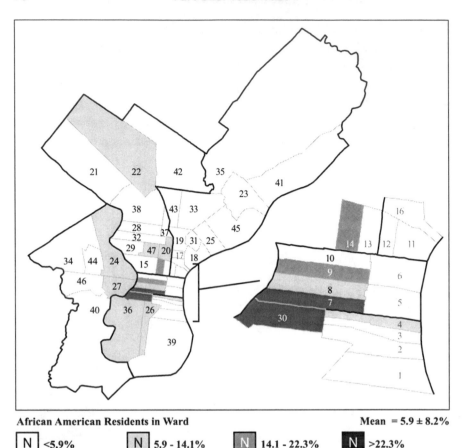

African American Residents in Ward   Mean = 5.9 ± 8.2%

| N | <5.9% | N | 5.9 - 14.1% | N | 14.1 - 22.3% | N | >22.3% |

Map 4.   Residential Segregation by Race in Philadelphia, 1910

Source: U.S. Bureau of the Census, *Thirteenth Census of the United States, 1910* (Washington, DC: U.S. G.P.O., 1913), vol. 3, *Population*, table 5, 605–8. 5.5 percent of Philadelphia residents were African American. The map, however, compares African American residency rates in each ward to the mean of all city wards, which was 5.9 percent ± 8.2 percent. The city was then divided into four categories: wards below the mean rate, wards within one standard of deviation above the mean rate, wards one to two standards of deviation above the mean rate, and wards above two standards of deviation above the mean rate.

16–19, 25, and 31). African Americans also lived close to available employment, especially near domestic service jobs in the wealthy homes around Rittenhouse Square (ward 8).[18] Not only did housing cost less near these clusters of semi-skilled and unskilled jobs, but the working class needed to live within walking distance of work because of the prohibitive cost of public transportation.[19]

Residential segregation, though, was not just driven by the concentration of working-class housing and employment opportunities in a handful of city wards. By the turn of the century, the city expanded beyond its densely settled core, connecting central Philadelphia with formerly remote satellite villages such as Germantown (inner portion of ward 22), in the outer reaches of Philadelphia County. But new real estate development and faster transportation also opened up previously unsettled or remote parts of the city, especially to the middle class who could afford new houses in these areas.[20] Although new development was necessary in order to make outer wards accessible and appealing to middle-class residents who still worked in Center City, affordable homes and better transportation only partly explain this first wave of suburbanization. In addition, the middle class wanted to leave behind the perceived nuisances of modern city living, and this desire fueled early suburban development in West Philadelphia and in parts of Northwest Philadelphia (especially ward 22).[21] Middle-class residents objected to loud and unsightly factories and feared the filth, disease, and crime assumed to plague the impoverished immigrant ghettoes near unskilled and semiskilled worksites.[22] Thus, residential segregation formed primarily along occupational and social-class lines, reflecting Philadelphia's opportunity structure as well as middle-class preferences and prejudices. Like Boston and New York, middle-class (especially white) flight to the suburbs was well under way by the turn of the century in Philadelphia, decades ahead of mid-century suburbanization found in cities like St. Louis or Los Angeles.[23]

Besides residential segregation, spatial differentiation also affected the medical marketplace. Classic analysis of early twentieth-century Philadelphia divides the city into five districts—downtown (or Center City), south, northeast, west, and northwest Philadelphia (see map 2). These five "specialized districts" had distinct functions, and closer examination of each district reveals the new and diverse locations in which doctors could practice medicine.

By the turn of the century, downtown Philadelphia had become the center of middle-class employment, shopping, and recreation. Mass transit enabled residents from Philadelphia and neighboring counties to travel to the central business district (CBD), which occupied most of the downtown west of Eighth Street. Besides being the center of municipal government, with City Hall at its center (Broad and Market Streets), the downtown also contained the metropolitan offices for a host of large firms such as regional banks and insurance companies. White-collar professionals and a sizable clerical workforce also found jobs in the district's many smaller businesses and professional offices. The CBD was also home to the largest retail department and clothing stores as well as many hotels and tourist attractions, from museums to theaters to historic monuments. While relatively few people lived downtown, the district was home to a range of social classes, from immigrant industrial workers, to African American domestic servants, to the wealthy residents of Rittenhouse Square (ward 8), which was one of the oldest and most affluent residential neighborhoods.[24]

South Philadelphia could not have been more different from the downtown. The district served as the primary destination for new arrivals to the city, especially to foreign immigrants. Many ethnic communities formed in the district, most notably Little Italy, though there were also Russian Jewish enclaves. In addition, many African Americans lived in South Philadelphia (especially ward 30), which was still within the orbit of the domestic service and manual labor jobs in great supply downtown. South Philadelphia was notorious for having the poorest housing and health conditions in the city, with rampant overcrowding and inadequate sanitation. Many urban housing and health reformers, such as the Octavia Hill Association, focused attention on improving the conditions of the working class in early twentieth-century South Philadelphia.[25]

Parts of the inner district of Northeast Philadelphia resembled South Philadelphia, with immigrant ghettoes that surrounded the many factories, workshops, and mills that clustered there. Even those wards having low immigrant residency rates in the inner northeast district (wards 18, 19, and 31) were still predominated by the working class. Unlike the factory district, the outer northeast district was quite remote, inaccessible, and sparsely populated, with large swaths of land that were entirely rural or altogether undeveloped (wards 35 and 41).[26]

Both the western and northwestern districts stood in stark contrast to the residential and economic characteristics of the south and the inner northeast districts in the early twentieth century. West Philadelphia, especially along Market Street, sprouted bedroom communities filled with middle-class residents who commuted to the downtown to work, shop, and recreate. The middle-class suburbs that formed along the "Main Line" of the Pennsylvania Railroad (heading west-northwest into Montgomery County) and along the new, rapid transit, Market Street elevated subway were primarily populated by native-born whites. Although portions of West Philadelphia such as Kingsessing (ward 40) and Overbrook Farms (ward 34) remained pastoral, the rest of the district was growing rapidly.[27]

Like West Philadelphia, Northwest Philadelphia was comprised of many middle-class suburbs, particularly near Fairmount Park and in the commuter railroad suburbs of Germantown, Mount Airy, and Chestnut Hill (ward 22). Some portions of Northwest Philadelphia were still undeveloped (especially ward 42), and one mill town—Manayunk—remained fairly isolated and distinctly working class (ward 21).[28] In general, though, real estate and infrastructure development in the west and northwest districts represented the first wave of sustained middle-class suburbanization in twentieth-century Philadelphia. Although these two districts were economically dependent upon the downtown, they were defined as much or more by their social and spatial separation from urban life.[29]

Given Philadelphia's growing residential segregation and spatial differentiation, how did doctors fit in to the changing social geography of the city? In 1910, there was one doctor for every 431 residents in Philadelphia, but the social backgrounds of Philadelphia doctors and residents differed considerably: 77 percent of doctors as compared to 44 percent of all occupied persons were native-born, white men (see table 5).[30] Philadelphia doctors therefore resembled middle-class commuters from suburbs in the west and northwest districts, while having little in common with the working class, immigrant, and African American residents in the south and inner-northeast districts. Knowing the social geography of Philadelphia matters because doctors selected locations to practice medicine based upon what they perceived to be good business locations in an increasingly diverse and segregated city. These perceptions, and the location behaviors that they elicited, were necessarily value-laden and further contributed to the social and spatial segregation of the city.

Finding a Good Location

Before a doctor could pick commercial or home office space, he or she first had to select a district and neighborhood in which to locate. This business decision had high stakes, and advice author Dr. Daniel Cathell warned that "many big blunders are made at the outset by locating in the wrong place; therefore take care to look before you leap." He advised doctors to "use your best judgment on yourself, and after giving the subject your best thought, then decide with great care, and only after considering your own qualities and qualifications, as well as the different locations."[31] Upon closer examination, social and economic factors, much more than professional factors, explain why Philadelphia doctors selected certain areas of the city in which to practice medicine.

By the early twentieth century, unevenly distributed doctor's offices had emerged as the central feature of the geography of private medical practice (map 5). Based upon a snapshot of 1909–1910 office locations, there were 226 private medical practices per 100,000 residents (PMP/100K) in the city as a whole, but individual wards had practice concentrations ranging from nearly zero in the fourth and eleventh wards to 3,867 and 3,352 in the eighth and ninth wards, respectively.[32] When compared to the city, 33 of 47 wards had relatively

few private practices, and 18 of these wards had less than *half* the citywide concentration. On the other hand, only a handful of wards had more than twice the
citywide practice concentration. As is evident in map 5, there were two important patterns to the uneven distribution of private practices: practices were clustered in central areas and in a handful of suburbs; and large swaths of the city,
including all of South and Northeast Philadelphia, had remarkably low concentrations of practices.

The location behavior of Philadelphia doctors in 1909–1910 indicates that
factors beyond residential density attracted doctors to some wards and not

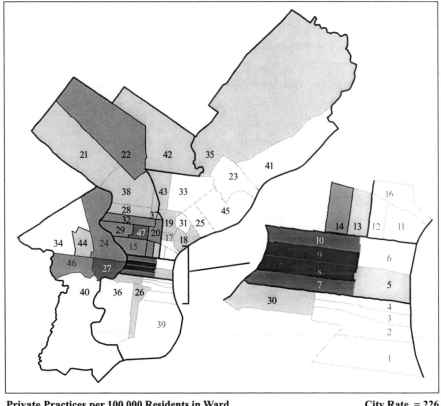

Private Practices per 100,000 Residents in Ward   **City Rate = 226**

| N | 0 - 113 | | N | 114 - 226 | | N | 227 - 452 | | N | 453 - 2260 | | N | >2260 |

Map 5.   The Distribution of Private Medical Practices in Philadelphia, 1909–1910

Sources: U.S. Bureau of the Census, *Thirteenth Census of the United States, 1910* (Washington, DC: U.S. G.P.O., 1913),
vol. 3, *Population*, table 5, 605–8, and the *AMD* (1909) sample. Doctors not in private practice (32 of 664 in the
sample) were excluded. There were 724 practice addresses for 632 sample doctors in active practice. 701 could be
ward-coded. The total number of practices in each ward was extrapolated from the sample number in each ward by
multiplying by five. See appendix for details.

others; otherwise doctor's offices would have been distributed evenly through-out the city with respect to the population, or at roughly 226 PMP/100K in every ward. Evidence from advice literature, from commercial real estate advertise-ments, and from the memoirs of individual Philadelphia doctors explains the pronounced variation in practice concentration. As with any business, finding a "good location" was one of the keys to success in private practice, and con-temporary advice on locating an office revealed some of the perceived market features of a good location. In *The Physician Himself*, Cathell summarized the general desiderata, stressing that office location and appearance would "affect your progress." He urged doctors to find neighborhoods that were "of easy access" and where "the rich are neither too rich or the poor too poor." Impor-tant features included adequate transportation networks as well as proximity to "a thickly populated, old section or a rapidly growing new one." Above all, he warned his large readership "do not locate among the common-place people in a run-down, going-to-wreck section, or where there is an overwhelming major-ity of the great unwashed. The more convenient to a large section of genteel, well-to-do business people, mechanics, etc., the better your chances to succeed, and the better for your purse."[33] His words are important, because many doctors heeded this and similar advice.[34]

The business advantages of having a centrally located office were obvious to Philadelphia doctors, who located disproportionately in the highly acces-sible central business district (CBD) of the downtown (wards 7–10), but also in a handful of central, yet prosperous, residential neighborhoods within walking distance of the CBD to the west (wards 24 and 27) and or a short trolley ride away near Fairmount Park (especially wards 15, 29, 32, and 47—see map 5). Real estate agents kept tabs on the location trends of doctors. In one sales pitch from 1915, entitled "What Doctors Want," the advertising copy defined the ideal location: "an office in town, with all [street] cars handy, afternoon hours, with heat, light, phone and service."[35] By locating centrally, Philadelphia doctors could remain accessible to the greatest number of clients even as city residents began to decentralize.

Traditionally, urban doctors had worked out of home offices in neighbor-hoods having middle-class residents from which they could build a lucrative practice. But the residential locus of private medical practice began to disap-pear as the middle class began to leave Center City for suburbs on the outskirts of Philadelphia. For urban doctors whose local clients were moving away, relo-cating to a central office made good business sense because scattered clientele still worked, shopped, and recreated in the CBD.[36] Real estate agents detected this market trend. As a 1915 advertisement for "Central Offices for Physicians" asserted, "Due to the shifting population of Philadelphia, general practitioners are adopting the custom of other cities by having convenient offices in the central section, and so being better able to hold their clientele."[37]

Besides relocating to a central office, the other advice for keeping middle-class clients was to relocate to a developing suburb, and some doctors were early adopters of this business strategy in 1909–1910. As map 5 shows, doctors concentrated in streetcar suburbs that were forming in West Philadelphia along Market Street (esp. wards 24, 27, and 46), as well as in the affluent commuter railroad suburbs of Germantown, Mount Airy, and Chestnut Hill (ward 22) in Northwest Philadelphia. Real estate agents again picked up on this development, with one advertising service seeking doctors who wanted "offices in the first-class neighborhoods, with best of references."[38] Only residential affluence, though, could lure doctors away from the accessibility and commercial vitality of Center City, as is evident from the low concentration private practices in undeveloped regions of the city (wards 34, 35, 40, and 41) and in the outer mill town of Manayunk (ward 21).

Besides favoring central locations and emerging middle-class suburbs, Philadelphia doctors generally followed advice to steer clear of the working-class neighborhoods of the inner city, especially immigrant ghettoes. The stark residential segregation of unskilled and semiskilled workers from skilled workers, clerical workers, and professionals meant that doctors could easily avoid working-class neighborhoods, and many did. Wards with above-average levels of immigrant residency (or higher than the city average of 24.7 percent) had only one-third the concentration of practices found in wards with low levels of immigrant residency. Most doctors shared white middle-class aversions to immigrant ghettoes, perhaps because most doctors were native-born and white. For example, in the second and third wards, where 53.9 percent of residents were immigrants (the highest level in the city), relatively few doctors were native-born and white: only 30.3 percent (versus 77.0 percent for the city as a whole). By contrast, nearly 70 percent of second and third ward doctors were immigrants themselves, as compared to just 11.7 percent citywide (tables 7 and 8). In other words, Philadelphia doctors in general, but native-born white doctors in particular, avoided immigrant ghettoes.

Different spatial relationships existed between African American neighborhoods and doctor's offices. Wards with high levels of African American residency (or higher than the city average of 5.5 percent) had three times the concentration of practices found in areas with low levels of African American

Table 7. The Nativity and Race of Doctors and Residents in Select Philadelphia Neighborhoods, 1909–1910 and 1940

	Ward 30		Wards 2–3		Ward 8		Ward 22		Ward 47		City	
1909–1910:	Doctors	Residents	Doctors	Residents	Doctors	Residents	Doctors	Residents	Doctors	Residents	Doctors	Residents
% Black	25.6	34.2	3.0	3.3	0.0	13.2	0.0	6.8	2.8	12.9	2.4*	5.5
% FBW	5.1	17.5	69.7	53.9	2.3	24.1	0.0	18.1	8.3	15.5	12.8*	24.7
% NBW-FBP	28.2	27.2	18.2	36.7	12.8	17.8	21.2	27.6	30.6	26.9	N/A	32.1
% NBW-NBP	41.0	21.0	9.1	6.0	84.9	44.7	78.8	47.4	58.3	44.6	N/A	37.7
1940:	Doctors	Residents	Doctors	Residents	Doctors	Residents	Doctors	Residents	Doctors	Residents	Doctors	Residents
% Black	25.0	80.4	11.1	16.0	0.0	4.9	2.4	9.3	21.1	57.0	3.2*	13.0
% FBW	0.0	2.8	55.6	23.0	6.6	15.4	4.9	10.9	0.0	6.1	N/A	15.0
% NBW	75.0	16.7	33.3	61.0	93.4	79.5	92.6	79.8	79.0	36.7	N/A	71.9

* The race and nativity of Philadelphia doctors for the city as a whole in 1910 and 1940 include only male doctors. Women doctors were not disaggregated by race or nativity in 1910.

Sources: Doctors in wards 30 and 2–3 in 1910 were collected from the street directory of *The Professional Directory* (1910). All other doctors were collected from the *AMD* (1909) and *AMD* (1940) samples. The nativity and race of individual doctors in each ward were identified in the manuscript census for 1910 and 1940 available at http://www.ancestry.com. Data on the race and nativity of doctors and residents for the city as a whole were collected from U.S. Bureau of the Census, *Thirteenth Census of the United States, 1910* (Washington, DC: U.S. G.P.O., 1914) vol. 4, *Population*, 181, 193, 428–29, 588–89; U.S. Bureau of Census, *Thirteenth Census of the United States, 1910* (Washington, DC: U.S. G.P.O., 1913), vol. 3: *Population*, table 5, 605–8; U.S. Bureau of Census, *Sixteenth Census of the United States, 1940* (Washington, DC: U.S. G.P.O., 1943), vol. 3, *Population*, "The Labor Force," table 11, 29–31 and table 13, 48–53; and the Historical Census Browser at the University of Virginia, Geospatial and Statistical Data Center, http://mapserver.lib.virginia.edu. "Black" includes census designations of "black," "negro," and "mulatto." "FBW" are foreign-born whites; "NBW-FBP" are native-born whites of foreign-born parentage; "NBW-NBP" are native-born whites of native-born parentage; and "NBW" are native-born whites. Native-born whites were not disaggregated by parental nativity in the 1940 census for Philadelphia doctors as a whole. Whites were not disaggregated by nativity in the 1940 census for Philadelphia doctors as a whole.

Table 8.   **The Distribution of Private Medical Practices by the Nativity and Race of Residents in Philadelphia, 1909–1910**

	Percent of Residents	PMP/100K
Wards with high immigrant residency rates	39.7	91
Wards with low immigrant residency rates	19.2	276
All city wards	24.7	226
Wards with high African American residency rates	12.3	389
Wards with low African American residency rates	1.9	141
All city wards	5.5	226

Sources: U.S. Bureau of the Census, *Thirteenth Census of the United States, 1910* (Washington, DC: U.S. G.P.O., 1913), vol. 3, *Population,* table 5, 605–8, and the *AMD* (1909) sample. Wards with residency rates above the city average were classified as "high," and wards with residency rates below the city average were classified as "low." "PMP/100K" is the number of private medical practices per 100,000 residents in these wards. There were 724 practice addresses for 632 sample doctors in active practice. 701 could be ward-coded. The total number of practices in each ward was extrapolated from the sample number in each ward by multiplying by five. See appendix for details.

residency (see table 8). But did doctors really prefer to locate their offices in African American neighborhoods, in contrast to contemporary racial prejudice generally found in the social and spatial organization of large cities? A closer examination of the opportunity structure in Philadelphia at the time explains this geographical coincidence.

Newly arrived African Americans, like foreign immigrants, tended to settle near available employment. Finding work mostly in domestic service and manual labor, African Americans typically settled near the affluent neighborhoods that provided these jobs, often in the same ward as their employers. This explains why the largest African American settlement in 1909–1910 (wards 7, 8, 30) formed within walking distance of perhaps the most affluent neighborhood in the city—Rittenhouse Square (ward 8). Although the average cost of housing was quite high in some of the wards having high African American residency (especially ward 8), African Americans found cheap housing either in the overcrowded back alleys of these wards, or in the dark, cold, and poorly ventilated basements of their employers.[39] Thus, the apparent link between African American residency and the location preferences of doctors is a red herring. For example, wards with high African American residency in the poorest district of the city—South Philadelphia—had very low concentrations of private practices relative to the population (see maps 4 and 5). Nearly 34 percent of the residents in the thirtieth ward were African American, and yet the ward had only 154 practices per 100,000 residents—roughly two-thirds of the citywide concentration of doctor's offices.[40] An unusually high percentage of these doctors were either African American or biracial (25.6 percent—see table 7). Besides racial prejudice, economic self-interest led the majority of white doctors away from neighborhoods like the thirtieth ward. In one of the earliest studies of urban health care spending—conducted by the Bureau of Labor Statistics beginning in 1917—African American families spent significantly less money than whites on doctors, even after controlling for income differences.[41] Market demand rather than patient need directed the location decisions of many doctors.

Doctors were aware of the different composition of city neighborhoods, and it would not have been uncommon for doctors, the vast majority of whom were middle class, native-born, and white, to share Dr. Cathell's aversion to "the great unwashed."[42] For example, during her hospital internship in Philadelphia from 1897 to 1898, Dr. Edith Flower Wheeler complained that there were times when her "scientific and missionary enthusiasm dimmed temporarily when working in the slums," and she came to the conclusion that "what they [the residents] needed more than anything else was to be washed. They certainly did seem to have a decided aversion to water on their bodies." Dr. Wheeler also complained that her working-class patients "do not always obey the doctor's orders or take their medicine as they are told."[43] Wheeler's views of Philadelphia ghettoes display the admixture of pity, disgust, condescension, and frustration felt by many doctors and urban reformers who served the working class in this period. For some, health work in urban slums provided an opportunity to fulfill missionary impulses (and assert middle-class identity), but most doctors ultimately opted to practice medicine elsewhere.[44] By the end of her internship, Dr. Wheeler had reached her limit. Between her experiences with the urban poor and the stifling summer heat of inner-city Philadelphia, she decided she "would never practice medicine in a big city," and promptly relocated to upstate New York.[45]

Besides their own race and class prejudices, doctors also avoided working-class neighborhoods because they argued that some residents therein refused to consult with outside doctors from different social backgrounds. For example, Cathell urged doctors to "bear in mind that unpopular opinions in politics or religion injure, and that, all else equal, you will be more likely to succeed and be contented in a community where your views, habits, and tastes are in harmony with the bulk of the people, morally, socially, and politically; where there are people you could respect and love, and where you will probably get the warm hand instead of the cold shoulder of good patients, and not have to hide your religion or your principles to get bread."[46] Other advice got far more specific about the importance of understanding the social geography of nationality and faith in prospective neighborhoods. According to one source, "Norwegians and Germans are the most clannish of any foreign element in this country. The Irish are always hard to handle and not very good pay. The French always prefer one who speaks their language, and are also very clannish. The other nationalities are as apt to employ an American doctor as they are one of their own nationality."[47] Other advice manuals insisted that religion mattered as much nationality. In *Building a Profitable Practice* (1912), author Dr. Thomas Reilly claimed that "orthodox Hebrews," Roman Catholics, and Methodists tended employ "one of their own," but suggested that writing letters to local religious leaders might open doors in these communities.[48] In select Philadelphia neighborhoods studied (see table 7), local doctors tended to resemble the residents in the surrounding neighborhood, especially in an immigrant ghetto (wards 2 and 3), an inner-city African American neighborhood (ward 30), and an affluent white suburb (ward 22).

Apart from class and race prejudice and fear of rejection, the main reason why doctors avoided locating their practices in poor inner-city neighborhoods boiled down to economic self-interest: doctors believed they could earn more money and have fewer hassles collecting fees elsewhere. As advice author Dr. Mabee put it, "There is no farmer who can succeed when he farms a poor farm, and there is no physician who can rise to fame in a poor location, among poor people."[49] This did not necessarily mean one shouldn't practice in working-class neighborhoods, and some advice authors tried to specify what kinds of returns a doctor could expect from different kinds of working-class residents. Dr. Reilly claimed that "race frequently makes a difference in fees." He specified further: "From the lower class of Italians you will seldom be able to collect more than a dollar a visit. If they ask for your advice for several [family members] on the same visit, charge a dollar apiece. They always pay cash." Reilly contended that poor Germans did not like to pay for house calls, but that with "Hebrews . . . if the disease be at all serious, you can scarcely make too many [house] visits. The pay is generally safe." By contrast, "the people who give you the most trouble are the oily-tongued natives, who pay you in compliments."[50] At the very least, this advice encouraged doctors to survey the social geography of a city when making location decisions. The distribution of private practices in Philadelphia indicates that most doctors concluded that locating in a working-class ghetto would be financially imprudent. For doctors who expected to earn two dollars or more per home visit in other parts of the city, working-class clientele, whether in the inner city or in a milltown like Manayunk (ward 21), simply would not do.[51]

The few geographical studies of private practice in other cities during this time period confirm that doctors preferred central business districts or middle-class suburbs, but which location took precedence depended on the social geography of the city studied. For example, San Francisco doctors began to separate their offices from their homes and to rent new commercial office space in the highly accessible CBD of the downtown: the number of doctors whose offices were located within one-half mile of the intersection of Market and New Montgomery Streets doubled from 1881 to 1911, even though the city began to decentralize residentially.[52] The geography of private practice in Brooklyn, New York, differed. Brooklyn's inner-city doctors dispersed as new foreign immigrants populated coastal neighborhoods along the East River in the early twentieth century. Most Brooklyn doctors headed inland in order to follow the departing middle class. In addition, many Brooklyn doctors left coastal neighborhoods because they could not afford the high cost of office space in the few business districts that formed there.[53] In Brooklyn, at least, class prejudice trumped the business efficiency driving office relocation in San Francisco, which had a singular, thriving CBD. In Philadelphia, the social geography of the city fell somewhere in between San Francisco and Brooklyn at this time, with social and economic changes driving some doctors into (certain) central areas while driving other doctors to affluent new suburbs.

The location behavior of Philadelphia doctors indicates that doctors made calculated choices based on their understanding of contours in the social geography of the city and of opportunities they envisioned in the medical marketplace. To be sure, Philadelphia doctors probably weren't consulting federal census reports in order to figure out where to locate, but most had developed their own understanding of the city during medical school, as 90 percent of Philadelphia doctors had graduated from one of the city's six medical schools.[54] Having an understanding of where different people lived, worked, shopped, and recreated helped doctors to make informed (even if self-interested and prejudiced) decisions about where to locate their private practices.

Moreover, doctors were accustomed to thinking about medical practice at the local level in the early twentieth century. Although Philadelphia doctors could discuss the heady topic of professional reform at the annual meeting of the Pennsylvania State Medical Society or, on occasion, at meetings of the Philadelphia County Medical Society, local meetings of the half-dozen or so neighborhood medical associations throughout the city focused on workaday issues affecting doctors in the immediate area.[55] As one doctor explained, "Here [at local branch meetings] each doctor greets the men from his own part of town—who are treating the same kinds of cases, meeting the same obstacles and overcoming the same difficulties with which he himself is contending. Some Branches have added social features that have proved popular and of value in cementing friendships among brother practitioners."[56] Doctors in private practice valued local business knowledge, and tips about the best office locations were no different. Doctors may have heeded general location advice in circulation at this time, but every locality had unique, ground-level market features that doctors had to consider.

Market Niches for Private Practice

When it came to locating their private medical practices, most Philadelphia doctors followed normative business advice favoring the central business district and wealthy suburbs in West and Northwest Philadelphia (see map 5 and table 9). Some doctors, however, clearly adapted to practice in suboptimal locations, otherwise there would have been no doctor's offices at all in working-class or in remote wards of Philadelphia. The social background of a doctor determined office location to some degree, and the handful of immigrant and African American doctors in Philadelphia worked primarily in immigrant and African American inner-city neighborhoods (see table 7). But so did some white doctors, who represented the vast majority of the city's profession (see table 5). What led these and other doctors to locations other than the CBD or wealthy suburbs? In particular, did different *kinds* of doctors practice medicine in different parts of the city—specialist versus GP, experienced versus young? Closer analysis of Philadelphia's medical marketplace reveals the relationship between urban space, medical careers, and the business of private practice in the early twentieth century.

As the city became socially and spatially stratified, distinct market niches for private practice were created, and these niches selected for doctors with particular combinations of specialization and experience. Specialists overwhelmingly preferred downtown offices: the district claimed 63 percent of all Philadelphia specialty practices. Moreover, doctors in downtown practices were the most likely to have limited their practice to a particular specialty: over 30 percent of downtown practices were specialized—roughly twice the citywide specialization rate (table 10). Furthermore, the majority of city wards (25 of 47) had no specialty practices at all, whereas GPs could be found in every

Table 9.   **The Distribution of Private Medical Practices and Medical Institu-**
tions by City District, Philadelphia, 1909–1910

	DT	S	NE	W	NW
Percent of Philadelphia population	5.8	21.7	25.4	16.0	31.2
Percent of private medical practices (PMPs)	31.1	8.0	8.8	15.1	37.0
PMPs per 100,000 residents	1,221.1	83.3	78.9	213.8	268.2
Percent of hospitals	21.6	15.3	13.5	18.9	15.3
Hospitals per 100,000 residents	26.9	5.1	3.8	8.5	7.0

Note: Abbreviations for the five districts are as follows: DT (downtown), S (south), NE (northeast),
W (west), and NW (northwest). Percentages in the table are rounded to the nearest tenth of a percent, and therefore do not necessarily total 100.0 percent.

Sources: For sources on population and private medical practices at the ward level, see source
note in table 8. Hospital data were collected from *AMD* (1909), 970–72; *The Professional Directory*
(1910), 209–66; U.S. Bureau of the Census, *Benevolent Institutions, 1910* (Washington, DC: U.S.
G.P.O., 1913), 142–45, 170–71, 240–45, 346–49, 390–93, 408–9; and under "Hospitals, Asylums,
Dispensaries, and Homes" in the *Philadelphia City Register* (Philadelphia: C. E. Howe Co., 1910).
See the appendix in this book for details.

ward but one.[57] Doctors with different experience levels also located in different districts of the city: downtown doctors had the highest average experience
level (20.5 years in practice) while South Philadelphia doctors were the youngest and least established, with an average of only 12.8 years in practice (table
10). To some degree, the collocation of specialists and the most established
doctors in the downtown district merely reflected the association of specialization and experience in medical careers at this time: most doctors waited until
mid-career before limiting their practices to a specialty (see figure 2).[58]

These distinct patterns of private practice location resulted not by accident but rather from the careful adaptation of different kinds of doctors to distinct market niches in Philadelphia. Professional factors (proximity to medical
schools, hospitals, and colleagues), spatial factors (accessibility of office locations to prospective clientele), and social factors (race, nativity, and class of
prospective clientele and area residents) distinguished each niche. A comparison of the two most distinct niches—downtown and South Philadelphia—
reveals how social geography shaped the medical marketplace at this time in
American urban history.

The downtown district was the most attractive market in which to locate
a doctor's office: the district had far and away the highest concentration of
practices (1,221 PMP/100K), with nearly one-third of all city practices to fewer
than 6 percent of city residents (see table 9). Downtown doctors, however, were

Table 10.   **The Experience and Specialization Rate of Philadelphia Doctors by City District, 1909–1910**

	DT	S	NE	W	NW
Percent of Philadelphia population	5.8	21.7	25.4	16.0	31.2
Percent of Philadelphia's specialty practices	63.5	3.9	1.9	8.7	22.1
Specialization rate in district (%)	30.1	7.1	3.2	8.5	8.8
Average experience level (years)	˙20.5	˙12.8	16.8	14.2	18.1

Note: Abbreviations for the five districts of Philadelphia from table 9. Percentages in the table are rounded to the nearest tenth of a percent, and therefore do not necessarily total 100.0 percent. ANOVA indicated that the variation in experience levels of doctors was significantly greater between districts than within a district (p < .01). Data not shown.

˙Difference in the mean experience level of downtown and South Philadelphia doctors differed significantly when measured by Student's t-test (p < .01).

Sources: For sources on population and private medical practices at the ward level, see source note in table 8. Data on specialization and experience of sample doctors in active practice were collected from the *AMD* (1909). See the appendix in this book for details.

concentrated in the CBD west of Eighth Street (wards 7–10) and around Rittenhouse Square (ward 8). Bounded by Chestnut Street, the Schuylkill River, Walnut Street and Seventh Street, the eighth ward in particular functioned as a kind of "Doctor's Row," with one-fifth of all city practices located in the eighth ward or on its border streets.[59] A 1915 advertisement for office space near Rittenhouse Square promised "a fine office for a good doctor" and described the area as "the best neighborhood in the city."[60] However, this market niche was not open to all, as eighth ward doctors were disproportionately native-born and white (96.5 percent—see table 7). Thus even within the highly desirable downtown district, doctors flocked to the most accessible, commercial, and affluent wards to the west and shunned the inconvenient, industrial, and working-class river wards to the east.

Because of the high concentration of doctor's offices in the CBD and around Rittenhouse Square, young doctors found the downtown district a particularly daunting place to first hang a shingle (see table 10). For example, when Dr. Howard Kelley began his private practice in the late nineteenth century, he decided to locate near the mills in northeast Philadelphia. As he explained, rather than "settling downtown, where my family lived, and waiting for some older doctor to adopt me, and to die and leave me his practice, I took up my quarters in a weaver's family, in a little two-story house, at 2316 N. Front Street" (ward 19).[61] Concern about stifling levels of competition led some Philadelphia medical faculty to advise their students to avoid large cities altogether. In her 1912 address, entitled "Timely Advice to the Recent Graduate," Dr. Ella B. Everitt, a professor of gynecology at Woman's Medical College, claimed that when it came to selecting a location, "many young graduates make a fatal error at the outset. For various reasons too many remain in the large cities." The danger was that the young graduate would, as she put it, "fail to recognize their own limitations or to appreciate the fierce competition of city life, and therefore remain where they are inherently unable to rise beyond mediocrity and obscurity."[62] Besides having higher levels of competition, the high cost of overhead for downtown offices was a barrier for younger doctors. Young doctors like Kelley, who needed to economize by combining home and office, simply could not afford such prime real estate.

Established doctors and specialists, however, proved better able to compete in the crowded and expensive downtown market niche (see table 10). These doctors had made it through the early lean years of private practice and were therefore more likely to have built up the necessary income to rent a downtown office. Relocation to a downtown office even signaled that one had arrived in the profession. For example, in 1910, among the fellows of the College of Physicians of Philadelphia—the city's elite medical society—71 percent had downtown offices, as compared to just 31 percent of Philadelphia doctors altogether.[63]

Some established doctors and specialists transitioned into the downtown niche by keeping their original neighborhood office while opening a second office downtown. This business strategy allowed the cultivation of new clientele but also the retention of old clients, including those who had moved away from the doctor's original neighborhood office but who lived a short commute from downtown.[64] Having a second office in downtown Philadelphia also made sense for established GPs who specialized in mid-career. These mid-career specialists could depend upon income from their residential general practice while slowly building up their specialty practice in downtown Philadelphia, where they could attract more specialty cases than in their original location.[65]

Besides having the level of establishment (and income) needed to afford the increased overhead of a downtown office, specialists were also unaffected by the crowded market. Specialists used vastly different business models from GPs, who typically resided in areas in which they hoped to build a practice and often combined home and office in order to cut costs. To be sure, plenty of GPs centralized their offices during this period, but GPs had the ability to make a living in more residential areas as well. In addition, GPs, especially young doctors fresh out of medical school, depended upon passersby and walk-in business in the early days of practice, not unlike a grocer at a corner store. As such, it was sheer folly to locate a first practice in a neighborhood having lots of other (more established) doctors. Even after establishing a practice and earning a good reputation, GPs still depended upon walk-in business to some degree, and plenty of advice books counseled GPs on how to situate their offices for greatest visibility.

Specialists, on the other hand, depended upon different sources of income in private practice: fees from consulting with other doctors (often GPs) on a specialty case and fees from specialty cases that were referred to the specialist from other doctors (usually GPs). Because of its centrality and accessibility, downtown offices were ideally suited to the specialist's business model. Furthermore, because specialists did not compete with other doctors for walk-in business, they were somewhat immune to competition from nearby practices. It was even common for a specialist to have an office in the same building as other doctors in his or her specialty. For example, six ophthalmologists, four surgeons, two ear-nose-and-throat specialists, and two dermatologists could be found among the twenty-nine doctors who located their offices in the ten-story Professional Building (1831–1833 Chestnut Street—ward 9), which was one of the first high-rise medical and dental office buildings constructed in downtown Philadelphia in the early twentieth century.[66] This kind of clustering in a single office building could only have occurred if these doctors did not compete directly with one another for patients in private practice.

Besides spatial factors, professional factors also distinguished the downtown from other market niches in the city. Specialists, who remained closely associated with medical institutions throughout their careers (see figure 3), benefited by locating their practices near hospitals, and the downtown district had the highest concentration of hospitals per residents in the city (see table 9). By locating downtown, specialists not only took advantage of the convenience and accessibility of the district, they also reduced the time lost in transit while shuffling between various worksites: from office hours in private practice, to lectures at medical schools, to clinical rounds or surgical duties in hospitals. Indeed, over half of downtown doctors (55 percent) held at least one position in a hospital, medical school, dispensary, or clinic—the highest position-holding rate in the city.[67]

The market niche for private practice in South Philadelphia could not have been more different. Unlike the densely packed doctor's offices in the CBD, all of South Philadelphia had well below average ratios of private practices to residents (see map 5): as a whole, the district had only 8 percent of the city's practices but 22 percent of its residents (see table 9). In terms of market features,

South Philadelphia lacked what most doctors preferred in the way of office locations: the district was not centrally located, did not have great accessibility, and
had some of the poorest residents: Italian, Polish, and Russian immigrants and
African American migrants. A combination of social, spatial, and professional
factors made South Philadelphia unappealing for most doctors (see map 5), particularly for specialists and established doctors. As table 10 shows, the few doctors who located in South Philadelphia were, on average, the youngest doctors
in the city, nearly all of whom were in general medical practice.

To a limited degree, hospital outpatient departments, dispensaries, and
clinics compensated for the lack in private medical care in South Philadelphia.
Many of these charity medical institutions were founded by or for immigrants
or African Americans and had immigrant or African American doctors on staff.
For example, residents near Little Italy could seek inpatient care at the Fabi-
ani Italian Hospital (ward 3) or outpatient care at the Italian Dispensary just
two blocks south (ward 2), or from the 24.2 percent of local doctors who were
Italian-born.[68] Similarly, African American residents in western South Philadelphia could see African American doctors at Mercy Hospital (ward 30) or
at Frederick Douglass Hospital (ward 7), both of which were established by or
for African American doctors, who comprised 25.6 percent of thirtieth ward
doctors.[69] Urban reformers, city public health officials, and hospital administrators in the early twentieth century also established a network of children's
health clinics in South Philadelphia.[70] Despite these institutional resources for
outpatient care, South Philadelphia nevertheless had a small ratio of medical
institutions to residents by comparison to other city districts (see table 9). In
other words, institutional care by no means eliminated the deficit of private
practices.

The low appeal of South Philadelphia made this niche a safe haven for
certain doctors. For starters, the low concentration of private practices meant
that there was little in the way of competition, which mattered greatly to young
doctors and GPs, both of whom needed room to breathe if they were to capture
enough business from walk-ins and passersby to earn a living. Furthermore,
real estate cost considerably less in or around working-class neighborhoods,
and thus young doctors and GPs could save money on the cost of both office
and home in South Philadelphia. Besides enjoying lower competition and overhead, doctors in South Philadelphia could use payment protocols normally
considered repugnant in middle-class markets: they could demand payment,
in cash, up front without offending their clients. As one classified advertisement for a "desirable office and home" in a "thickly populated foreign section

of the city" claimed, the area provided a "good opportunity to acquire a cash practice."[71] Not only was South Philadelphia so densely populated that a young doctor could make up for lower fees by having higher volume, but the working-class foreign immigrants and migrant African Americans who lived there were also accustomed to cash transactions. As Dr. Thomas F. Reilly advised in *Building a Profitable Practice* (1912), "If you decide to locate in a large city, unless you have a large circle of friends, it is better to go into a tenement quarter or near one." Unconnected young doctors benefited from working-class neighborhoods because of the nature of the wage labor economy in such areas. As Reilly elaborated, "A city, containing a number of factories of different kinds, makes a good location for the beginner. In such places, money is usually in circulation, and if one class of work is slack, there will always be other factories running. This makes for ready money."[72] Whether in textile mills, in garment sweatshops, in factories, or on the docks, wage labor fueled enough of a cash economy in the "river wards" from the South to the inner Northeast districts of Philadelphia to support the few young GPs, along with immigrant doctors, who located their offices there.

Besides featuring lower competition, less overhead, a dense population, and a cash economy, South Philadelphia also had valuable professional features for young doctors and GPs—namely, there weren't too many medical institutions. For most doctors, especially those with specialty aspirations, this would have been problematic. But GPs preferred this arrangement because medical institutions, and dispensaries in particular, provided low-cost or free outpatient care to working-class patients in exchange for the opportunity to use these patients as clinical material for teaching purposes. As we have seen, established GPs objected to dispensary care because it threatened to undermine the market value of private medical care, especially for doctors located in close proximity to a dispensary. The relatively low concentration of medical institutions in South Philadelphia partly explains why GPs might have preferred to locate there.

On the other hand, some young doctors couldn't resist the benefits of dispensary work, which helped to augment income at first, to build a reputation in a neighborhood and to attract loyal clientele for private practice. Some young doctors in South Philadelphia found work in the handful of area dispensaries while trying to build a neighborhood general practice. For example, after finishing a hospital internship in 1916, Dr. Rita S. Finkler found institutional work in a Child Federation clinic in Little Italy. She decided to learn some Italian in order to communicate with her patients who, as she characterized them, "usually settled among their relatives and friends, spoke their native tongue for many years after their arrival, and sometimes never learned English."[73] She worked from 9:00 A.M. until 5:00 P.M. in the clinic, and used one large room in her apartment for her private practice in the evenings and on weekends. As she explained, "This room served as a waiting room and an examining room; the two being separated by a large screen. The equipment was modest to say the least, but the patients began to flock in, mostly the Italians, because I was already known in Little Italy and because I knew the language."[74] Dr. Finkler's dispensary work afforded her the opportunity to build a small practice while earning a modest salary, and because she located in a low-rent district, she could afford to combine her home and office.

By locating in a working-class neighborhood, young doctors and GPs could also cultivate the kind of familiarity with their patients and neighbors that downtown doctors, whose patients came from all over the city, could not. On occasion, familiarity even inspired loyalty between doctor and patient in working-class neighborhoods. As Dr. Howard Kelley explained about the advantages to the location of his first general practice near the textile mills of Kensington (ward 19 in Northeast Philadelphia): "the pecuniary returns of my work were good; my mill people paid their bills promptly, and always added a big debt of gratitude which they held onto and kept returning in interest to me as long as they lived."[75] Dr. Finkler found that loyalty paid similar dividends in her South Philadelphia practice: "Gradually 'Little Italy' realized that I was also available for making house calls after 5pm and on weekends. I was happy to receive such calls and get the foretaste of deep satisfaction in knowing that you are needed, wanted, and trusted."[76]

Despite all of these advantages, young doctors probably hoped to use a first practice in South Philadelphia as a stepping-stone to practice elsewhere in the city. Although young doctors may have fought hard to earn the trust of their South Philadelphia patients, most either wanted or needed to move on to more lucrative market niches despite missionary proclamations to the contrary. Even though Dr. Charles R. Mabee advised young doctors in *The Physician's Business and Financial Adviser* (1900) to "adapt [yourselves] to all circumstances and all classes of people," even he suggested there were limits to social opportunism in practice. "When you are with the upper ten, you must be one of them, when you are among the middle class, you must be one of them, and when you are with the lower classes, you must suit yourself to their ways at least for the time being."[77] The fact that young doctors left South Philadelphia after only a few years partly explains why the average number of years in practice was lowest in that niche (see table 10): other than immigrant and African American

doctors, very few doctors remained there past their early career. South Philadelphia may have been a good place to start a practice, but a young doctor had
to move elsewhere if he or she aspired to specialty practice or a middle-class
lifestyle. Dr. Kelley, for example, climbed institutional ladders in Philadelphia
and later moved to Baltimore where he became a professor of gynecology at
Johns Hopkins University. Similarly, after three years in South Philadelphia,
Dr. Finkler moved to Newark, New Jersey, in 1919 in order for husband to be
close to his new job in New York City. There she focused on making the institutional connections she needed in order to specialize.

Given that the career, business, and personal circumstances of every doctor changed over time, it was also not uncommon for a doctor to migrate from
one niche to another in the medical marketplace. Returning to the example that
began this chapter, Dr. Catherine MacFarlane relocated three times in her first
ten years of practice from 1899 to 1908 (see map 2). After finishing her internship, she undertook clinical and teaching duties in a maternity outpatient service at 335 Washington Avenue (ward 2), in the heart of the immigrant ghettoes.
Dr. MacFarlane was well aware of the residential and occupational character of
South Philadelphia, remembering, with an outsider's detachment, "the lives of
the recent immigrants in the narrow streets and quaint little houses was a rev-
elation to me. Poles, Italians, Jews, Negroes, all treated the young doctors with
great respect." She continued,

> at the waterfront, the strange foreign people fascinated me. Some were so
> poor they had nothing to wrap the baby in. The thrifty Italians wrapped
> the baby tightly in wide muslin bandage, binding fast arms and legs, as
> we looked on astonished. The Jews, when the baby was a boy, invited us
> to the circumcision party and offered us wine and cakes. The long night
> vigils, the view of the shot tower against the rosy dawn, the gratitude of
> our simple patients, were the warp and woof of my initiation into the
> practice of medicine. I learned that being a doctor was more than driving
> a horse and carriage over country roads.[78]

For MacFarlane, her work as an instructor and outpatient doctor in South Philadelphia gave her valuable experience and a sense of moral purpose, but little
financial reward.

After two years of earning but $150.00 in salary, Dr. MacFarlane was eager
to hang out her shingle and begin her private practice. She settled on Germantown, where her parents had recently retired. There, MacFarlane purchased
a home and office at 6112 Germantown Avenue (ward 22) where she kept up

appearances while "waiting for patients." After a few lean years in general practice, during which she earned barely more than she had as an instructor, MacFarlane built a steady practice and cultivated new career opportunities. In 1908, she took her first major step on a lifelong specialty career path when she secured an appointment to the Gynecological Staff at Woman's Hospital. This career change, though, necessitated yet another location decision. As she put it, "As a budding specialist, I felt the need of a city office." MacFarlane kept her Germantown home office and practice but shared Center City office space with another doctor at 132 South Eighteenth Street (ward 8), one block from Rittenhouse Square, where she saw patients with gynecological complaints. By this point in her career, her annual income was $2,200, though she still felt like "a continual financial burden to [her] parents."[79]

In the case of Dr. MacFarlane, a number of factors influenced her location changes from market niche to market niche in her first ten years after medical school. Her location decisions were influenced by personal factors (such as where she had family support networks) and professional factors (such as where she could get hospital appointments), but also by larger social and economic forces (such as where she could support a gynecological practice versus a general practice). These factors ultimately led Dr. MacFarlane to relocate her practice several times in the city: from initial charity work in the ghettoes, to general practice in a suburban home office, and finally to specialty practice in a Center City office.

Altogether, Dr. MacFarlane's career illustrates the diversity of market niches for private medical practice in Philadelphia in the early twentieth century. These market niches had distinct features that selected for different kinds of doctors. Specialists required the centrality and accessibility of the downtown, as well as its many medical institutions, but established doctors were among the only doctors who could afford the high cost of office space in and around the central business district. GPs, on the other hand, were adaptable to many market niches in the city. Young doctors preferred to locate where they would not be stifled by competition or bankrupted by the cost of overhead. This explains why South Philadelphia, with its low concentration of private medical practices, cheap housing, and working-class residents, proved to be an appealing market niche for certain young doctors. Immigrant and African American doctors had the fewest choices of location. Institutional discrimination prevented access to all but a few hospitals, thereby inhibiting specialization and specialty practice downtown; patient prejudice made it difficult for immigrant and African American doctors to build a practice across the patrolled borders of white suburbia, thereby limiting office locations to South and inner Northeast Philadelphia.

That doctors like Catherine MacFarlane acted out of economic self-interest in the early twentieth century is not particularly surprising, nor does this fact diminish the very real contributions doctors made to the health of cities in this time period. But by placing career advice and economic self-interest in the context of broader social and economic changes in American cities, we can begin to understand how and why private medical practices became unevenly distributed across city neighborhoods. Doctors, like any other small business owners, necessarily made location decisions based upon economic self-interest, but in an increasingly balkanized urban setting, these location decisions reinforced underlying structural inequality. Career and financial motives in medicine incentivized the location of doctor's offices in the central business district and in select wealthy suburbs just as other components of the city's opportunity structure—good education, affordable and safe housing, high-paying jobs, and well-developed infrastructure—became unevenly distributed. The geography of private medical practice replicated the larger social and spatial order of the growing American metropolis.

Doctors were well aware of different business opportunities in the new urban medical marketplace, and they carefully crafted business strategies to achieve social, economic, and professional goals. In this market, specialization served as a business strategy suited to the doctor on the make, though limiting a private practice to a particular specialty took planning and strategic office relocations. Read through the lens of urban history, the growth of specialization in the early twentieth century was fueled by the diversification in medical marketplaces as cities became racially segregated and economically stratified. GPs by no means disappeared overnight, but it became more difficult to succeed in urban general practice as time went on. When examined in this fashion, both the maldistribution of urban private practice and the growth of specialization among urban doctors reflected the same process—the entrenchment of new patterns of social inequality in modern American society.

Part II

1920–1940

Chapter 4

New Career Paths, New Business Methods

When Dr. Carl C. Fischer finished his internship year at Hahnemann Hospital and then passed his state board examinations in 1929, his career was no different from all of the other newly minted medical doctorates in Pennsylvania after 1914, the year in which the state became the first to require internship for licensure. Young doctors no longer entered private practice directly, but rather took a year of additional clinical training in the form of the general rotating hospital internship. Dr. Fischer, though, had ambitions to specialize in pediatrics. Unlike earlier generations, who first spent several years in general practice, Fischer belonged to an intermediate generation that came of age when hospitals had become mainstream health care institutions and when pre-specialists felt justified in skipping general practice, instead heading straight into early residency programs that promised to produce full-fledged specialists in just a few years after medical school. Given that the growth of hospital care and specialization are two of the most significant changes in the structure of American medicine during the mid-twentieth century, it is vital to examine Dr. Fischer's generation in order to uncover the motives behind their career choices and the effects of these structural changes on the business of private medical practice.

What place did private practice have in a medical marketplace in which medical labor had become more divided and more dependent upon medical institutions? Was private practice still the ultimate career goal for doctors? How did the expanding role of the hospital in medical education and patient care change the relationship between private practitioners and hospitals? In terms of business practices, how did the business goals and methods of GPs and specialists change with the growing market share of hospitals? And finally, to what extent did the ever more divergent business interests of GPs and specialists reinforce intra-professional stratification and conflict found in earlier decades? This chapter examines each of these questions in turn.

Walking the Wards before Setting Up a Practice

As we have seen, the process of becoming a doctor became increasingly standardized during the Progressive Era, as the medical profession gained regulatory control of an unruly marketplace for private practice. New or revitalized institutions—from state licensing boards to the reorganized American Medical Association—served as the levers by which the status and legitimacy of the profession were raised. During the 1920s and 1930s, the role of institutions expanded further. By 1940, nearly every medical graduate received additional training in internships and residencies, both of which revolved around institutions. In particular, the growing influence of hospitals and specialty certification boards on graduate medical education and the process of becoming a doctor during the 1920s and 1930s deserves closer inspection.

In the first few decades of the twentieth century, hospitals grew in number and importance.[1] From 1875 to 1928, the number of hospitals in the United States increased at least tenfold, from 661 to 6,852, with the rate of establishment averaging almost 200 new hospitals per year from 1900 to 1920.[2] In addition, many older hospitals expanded their facilities by adding new wards and more beds, especially well-established teaching hospitals in large cities. In Philadelphia, for example, hospital capacity continued to increase during the 1920s, even as construction of new hospitals declined. By 1930, one survey counted more than ten thousand beds combined in the forty-nine general and specialty hospitals in Philadelphia (figure 4).

As many historians have noted, rapid urbanization and massive immigration generated unprecedented demand for hospital care in the late nineteenth century. Traditionally, hospitals had been charity institutions of last resort. The vast majority of Americans instead relied upon domestic care networks during illness and could afford private medical care in the home when needed. But because new arrivals to cities often came alone, they had no family to care for them when ill, no family to pay for private medical care when illness or injury limited their ability to earn a living. In response to the emergent needs of the urban working class, many immigrant and religious communities, municipal governments, and philanthropists founded hospitals that became important social institutions for ever larger segments of urban populations.[3]

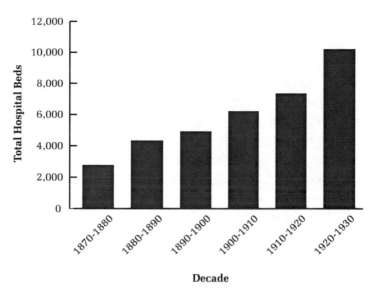

Figure 4. The Expansion of Philadelphia Hospitals, 1870–1930

Source: *Philadelphia Hospital and Health Survey, 1929* (Philadelphia: Philadelphia Hospital and Health Survey Committee, 1930), 566–73. This survey only counted beds in the forty-nine largest general and special hospitals within the city limits.

By the 1920s, the middle class further added to the growing demand for hospital care. With the development of anesthesia at mid-century and aseptic technique by the turn of the century, the range of surgical procedures expanded considerably, though most required sterile conditions. Individual doctors could rarely afford such facilities in office practice, but hospitals, which had also begun to place a premium on sanitary engineering and housekeeping practices, could afford to add new and modern operating rooms and buy equipment for sterilization. As a result of their economies of scale, hospitals became attractive surgical centers where doctors on staff could share operating facilities, as well as new diagnostic equipment such as X-ray machines.[4] Many doctors began to refer their middle-class patients to hospitals for new procedures such as appendectomies and tonsillectomies. Childbirth also moved to the hospital, as new interventions promising safe and pain-free parturition, like twilight sleep, were incompatible with home births.[5] In order to attract middle-class patients, to generate capital for new and expensive surgical facilities, and to remove the social stigma of hospital care, many hospitals began to charge patient fees, and even created wards with semiprivate and private rooms in order to separate patients by social class. With the growing consumer appeal and the increase in surgical admissions, hospitals changed from charity institutions for the long-term care of the chronically ill to profit-oriented institutions for the short-term care of surgical cases or acutely ill patients who came from an ever wealthier cross-section of society.[6] Admission rates continued to increase during the 1930s—from 51 to 70 admissions per 1,000 people per year—as hospitals became central to the American health care system.[7]

At the same time as hospitals gained public appeal, they also grew in importance for medical careers. With increasing patient demand, hospitals radically expanded their staffs. This was particularly evident in teaching hospitals, which included interns, residents, and additional supervisory staff.[8] Teaching hospitals had complex hierarchies wherein entry-level staff generally handled charity cases (for little pay) in the outpatient department or dispensary. A smaller number of doctors who had proven themselves in this capacity were then invited to join the admitting staff, which handled inpatient care. In exchange for clinical and surgical work in the free wards and a small salary, the admitting staff could also admit middle-class patients from their private practices and earn separate fees for their care (fees beyond the cost of the room, which the patient paid to the hospital). This arrangement generated extra income for doctors and added to their prestige in private practice, as well-connected doctors could promise their private patients continuity of care in the best hospitals. The most senior and well-respected of the admitting staff were eventually awarded consulting staff status, which relieved them of their duties on the charity wards and enabled them to focus on private inpatients. Ultimately, a hospital doctor might ascend to a leadership position as chief of a clinical department, though relatively few staff ever reached that level.[9] Because patient referrals increased hospital revenue, staff doctors began to wield new power, which they leveraged to gain greater control over hospital administration by the 1920s.[10]

With growing demand for inpatient services, hospitals gradually welcomed interns as a cost-effective solution to staffing needs. As we have already seen, by 1914 as many as three-quarters of doctors undertook a year of internship after graduation from medical school, but many hospitals provided little mentoring and simply used interns as cheap labor. Given the American Medical Association's ongoing involvement in medical school reform, which included advocating for better clinical training, the AMA endeavored to tackle the problem of internship standards. Beginning in 1914, the AMA's Council on Medical Education and Hospitals published an annual list of hospitals approved for internship—that is, hospitals with the minimum facilities and oversight deemed satisfactory for internship. By 1924, the number of internships in

AMA-approved hospitals exceeded the number of medical graduates for the first time; by 1940, a total of 7,998 internships were available in 732 AMA-approved hospitals, but only 5,097 graduates of American medical schools were available to fill these positions. These milestones reflected not only the overall expansion of hospital staff but also the gradual stabilization of internships and their concomitant integration into graduate medical education.[11] With the growing educational value placed on internship, licensing boards began to require a year of AMA-approved internship as a prerequisite for licensure. In 1914, Pennsylvania became the first state to enact such a law, and by 1940, twenty other states had enacted similar laws.[12] In practice, the internship had become a universal stop in the career paths of young doctors, with 99.7 percent of the graduating classes of 1935 and 1940 undertaking hospital internship (see figure 1).[13]

Despite the growing career importance of internships, most young doctors set their sights on private practice, not full-time institutional practice in a hospital, state asylum, or other clinical institution. Young doctors made important decisions about their careers and future practices during internship, and their options were influenced by the relationships established with hospital staff. If an intern ultimately wished to specialize in private practice, then it was advisable to get further graduate education, and hospital staff could facilitate the advancement of a promising intern into an informal "preceptorship" or (later on) into a formal residency program. If an intern wished to join the outpatient staff or admitting staff, whether to gain additional clinical experience or to supplement income while getting established in private practice, then it was necessary to make good impressions with senior staff. Finally, if a young doctor wished for the occasional discharged inpatient to be referred to his or her private practice for follow-up care, then it was necessary to establish good relations with the hospital staff during internship. As Dr. George Wolf summarized it in *The Physician's Business* (1938), a popular career advice book, "It is during the period of internship that the young doctor lays a foundation for future professional contacts," and these contacts greatly affected the career paths available to young doctors. Dr. Wolf elaborated further: "Hospital alumni are rather clannish, and often influence the professional careers of their fellow alumni."[14]

For example, during his internship at Hahnemann Hospital, Dr. Carl Fischer must have impressed the senior staff, because several department chiefs offered him preceptorships in pathology, pediatrics, and obstetrics and gynecology. Dr. Fischer accepted the offer from Dr. Sigmund Raue, a Center City pediatrician. In exchange for a small salary, Dr. Fischer assisted Dr. Raue in office practice. In between patients, Dr. Raue would "discuss questions of pediatric interest," which Dr. Fischer found to have been "a most valuable experience." In addition to his office duties, Dr. Fischer also worked several afternoons a week in the Pediatric Outpatient Clinic at Hahnemann Hospital, "for which the only reward," Dr. Fischer recalled, "was the privilege of working with my seniors and seeing all kinds of cases! What spare time I had I was permitted to see private patients—if I could find any at all!"[15] Eventually, Dr. Fischer finished his preceptorship and established his own private practice in pediatrics. His experience illustrates how the internship year functioned as a critical period during which young doctors made choices about further graduate training and specialization, both of which affected opportunities in private practice; these choices were constrained by the professional contacts made during the internship year.

By the time that Dr. Fischer began his preceptorship in 1928, a new system of graduate training was forming—hospital residency training—that would become the dominant form of education for specialists by 1940.[16] Graduate medical education in the specialties was relatively rare at the turn of the century, and the program design varied considerably even as specialty training came into vogue in the 1920s: some doctors merely took a six-week course and declared themselves specialists; others, like Dr. Carl Fischer, worked closely with a single specialist in a preceptorship; and yet other doctors enrolled in a handful of newly established graduate medical schools, like the one at the University of Pennsylvania, which involved years of coursework, clinical duties, and research, culminating in a thesis and a formal graduate degree. The hospital residency system that prevailed by 1940 combined elements of each of these precursors and generally involved one to three years of graduate education (after internship) with supervised training and research in a hospital, culminating in examination and certification by the board of a national specialist organization in the doctor's chosen field.[17]

The American Board for Ophthalmic Examinations was the first specialty certification board established in the United States (1917). The next specialty certification boards were founded after the first world war, which for many reformers had first exposed the need for more rigorous specialty training.[18] By 1940, national boards had been established in fourteen AMA-recognized specialties, and an estimated 40 percent of the full-time specialists in these fields were board-certified.[19] Although specialty boards did not teach doctors directly, they defined the minimum training needed to pass examination and become certified. The AMA's Council on Medical Education and Hospitals also participated in defining residencies after 1924, when the council began to inspect and approve hospital residency programs. Between 1927 and 1940, the number of AMA approved residencies increased from 1,776 to 2,589.[20] In essence, the new institution of specialty boards in concert with the AMA had systematized the process of becoming a specialist by 1940, though there were still issues of coordination and overlapping jurisdiction between specialty boards.

Although there were no legal barriers to specialty practice like there were for medical practice in general, the growing systematization, if not full standardization, of residency training made graduate medical education more appealing to young doctors with every graduating class.[21] Dr. H. G. Weiskotten's classic survey of the classes of 1935 and 1940 in American medical schools, for example, found that 89 percent of full specialists and 55 percent of partial specialists had undertaken residency training; by the class of 1950, the number of full specialists who had received residency training had increased to 97 percent. Residency programs appealed primarily to pre-specialists: only 34 percent of GPs in the classes of 1935 and 1940 undertook residency training, likely because board certification offered few benefits over immediate entry into private general medical practice following internship.[22] The appeal of graduate education for specialists began even earlier in large cities. In Philadelphia, as early as 1929 the average full specialist had 1.7 years of graduate medical education as opposed to 1.2 years for the average GP, and 37 percent of full specialists as opposed to 14 percent of GPs had pursued graduate medical education beyond internship.[23] In effect, the institutions of hospital residency and board certification lengthened the process of becoming a specialist in the United States, and the expansion of training only continued: the median number of years full specialists spent in residency training increased from 2.9 to 3.6 years from the class of 1935 to the class of 1950.[24]

The advent of residencies and the expansion of graduation medical education, however, did little to change the ultimate agenda for doctors: to establish a lucrative private medical practice. Because they had sacrificed immediate entry into private practice for low salaries during their graduate medical education, residents needed to make up for lost time once in practice. For specialists, though, residency was not a huge career gamble as they stood to earn much more, on average, from private practice than the GPs who entered private practice after internship. If anything, the hospital residency functioned as a prolonged job interview for the pre-specialist who ultimately wished to join the admitting staff of a hospital, to be hired as a faculty member of a prestigious medical school, and to be invited into the group practice of an established specialist.

For example, during his residency at the University of Pennsylvania Hospital (1937–1940), Dr. Harold Scheie worked closely with Dr. Francis H. Adler, a renowned Philadelphia ophthalmologist and faculty member at the Graduate School of Medicine. His residency combined coursework, some teaching to undergraduate medical students, and clinical work in the "eye ward" and outpatient department of University Hospital.[25] After Dr. Scheie had proven himself, he was asked to become an assistant in Dr. Adler's practice, where he began to develop a clientele of his own. Dr. Adler even arranged for some hospital patients to be referred to Dr. Scheie, who was most grateful. As Scheie put it in a letter to his parents,

> While trying to complete my training, complete some papers and the like I am gradually starting private practice. I have a few patients of my own, who aren't clinic patients, every week, which means by the time I finish my fellowship in two years I should be able to support myself. Starting in a specialty is hard here, for [in] the city in large, I know few people, and there are several hundred specialists. . . . Dr. Adler sends cases to me, my friends, some doctors, and I get all the [workmen's] compensation and accident eye work from the hospital including the Philadelphia railroad. . . . Dr. Adler's idea is that by starting me early I will have my own practice worked up by the time I no longer get a fellowship salary. A year from now I will go into his private office as his assistant, [which is] also a help.[26]

Once the assistantship began in 1939, Dr. Scheie was delighted, noting to his parents, "it is a phenomenal break. He will have me help him, I will take care of my own practice, and he will send me what patients he can. No one has ever been more fortunate. It means that I can go as far as my ability will take me for he is absolutely unselfish, has the prestige and connections to boost me, and will."[27] Dr. Scheie finished his residency in 1940, passed his examination by the American Board of Ophthalmology, and landed several hospital and faculty appointments. At that time, Dr. Adler invited Dr. Scheie to become partner in his group practice. Dr. Scheie was ecstatic, convinced that his new partnership "will mean that we keep on together and eventually in years to come I will fall heir to the practice. My income should be beyond all hopes that I have entertained in addition to the honor involved."[28] With only a handful of exceptions for purely research or hospital-based specialties such as pathology, radiology, or bacteriology, most residents hoped to use their graduate education like

Dr. Scheie—to make a favorable impression upon older specialists in order to get a leg up in private practice.

Indeed, despite the growing role of hospitals for patient care and medical education, private practice still served as the primary locus for patient care and as the cornerstone of medical careers and livelihoods from 1920 to 1940. Although 65 percent of Philadelphia doctors held staff positions in hospitals or clinics in 1929, the vast majority of these positions were part-time positions, unpaid positions, or both. Even with hospital and clinic duties, the average Philadelphia doctor, even the average specialist, devoted the majority of the workweek to private practice. Furthermore, whether they paid directly through fee-for-service or paid indirectly through charitable donations and state and local tax disbursements, the people of Philadelphia spent a far greater share of total health expenditures on care from private practitioners than on care in hospitals and sanatoria—or 45 to 27 percent of the total, respectively. Together, these data confirm the enduring primacy of private practice for patient care during the 1920s and 1930s.[29]

Private practice also continued as the main source of income for American doctors from 1920 to 1940. A nationwide survey conducted in 1929 found that 86 percent of American doctors were "in independent private practice" whereas only 12 percent "held full-time positions from which they derived a salary."[30] A later study of California doctors found that while nearly every doctor spent at least some time each week in office practice, less than half that many spent any time in paid or free hospital service.[31] To be sure, the tendency to accept salaried work did increase during the 1920s and 1930s, particularly among specialists who combined hospital and office practice, but the increase was slight.[32] Curiously, only 5 percent of Philadelphia doctors were in full-time institutional practice in 1940. Of the remainder, 79 percent were in active private practice, 13 percent were in internships or residencies and thus headed into private practice, and 3 percent were retired.[33] Hospital work, though of greater importance to medical education and health care in 1940 than in 1909–1910, had not displaced the ultimate goal of becoming a doctor—to establish a private medical practice.

Persistent Sources of Stratification and Conflict

Given that doctors began their careers more or less the same way after the advent of state-mandated internship, one might assume that career paths remained undifferentiated thereafter. As with medical careers earlier in the century, nothing could be further from the truth. A number of features could distinguish career paths: some doctors undertook residency while others entered directly into private practice after internship and licensure (see figure 1); some doctors sought salaried positions while others did not; some doctors associated closely with hospitals and clinics throughout their careers while others were content in office practice; and some doctors reaped great financial rewards from private practice while others did not. In order to understand the relative value of private practice, we must examine the different factors that shaped career paths and financial success. Attention will be directed to describing how career paths diverged, to determining the extent to which divergent career paths separated doctors into distinct occupational strata, and to explaining the major sources of stratification in private practice.

As we have just seen, the process of becoming a doctor required institutional access: to colleges, to medical schools, to hospital internships, and (for specialists) to residencies. Although formal qualifications or technical ability no doubt helped applicants gain access, factors external to applicants also played a role. Just as in the early twentieth century, discrimination on the basis of social background, race, and gender limited access to institutions, and therefore determined the demographic composition of the medical profession. It is difficult, if not impossible, to identify the social class or ethnicity of individual doctors from historical sources, let alone the social class or ethnicity of unsuccessful applicants to the institutional entry points for medical practice.[34] Therefore, the following analysis will focus mostly on racial and gender barriers.

At least one contemporary study of the organization of the medical profession in Providence, Rhode Island, however, suggested that ethnicity partially determined the career paths of doctors in 1940, where an "inner fraternity" of doctors controlled access to hospital positions. This fraternity consisted of "Yankee" doctors who resided in the upscale East Side, had lucrative private practices in the most fashionable East Side medical office buildings, and hoarded the highest hospital staff and leadership positions in the largest, and most coveted, general hospital. This close-knit fraternity united around social, ethnic, and religious bonds, and severely restricted access to the members of Providence's other main ethnic groups—Irish doctors, Italian doctors, and Jewish doctors. To some degree, Irish and Italian doctors could secure staff positions in the city's one Catholic hospital, and Jewish doctors in other smaller secular hospitals, but these positions paled in comparison to the career advantages gained through internship, residency, and staff positions in the main general hospital. Because of their greater institutional access, Yankee doctors were specialized to a much higher degree than doctors from any of the other ethnic groups, who were more often relegated to general practice outside of institutions, typically in neighborhoods where clientele of similar ethnic backgrounds lived, worked, or shopped. This single study suggests that although the formal qualifications and technical ability of "new recruits" to the inner fraternity still mattered in Providence, ethnicity placed limits on the ability of a young doctor to get "sponsorship" from the Yankee cabal.[35]

The applicability of this study to larger cities, however, is uncertain. By comparison to Philadelphia, for example, Providence had but 13 percent of the population, 13 percent of the doctors, and 13 percent of the hospitals.[36] It may have been easier for an inner fraternity of doctors defined by ethnic, social, and religious affiliation to rule a small town like Providence than a large metropolis like Philadelphia. Nevertheless, there is evidence that larger anti-immigrant sentiment that took hold during the 1920s and 1930s manifested itself in medical institutions, thereby limiting the career potential of "white ethnics." For example, many medical schools, including Woman's Medical College in Philadelphia, enacted admissions quotas for Jewish applicants during this period.[37]

Unlike discrimination on the basis of social class or ethnicity, it is sadly very easy to demonstrate race and gender discrimination in Philadelphia medical careers (table 11).[38] A series of institutions throughout the American education system discriminated against African Americans and women, beginning in primary and secondary schools. It was especially difficult for African Americans to get the primary and secondary education required for college admission, where discriminatory admissions committees were all too eager to find reasons to exclude African American applicants. Even if African Americans and women succeeded in getting all of the education required for admission to medical school, discrimination severely restricted matriculation and retention as many schools were integrated or coeducational through symbolic inclusion only, providing little encouragement to African American or women students.[39] Because of sex discrimination and the unique family demands of women medical students, their drop-out rates were much higher than for men.[40] In 1940, as a result of quotas and hostile learning environments, most African American doctors in Philadelphia (around 60 percent) had attended one of the two remaining black medical colleges in the United States—Howard University School of Medicine or Meharry Medical College—and most women doctors in Philadelphia (around 75 percent) had attended the one remaining female medical college—Woman's Medical College.[41]

Institutional discrimination did not end with graduation. African American doctors, in particular, had difficulty gaining access to hospitals for further

Table 11. **The Gender and Race of Doctors versus All Occupied Persons in Philadelphia, 1940**

Category	Percent of Physicians & Surgeons	Percent of Occupied Persons
White Men	90.1	62.8
African American Men	3.2	6.0
Other Men	0.2	0.1
White Women	6.2	26.7
African American Women	0.2	4.4
Other Women	0.0	0.0

Sources: U.S. Bureau of the Census, *Sixteenth Census of the United States, 1940* (Washington, DC: U.S. G.P.O., 1943) *Population*, vol. 3, "The Labor Force," table 11, 29–31 and table 13, 48–53. Unfortunately, the nativities of occupied persons were not recorded in the 1940 census. Percentages are rounded to the nearest tenth of a percent, and therefore do not necessarily total 100 percent. See appendix for details.

training and for staff positions during the 1920s and 1930s. African American doctors were only able to undertake internships or to secure staff positions at the two African American hospitals in the city—Mercy Hospital in West Philadelphia and Frederick Douglass Hospital in South Philadelphia. As a result, the percentage of African American doctors who undertook residencies or who held clinical or teaching positions was far lower than for white doctors in Philadelphia. As a result, only 14 percent of African American doctors were specialists in 1938, as opposed to roughly 41 percent of white doctors; furthermore, most African American specialists were only part-time specialists.[42] With the exception of public health clinics, where the white doctors solicited help in addressing the growing health problems of African American migrants during the 1920s and 1930s, the medical world of African American doctors—both in private practice and in medical institutions—was completely segregated from that of white doctors.[43]

By comparison to African Americans, women doctors fared only slightly better after graduation. Although the number of available internships in the United States exceeded the number of medical graduates after 1924, most hospitals with internships were closed to women applicants, and at the start of World War II, only 15 percent of the hospitals with AMA-approved internships accepted applications from women. As a result, the number of women medical school graduates often exceeded the number of AMA-approved internships available, meaning that some women doctors had to forgo internship or else take an internship in a low-status hospital.[44] Women doctors had similarly low access to residencies, with only 6.5 percent of American hospitals with residency programs enrolling women in 1940. Although women only represented about 4.6 percent of practicing doctors in 1940, women residents had fewer options than men (in terms of hospitals and cities). To make matters worse, many specialty medical societies excluded women until the 1930s, and women had fewer and lower-status faculty positions by comparison to men. It was therefore difficult for women specialists to recruit more women doctors into specialties.[45] Despite institutional discrimination, women doctors did manage to specialize at relatively high rates in some cities, like Philadelphia, where internships and residencies were more readily available to women: of Philadelphia doctors in 1940, 33 percent of women versus 39 percent of men doctors were specialists.[46] Women, though, were more likely to be found in certain specialties in which women were thought to have gender-specific expertise, especially pediatrics.[47] What institutional access women doctors did achieve during the 1920s and 1930s was in spite of gender discrimination, which continued to limit their career opportunities through the mid-twentieth century.

Discrimination on the basis of social background—ethnicity, class, race, and gender—limited the career choices for many doctors to private general practice, and made it so that specialists were not a representative sample of all doctors in the 1920s and 1930s, despite the fact that specialization increased significantly during this period.[48] As specialists tripled from 1909 to 1940—from 13 to 39 percent of all Philadelphia doctors (figure 5)—the medical profession became more stratified than ever before along the lines of specialization. Besides having different social backgrounds, specialists and pre-specialists diverged from GPs in terms of their career paths, institutional tenure, workweek activities, income, and financial aspirations.

As measured by the timing of the specialization decision, career paths in private practice had changed significantly, with specialization stratifying doctors at a much earlier career phase than earlier in the century. As residency training and board certification became the recognized hallmarks of expertise in many specialties by the late 1930s, pre-specialists had a new career path that traded the five to ten years of preparation in private general practice required of their forebears for one to three years of specialty training in a residency (after hospital internship).[49] Unlike for medical practice as a whole, there were no legal barriers to specialty practice, which meant that it was still possible for doctors to specialize gradually over the course of a career in private general practice, as was common earlier in the century. It was also possible for doctors with no specialty training or certification whatsoever to declare themselves

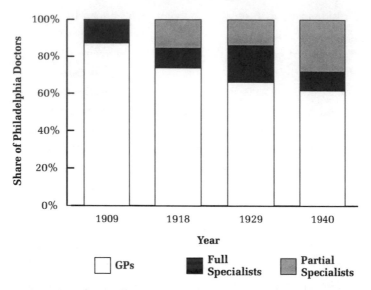

Figure 5. The Decline of General Practitioners in Philadelphia, 1909–1940

Source: AMD (1909) and *AMD* (1940) samples. This tabulation included all doctors listed, including those in internships, residencies, or otherwise not in private practice. Partial specialists were not listed in the *AMD* (1909). See appendix for details.

specialists and to practice as such. There were, however, market barriers to specialty practice, as doctors could only succeed in specialty practice so long as their claims to specialty expertise were recognized by peers and affirmed through consultations and referrals.

In their 1940 report, the Commission on Graduate Medical Education explained the effects of residency on the timing of the specialization decision and on the hierarchy of expertise in the medical marketplace:

> Will the young graduate of today, after the completion of his internship, enter general practice as did the graduates of older generations and eventually develop a specialty through the types of cases he elects to see and treat? Perhaps he will, but the barriers to such a course are greater than they ever have been. First, each specialty is developing so fast scientifically that the active general practitioner will find it difficult, if not impossible, to keep abreast of all of his needs for general practice and at the same time master the constantly expanding technics of a specialty. Second, the general practitioner will find himself in competition with specialists who have already mastered the technics of the specialty through their long period of graduate training and are relieved of the

necessity of keeping up with the details in those other fields that must be followed by the general practitioner. The properly trained specialist will have been certified by his specialty board and this added prestige will affect his standing with the public. Medical colleagues, too, will turn to him rather than to the general practitioner for consultations.[50]

Instead of undertaking general medical practice after internship, with all of the career uncertainty and financial hardship of hanging a shingle and waiting for patients, the pre-specialist resident could gain, inside the hospital, the experience necessary to be recognized as a specialist and could establish the consultation and referral networks necessary for later success in private specialty practice (see figure 1). In addition, many hospitals began to restrict surgical privileges and staff promotions to board-certified specialists, making it even harder for GPs who had specialized their practices gradually to prove their skills or gain further specialty training in hospitals.[51] Thus one central explanation for the decline of general medical practice as the default career path for American doctors is that it became more difficult for established GPs who had specialized gradually to compete with younger specialists who had completed residencies. It therefore behooved the pre-specialist to follow the direct path to specialization via residency training rather what had become a dead-end career path in general practice.

The career paths of Philadelphia specialists and GPs reflected these national trends. In 1909, when residency training in specialties was both informal and rare, full specialists were significantly more experienced than GPs— 3.7 years—an indication that specialization was a mid-career phenomenon. By 1940, difference in the average experience of full specialists and GPs persisted, but the gap had narrowed to 2.5 years, reflecting the expanding representation of young doctors among the ranks of specialists.[52] Not only did the overall specialization rate increase from 1909 to 1940, but the youngest cohorts of doctors had higher specialization rates as well (figure 6). Other cities had comparable trends. A longitudinal analysis of the 1915, 1920, 1925, 1930, and 1935 graduates of the University of Buffalo School of Medicine also found that the trend to limit medical practice to a specialty increased with each class, and that each class specialized, on average, earlier in their careers than had the previous class.[53] The career paths of specialists and GPs in the 1920s and 1930s diverged sooner after medical school than ever before.

Once specialized, the career paths of specialists became even more distinctive. Because of their dependence upon institutions for specialty training, for career building, and for the establishment of referral and consultation networks,

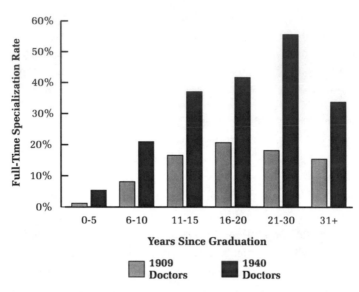

Figure 6. The Full-Time Specialization Rate of Philadelphia Doctors, by Experience, 1909 and 1940

Source: AMD (1909) and AMD (1940) samples. Doctors not in private practice were excluded. See appendix for details.

it is not surprising that specialists sought more institutional positions on average than did GPs; the same had been true earlier in the century (see figure 3). One nationwide survey of 1935 and 1940 medical graduates found that full specialists were far more likely to have undertaken hospital residencies than GPs (89.0 versus 34.1 percent), and that full specialists represented the largest share of doctors who held full-time salaried positions (81.4 percent) and part-time salaried positions (65.8 percent) in 1950.[54] Besides holding more salaried positions in hospitals, medical schools, or public health departments, other studies found that full specialists spent more time practicing medicine in hospitals and clinics than did partial specialists or GPs (figure 7). Full specialists still spent the majority of their time in private practice (51.9 percent), though barely more than in institutional practice; by contrast, GPs devoted the bulk of their workweek (84.4 percent) to private practice, whether in the office or on house calls (figure 8). Because of the greater amount of time devoted to institutional practice, specialists were more likely than GPs to reap financial rewards from institutional practice. A nationwide study in 1928 found that 20.4 percent of specialists versus 8.9 percent GPs earned most or all of their incomes from salaried work in institutions.[55]

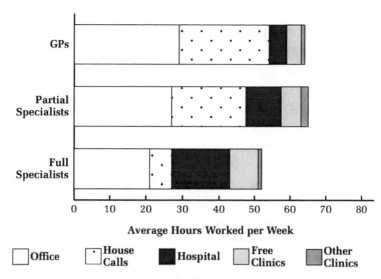

Figure 7. The Number of Hours Spent by Philadelphia Doctors in Private Practice versus Institutional Practice, 1929

Source: Nathan Sinai and Alden B. Mills, *A Survey of the Medical Facilities of the City of Philadelphia, 1929*, Publications of the Committee on the Costs of Medical Care, no. 9A (Washington, DC, 1931), 5, figure 1.

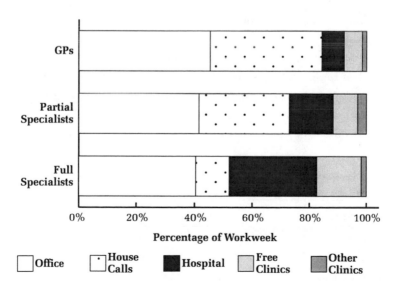

Figure 8. The Percentage of Workweek Spent by Philadelphia Doctors in Private Practice versus Institutional Practice, 1929

Source: Sinai and Mills, *A Survey of the Medical Facilities of the City of Philadelphia*, 5, figure 1.

Besides differing in their workweek activities, the financial success of specialists and GPs also diverged considerably when measured by income and fee collection. Specialists earned more income and collected a higher percentage of their accounts in 1940.[56] These disparities manifested in Philadelphia's medical marketplace, too: the average gross income, the average net income (the income after expenses), and the median net income of Philadelphia doctors in 1929 was highest for full specialists and lowest for GPs, with partial specialists in the middle (table 12). Even during the Great Depression, when the incomes of all doctors suffered as the market value of private medical care depreciated, specialists continued to earn more than GPs, despite the higher costs of specialty medical care for patients.[57] Greater financial rewards provided powerful economic incentives for doctors to specialize at an earlier career phase than ever before, and specialization rates increased throughout the early twentieth century, even during the Great Depression.[58]

Questionnaire-based analysis of career decisions confirmed the financial appeal of specialty practice. In one of the earliest such studies, 47 percent of first-year medical students at the University of Pennsylvania and Cornell University in the classes of 1955, 1956, 1957, and 1958 already planned to pursue a specialty career, and this number increased to 65 percent by the senior year. The study concluded that "lack of financial difficulties" and "high economic aspirations," among other factors, increased "the probability of choosing a specialty over general practice."[59] For example, when comparing first-year medical students whose fathers had blue-collar jobs with students whose fathers were white-collar professionals (physicians, other professionals, and businessmen), only one-quarter of the former planned to enter specialty practice as compared to one-half of the latter.[60] Besides having higher socioeconomic status when entering medical school, the financial aspirations of pre-specialists exceeded those of students who expected to become GPs, as measured by the "lowest satisfactory annual incomes" that members of these two groups of medical

Table 12. **The Relative Incomes of Philadelphia Doctors by Specialization, 1929**

Practitioner Type	Average Gross	Average Net	Median Net
Full specialists	$12,691	$6,797	$5,500
Partial specialists	$8,836	$5,265	$4,428
General practitioners	$6,413	$3,744	$3,197
All doctors	$9,056	$5,156	$4,207

Source: Sinai and Mills, *A Survey of the Medical Facilities of the City of Philadelphia*, 5, figure 1.

students found acceptable.[61] Studies like this strongly suggest that anticipation of greater financial rewards in specialty practice motivated the career decisions of students who switched their plans from general to specialty practice during medical school.[62]

By noting the economic incentives of specialization, we should not assume GPs at mid-century were uninterested in making a living. On the contrary, as will be explained, economic self-interest directed the conduct and organization private practice, regardless of the type of practitioner. Instead, we should conclude the following: specialization divided doctors at an earlier point in their careers in 1940 than in 1909; the growing pecuniary advantages of specialism contributed to this change in career structure; when specializing, the postgraduate education of incipient specialists diverged from that of incipient GPs, who entered private practice much sooner than pre-specialists; and, finally, once in private practice, the workweek activities and the income expectations and financial returns of GPs and specialists diverged substantially. When considered altogether, specialization generated such a stark and early bifurcation in career paths as to create altogether separate strata in American medicine.

Besides social background and specialization, experience continued to separate doctors into measurably different occupational strata in 1940, much as in 1909–1910. Not only did the likelihood of specialization increase with experience for all doctors (see figure 6), so too did the proportion of full-time to part-time specialists (figure 9). Because limiting a practice to a particular specialty required the establishment of consultation and referral networks, specialists who had been in practice longer were more likely to have established these networks; younger specialists, who could not (yet) depend on earning enough income from consultations and referrals, supplemented their income by accepting general cases and therefore only partially specialized their practices.[63]

In addition to differing in likelihood and degree of specialization, younger doctors also had different incomes and position holding patterns from established doctors in the United States. Once younger doctors entered private practice, they earned less money than more established doctors, because, irrespective of skill level, young doctors had not yet built the public and professional reputation needed for a steady client base. According to one national study, it took, on average, eight years for the median income of young doctors to equal the median income of all doctors combined. After that point, doctors entered their peak "income-producing period," which lasted until about thirty-five years in practice. After that point, median income declined, as older doctors eased into retirement by scaling back their hours.[64] Incomes for

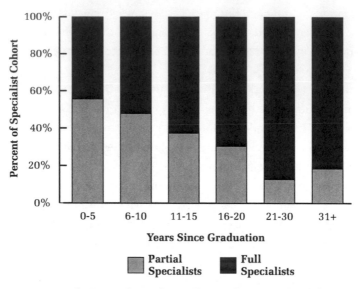

Figure 9.   The Ratio of Partial to Full Specialists in Philadelphia, by Experience, 1940

Source: AMD (1940) sample. Doctors not in private practice were excluded. The ratio of partial to full specialists in is expressed as a percentage of the total specialists in each cohort. See appendix for details.

Philadelphia doctors followed this pattern.[65] Because of the money lost due to idle early years of practice, because of the need to gain clinical experience, and because of the need to find supplemental income, younger doctors were far more likely than established doctors to derive most or all of their incomes from salaried work in institutions such as staff positions in hospitals, clinics, or public health departments: 28 percent of doctors less than five years in practice versus 7 percent of doctors more than thirty years in practice earned all or most of their income from salaried positions.[66] As doctors became more established, the earning potential of private practice far exceeded that of institutional practice, and many doctors, particularly GPs, scaled back their institutional engagements in order to capitalize on their peak income-producing period in private practice. In addition, because the majority of institutional positions were entry level, perhaps with the intention of exploiting the services of hungry young doctors, there were few prestigious middle- to upper-level staff positions to entice the services of established doctors.

Altogether, social background, specialization, and experience stratified doctors in many of the same ways as earlier in the century. Discrimination on the basis of social background, race, and gender limited the career options of individual doctors, including the ability to specialize. Specialization and experience, however, comprised even more fundamental sources of intra-professional stratification, even within groups of doctors harmed by discrimination. The career paths of women GPs and women specialists, for example, diverged considerably as gender discrimination influenced but did not fully determine career paths. As we shall see, the business strategies of specialists and GPs differed as well, as each group fought tooth and nail protect its economic self-interest in private practice.

Adaptation in the Business of Private Practice

Not only did private practice remain central to the careers and livelihoods of American doctors in the 1920s and 1930s, the fundamental nature of private practice remained unchanged. Despite new Progressive Era regulation and stabilization of supply, doctors still competed for patients. As with previous generations, mid-century doctors often disavowed the commercial underside of private practice, especially in professional rhetoric depicting doctors as humanitarians or as disinterested scientific experts. The rhetorical disavowal of commercial motivations became particularly florid during the 1920s and 1930s as the American Medical Association opposed popular legislative attempts at the state and federal level to create a system of compulsory health insurance for industrial workers, to fund maternal and child welfare clinics, and to entitle injured workers to medical care. Critics claimed that the AMA opposed these policy initiatives because doctors wanted to protect the high cost of their services; the AMA claimed to be defending the doctor-patient relationship against the imposition of government bureaucrats in treatment decisions.[67] Regardless of the rhetoric, private medical practices continued to function as small businesses, though in a rapidly changing medical marketplace.

Like their forbears, doctors in the 1920s and 1930s were avid consumers of published business advice in medical journals and in how-to manuals. For example, after its launch in 1923, the journal of *Medical Economics*, which devoted itself "to aid physicians in making medical practice pleasanter, easier, and more remunerative," reached a circulation of more than 100,000 doctors by the 1930s.[68] The journal, like other published advice such as *The Physician's Business* (1938), covered all of the early and mid-career business decisions familiar to doctors earlier in the century: whether to pursue graduate medical education, how to set up a practice, how to build clientele, how to make ends meet while waiting for patients, how to manage growth in a practice, and how to limit a practice to a particular specialty.[69] With the growth of specialization in the 1920s and 1930s, advisors paid particular attention to establishing and maintaining good relations with colleagues and institutions as specialists depended upon the referral and consultation networks they established with other doctors and with hospitals.[70]

Even the AMA published business advice, not only in the *Journal of the American Medical Association* but also in manuals authored by its Bureau of Medical Economics, such as *Collecting Medical Fees* (1938). In the introduction to this manual, the bureau's team of authors blamed the challenge of collecting fees upon the commercial innocence of doctors and the opportunism of some patients: "ethics and professional tradition have introduced so large an element of philanthropy into medical practice that debts for medical service seem to have lost the sharp sense of obligation that distinguishes commercial debts."[71] The more fundamental problem, as the manual later conceded, had more to do with economics—namely, that "the practice of medicine does not involve the transfer of a tangible material commodity" but rather consisted of "personal service." Because personal services were "not subject to resale," their price had "no basic exchange value." Unlike other professionals, such as lawyers, architects, and engineers, doctors could not usually secure fees in advance of services rendered, nor was it ethical to refuse to provide services "when life and death are at stake" or when a patient was too poor to pay. More to the point, "it would be foolhardy for a physician to pursue collection methods which antagonize his patients and cause them to discontinue his services. The ill will created by improper collection tactics may cause a physician to lose far more than the value of delinquent accounts collected."[72] The manual then detailed the costs and benefits of various methods of collection, including the details of contracts with collection agencies. Altogether, the manual reveals that many of the business concerns in private practice persisted from earlier in the century and that even the AMA acknowledged the business nature of private practice, at least to an insular audience of doctors.

The business concerns doctors faced in the 1920s and 1930s were perhaps most intense when first establishing a private practice. Despite the advent of state-mandated hospital internships, the challenges of setting up a first practice after licensure proved just as troubling as earlier in the century, especially during the period of waiting for patients. In one classic study of incomes in 1929, statistician Maurice Leven called particular attention to the plight of young doctors:

After years of purely professional preparation, he [the young doctor] is turned loose in a commercial world to compete for business as well as professional success. He is highly trained yet his first and primary concern after graduation must, of necessity, be that of a small-scale business man. At the age of 30 a man who has chosen a business career has, as a rule, long served his apprenticeship; at the same age the physician finds himself learning the rudiments of business and still struggling for an opportunity to exercise his professional skill. This period of struggle further shortens the productive period of physicians as compared with that of men in most other fields.[73]

In general, as Leven noted, it took seven to eight years in private practice before the average young doctor had attracted enough clientele to be fully occupied and before the average gross income of young doctors matched that of all doctors combined; data for Philadelphia doctors support these findings.[74] During these first seven to eight years of meager earnings, young doctors had to worry about the fixed costs of overhead—especially the cost of office space, which, as measured for Philadelphia doctors in 1929, consumed the largest share of gross income on average.[75] Although young doctors could economize by renting more modest offices in less convenient locations, overhead could not be reduced below a certain threshold. One study of California doctors in 1933 found that even doctors in the lowest gross income brackets nevertheless spent an average of $1,672 of their gross income on "professional expenses."[76]

In order to attract clientele and establish a private practice, doctors used a variety of business strategies, and specialization largely determined the particular strategy used. One study of Providence, Rhode Island, distinguished between strategies used by "institutional" doctors and "individualistic" doctors in 1940. Institutional doctors had specialized practices and their careers and incomes were inextricably linked to hospitals and sponsorship from "established men" who dominated the powerful positions therein. Established hospital specialists sponsored select younger doctors who inherited not only institutional positions but client lists and referral and consultation networks; in short, market competition did not affect the day-to-day world of established specialists and their protégés. By contrast, GPs in Providence tended to be "individualistic," with few hospital appointments let alone referral networks. Because GPs cultivated clientele from the immediate area in which they practiced, GPs in a given neighborhood competed with each other for patients. Competition undermined professional comity and association, hence the predisposition to individualism among GPs.[77]

The most obvious differences between business strategies formed in early career. Returning to the example of Dr. Harold Scheie, young specialists in Philadelphia had opportunities to build their private practices through referrals all the while holding down salaried positions in hospitals. Although Dr. Scheie did not have many patients in his first years of his private practice in ophthalmology, he had more than enough work as an assistant in his mentor's practice and as a hospital resident to keep himself gainfully employed. Within a couple of years, he became a partner in his mentor's practice, at which point his financial future brightened. By contrast, GPs were often left to their own devices, and they resorted to many of the same strategies to build clientele as earlier in the century. For example, after finishing several internships in 1938, Dr. M. Agnes Gowdey bought the general practice of Dr. Yetta Deitch, who was retiring in order to get married (a sacrifice expected of many women doctors). By buying a practice, a young doctor risked precious resources with the hope of retaining the clientele of the previous doctor. At first, Dr. Gowdey rented Deitch's North Philadelphia office but later relocated to a nearby home office when she could afford to buy a place of her own. In order to make ends meet, Dr. Gowdey accepted several entry-level clinical and teaching positions at Woman's Hospital, where she developed her budding interests in obstetrics and pediatrics.[78] Unlike specialists such as Dr. Scheie, GPs and marginalized pre-specialists such as Dr. Gowdey did not have patronage networks to cushion the transition from internship to private practice.

When setting up a practice, partial specialists fit somewhere in between specialists and GPs. After finishing his internship at Philadelphia General Hospital in 1926, neurologist Dr. Samuel B. Hadden initially ran a private general practice out of his home. Like most GPs, he too waited for patients, later recalling that his first case had come while he was shellacking the floors in his new home in Southwest Philadelphia. He "washed up in minutes" and treated his patient, a child who had fallen six feet onto a concrete walk. A local druggist had referred the child's parents to Dr. Hadden, a favor that Dr. Hadden appreciated greatly. Within a few years, Dr. Hadden became more established in practice and could afford to rent a separate office near the University of Pennsylvania in West Philadelphia, which was a much more convenient location given its proximity to medical institutions upon which neurologists relied.[79]

Although business practices remained relatively unchanged from the early century, both GPs and specialists developed new strategies in order to adapt to changing market conditions in private practice. For GPs, the most significant adaptation came in reaction to their declining market share in private practice. Not only were specialists and hospitals providing a greater share of medical services than ever before, but public health officials in health departments and clinics also began to duplicate some of GP services.[80] In Philadelphia, local doctors in many of the poorest neighborhoods initially supported the preventive medical activities of a wide network of charity clinics for children that had developed by the late 1910s. By the 1920s, however, local doctors began to resent the free services offered and withdrew their support for the clinics.[81] In response to the perceived threat posed by public health clinics, the AMA fought to protect the interests of private practitioners and successfully lobbied Congress to allow the expiration of funding for the Sheppard-Towner Act in 1927. The act had provided federal matching funds for prenatal and child health centers since 1921.[82] While opposing local clinics, GPs in Philadelphia and elsewhere tried to capitalize on the growing demand for preventive medicine by offering immunizations and periodic health examinations (PHEs) in their office practices.

The idea of PHEs first gained popularity in the United States among life insurance companies in the early 1910s. By 1922, the AMA also began promoting PHEs through state and county medical societies, and funded a massive advertising campaign to inform patients about the value of PHEs.[83] Publicity focused on the alleged health benefits of the PHE, but editorials in national, state, and local medical journals highlighted the many economic incentives for offering PHEs to patients in private practice.[84] For example, in a paper on "The Growing Importance of Preventive Medicine to the General Practitioner" read at the annual meeting of the AMA in 1924, Dr. James Dodson conceded that "the nurse, the social service worker and other outside agencies" had encroached on the "domain of the physician," but these encroachments were "due to the fact that the physician has neglected certain fields of activity which were important and in which work needed to be done." Dodson then urged doctors to become more educated about preventive medicine in order to prevent further encroachment. He also invited doctors to display issues of *Hygeia*, the AMA's new public outreach journal, in order to better educate office patients about the need to see a doctor for preventive medical care rather than a nurse or social service worker.[85]

Editorials and papers published in state and local medical journals, like *Pennsylvania Medical Journal* and *The Weekly Roster*, specifically noted the pecuniary advantages of PHEs for GPs. For example, one editorialist noted that "we [the editorial board] have stressed on many occasions the need for the general practitioner to realize fully that curative medicine though very essential and always a necessity is becoming less so. Preventive medicine is coming more and more to the front and is a big source of revenue if the physician would visualize it." In the editorialist's opinion, there were "acres of diamonds at the front door of every practitioner, but too many fail to see them." Instead, "many physicians bemoan their fate because preventive medicine is 'killing the goose that laid the golden eggs,' totally oblivious to the wealth in the field." The article then listed all of the diagnostic tests, immunizations, and vaccinations that could be billed during a PHE.[86]

Although some GPs had adapted their business strategies to include PHEs, others resisted. Many of the articles heralding the benefits of PHEs in the 1920s and 1930s were written by specialists, and they formed part of a larger discourse in which specialists sought to limit the role of GPs to primary care, to narrow the market niche for general practice, and to establish the intellectual and therapeutic limits of the rank-and-file doctor. The stated goal of this literature was to determine the appropriate stage at which the GP should refer a patient to the specialist.[87] Some GPs resented such outside attempts to limit their role, which partly explains the slow adoption of PHEs in private general practice. Furthermore, GPs were only willing to promote the PHE in private practice so long as the PHE added to the bottom line—their income—and some GPs were skeptical that an otherwise healthy patient would be willing to pay for a medical examination.[88] Although GPs had by no means universally adopted the PHE by 1940, the PHE movement shows that GPs, at the very least, deliberated about market changes affecting their private practices and considered how best to adapt their strategies accordingly.

Specialists were no different from GPs in surveying and adapting to changing market conditions—to manage their private practices, in other words, as businesses. As the diagnostic equipment and facilities upon which specialists depended became more complex and expensive in the early twentieth century, many specialists began to consider ways to cut overhead. One of the most logical ways was to share equipment, which specialists began to do by forming group practices. Most remained fairly small, though, and fewer than twenty large group clinics (or those having more than fifteen doctors on staff) existed in 1940.[89] Despite the greater efficiency of referrals and consultations and the less expensive and more effective patient care in private group clinics promised by some health care reform studies, such as the "Majority Report" of the Committee on the Costs of Medical Care published in 1932, most specialists simply did not wish to relinquish individual autonomy by joining a *large* group clinic, such as the Mayo Clinic, as a full-time salaried employee. The fear of corporatism motivated several members of the Committee on the Costs of Medical Care to write a dissenting opinion to the Majority Report. Backed by the AMA, "Minority Report Number One" rejected (large) group medical practice as a solution to the rising costs of medical care and promoted the economic status quo—or solo practice.[90] Individualism, in other words, continued to limit the appeal of the large business firm model in general, as well as the size of what few firms existed in private medical practice.

Although few doctors joined large group clinics, some doctors, particularly specialists, had indeed begun to form small group practices by 1940, though the full extent of this trend is difficult to measure.[91] Some small group practices consisted of formal arrangements wherein an older specialist added a younger partner in order to handle overflow cases and to share expenses, as was the case when Dr. Harold Scheie joined the practice of his mentor, Dr. Adler. In other cases, specialists from different fields shared office space and common equipment as a means to cut overhead. Such informal arrangements effectively constituted small mixed group practices, but they did not have consultation and referral as a raison d'être, unlike group clinics such as the Mayo, which had a wide variety of salaried specialists on staff.[92] Despite the "professional and economic advantages" of small and informal group practice, advice columnists cautioned readers about the "possibility of cramped quarters or incompatibility between the doctors."[93] Proscriptive advice such as this indicates that specialists contemplated new business strategies to adapt to novel market conditions.

Despite growing appeal to specialists, group practices had not yet become major sites for patient care by 1940. Instead, hospitals constituted the only corporate structure that enjoyed widespread popularity among American doctors. Like large business firms, hospitals had hierarchical bureaucracies, complex division of labor, and ever more scientific management of patient cases and records.[94] The key difference between hospital doctors and company employees was that hospital doctors had business interests outside of and at times in competition with the firm—namely their private practices. Hospital doctors therefore functioned more like private consultants or contractors, and it was common for doctors to have admitting privileges or staff positions at several hospitals. Apart from a handful of hospital- or laboratory-based specialties, such as pathology or bacteriology, there were very few full-time salaried doctors in 1940.[95] Individual office practice endured as the primary business structure and as the largest site for patient care.

When it came to hospitals, GPs and specialists had trouble finding common ground, much as they had earlier in the century. In part, this merely reflected the very different value of hospitals to each group: GPs depended very little upon hospitals for income or for career advancement beyond internship, whereas specialists built their entire careers and private practices around inpatient and outpatient hospital service. Even the very founding of a hospital could lead to intra-professional rivalry, as shown for rural demonstration hospitals funded by philanthropic organizations in the 1920s and 1930s. Rather than cooperating to meet health care needs in new demonstration hospitals, local doctors instead vied for staff privileges and for ways to exploit hospital equipment and surgical facilities in order to gain competitive advantage in the rural medical marketplace.[96] Like dispensaries earlier in the century, hospitals had the potential to sour collegial relations in medical communities that were otherwise unified around common professional goals such as the enforcement of licensing laws.

Although allegations of "dispensary abuse" per se quieted down in Philadelphia during the 1920s, GPs and specialists clashed over other hospital issues, such as admitting and surgical privileges. GPs fought for open staffing at hospitals and were angered when hospitals tried to limit the ability of local doctors to admit and treat their medical and surgical patients in hospitals. In the end, most hospitals opened their staffs to local doctors in order to maximize the number of paying patients referred from private practices in the area.[97] Hospitals with open staffs, however, continued to favor specialists over GPs, especially when it came to surgical privileges. For example, in the mid-1940s, Cincinnati GPs protested when one of the main hospitals in the city, Jewish Hospital, revoked their right to perform two lucrative surgical procedures, tonsillectomies and adenoidectomies, instead limiting these procedures to board-certified ear, nose, and throat specialists. Concerned that tonsillectomies and adenoidectomies would be the entering wedge for restricting all minor surgical procedures to board-certified specialists, Cincinnati GPs organized to promote their interests and applied considerable pressure on the medical staff of the hospital. Eventually, Jewish Hospital reversed its policy but retained the right to determine, on an individual basis, what surgical procedures any given doctor was competent to perform.[98] This confrontation and others like it in hospitals nationwide inspired GPs to form the American Academy of General Practice in 1947, which sought to elevate the status of GPs by creating a certification board comparable to that of many specialties, by standardizing the postgraduate education and surgical credentials of GPs and by securing adequate representation of GPs on hospital staffs.[99]

In Philadelphia, the issue of dispensary abuse or "hospital abuse" reemerged between 1929 and 1936, as the Great Depression took hold and patients struggled to pay for all manner of goods and services, including the doctor's bill. Because of its diverse industrial and manufacturing base, Philadelphia was not as hard hit as single-industry cities like Detroit or Pittsburgh, but unemployment nevertheless soared to 46 percent in 1933.[100] Unemployment in Philadelphia remained at 31 percent three years later, with another 8.8 percent only partially employed. Even professional workers such as doctors suffered from 11 percent male unemployment as late as 1936, though their hardship paled in comparison to the 43.3 percent male unemployment among unskilled workers.[101] A nationwide study of doctors published in *Medical Economics* confirmed that the average gross income of employed doctors declined from a peak of $9,329 in 1929 to $6,139 in 1935, and had not yet fully recovered to pre-Depression levels by 1939.[102] Philadelphia followed these nationwide trends, with doctors' net incomes decreasing nearly 50 percent from 1929 to 1932, and with 23 percent of doctors finding it "necessary to depend upon other sources of income to meet their expenses."[103] Dr. Carl Fischer, for example, recalled that many of his patients were unable to pay for his services, but "many men who had lost their jobs tried to eke out an existence by selling apples on street corners. On a number of occasions," Dr. Fischer recalled, he was "offered a few of these apples in payment for an office or house visit. Needless to say my wife and I soon came to look upon apples as a not too desirable delicacy!"[104]

CPs were harder hit by the Depression because they earned considerably less, on average, than specialists (see table 12) and held fewer salaried positions than specialists to soften the blow from declining returns in private practice. Although GPs and specialists experienced comparable percentage decreases in income, one California study concluded that "averages and proportions mean little until applied to the actual problems of individuals. Although [the Depression] has not changed the relative economic position of specialists and non-specialists, the depression has undoubtedly been most disastrous for the poorly-paid general practitioners, half of whom in 1933 had net professional incomes of less than $2,200."[105] In Philadelphia, editorials in *The Weekly Roster* pleaded for contributions to the Aid Association to help out-of-work GPs and their dependents. The primary beneficiaries, one editorial noted, "were not the big chiefs who read and write papers and run big free dispensary services with the aid of an army of subordinates, and everlastingly stress the importance of enlarging the free medical service of the hospital. No, they were just regular doctors."[106]

It was in this context of declining returns from practice during the Great Depression that the issue of "abuse" resurfaced. GPs began to wonder whether hospital outpatient departments were further depressing the market value of office fees by offering free or nearly free care to patients who could did not merit charity care. In 1932, 65 percent of doctors surveyed by the Philadelphia County Medical Society were "certain that they are losing patients who are fully able to pay."[107] At an open PCMS meeting on "medical economics" held on January 18, 1933, many GPs expressed their outrage at what they felt was blatant evidence of hospital abuse. One doctor claimed that in his neighborhood's clinic, "it was known that patients came within easy walking distance of the hospital door, in an expensive automobile, making the remainder of the trip on foot in order that the hospital authorities should not know their true financial standing."[108] Another Philadelphia doctor claimed that he had "known people making from $3,000 to $4,000 yearly with only two dependent upon that income to be allowed to have dispensary treatment by the payment of such small sums as are asked in many out-patient departments, ranging from $.10 to $.35."[109] The *Pennsylvania Medical Journal* published other such accounts, one of which alleged, "In the old days poor people were poor people; now the ward cases have boudoir caps and lace nighties."[110] The villains in these stories were hospital social workers who neglected to conduct means tests, as well as the hospital specialists who turned a blind eye to the harm their deceitful patients inflicted on the struggling family doctor.[111]

As a result of pressure from its membership and outrage by its rank-and-file members, the PCMS investigated a litany of pocketbook issues during the Great Depression, from the enforcement of licensing laws to the reimbursement of doctors under worker's compensation laws to yet another investigation of hospital abuse in 1933.[112] After extensive investigation, the PCMS issued a fourteen-point plan to curb such abuse, the central feature of which called on hospitals to increase the efficiency and oversight authority of their social service departments. The plan further suggested that these departments limit admissions to patients who had written referrals from local doctors who had personally ascertained economic need. Once treated, inpatients and outpatients were to be referred back to local doctors and only readmitted with similar referral.[113] In 1934, the PCMS reported that eight hospitals had already adopted the plan, which could be viewed as a minor success for the GPs incensed by alleged abuses.[114] In the end, though, after careful study of 1,036 cases in nineteen Philadelphia hospitals, the PCMS concluded that fewer than 5 percent of charity cases were fraudulent. Despite allegations, the PCMS concluded that abuse was infrequent, though hospitals and dispensaries were urged to strive for greater efficiency by coordinating their services with local doctors.[115]

Although the investigation ultimately determined that few patients took advantage of free or nearly free services in Philadelphia during the Depression, the festering issue of hospital or dispensary abuse reinforces the following points about changing career paths and business methods during the 1920s and 1930s. First, GPs and specialists had divergent business interests in private practice. These different interests led to different strategies for building a career, for establishing a private practice and for adapting to changing market conditions. Institutional discrimination limited the ability of ethnic minorities, African Americans, and women to specialize, thereby further separating GPs and specialists on the basis of social background. What resulted by 1940 was a medical profession stratified primarily by specialization, with doctors in each stratum fighting to protect their particular economic self-interests. Some of the interests of GPs and specialists overlapped, and led to cooperation on issues such as the enforcement of registration and licensing laws. When it came to hospitals and dispensaries, however, GPs and specialists clashed much as they had earlier in the century, with GPs resenting the specialists who attracted the wealthiest patients in private practice but who also treated many of the poorest patients for little or no charge in hospitals and dispensaries. Given their shrinking market share during the 1920s and 1930s, it is perhaps not surprising that GPs blamed their declining fortunes on closed staffing policies and on deceitful patients, even though evidence supporting these allegations was often wanting. In a medical marketplace increasingly dominated by specialists and their medical institutions, GPs fought to protect their business interests in private practice. Competition and market demand, rather than public health planning and patient needs, directed the evolution of health care services.

Chapter 5

From Center City to Suburb

Besides signaling new career paths and business practices, especially in large cities, increased specialization and hospital-based medicine also transformed patient care. Not only had traditional services been shifted from the home to the hospital, such as attendance at childbirth, but a variety of new surgical procedures and diagnostic tests were centered in hospitals, such as tonsillectomies or X-rays.[1] As technologically sophisticated care became the hallmark of "modern" scientific medicine in the early twentieth century, health care costs began to rise. Cost inflation forced structural changes in patient care, whether in the hospital or in the doctor's office. Hospital administrators built new semiprivate and private wards in order to attract more paying patients, thereby changing the charitable mission of hospital care.[2] Private practice doctors struggled to adapt as well, often debating whether to purchase expensive new diagnostic equipment. Most solo practices could not afford an X-ray machine or laboratory facilities and staff in the 1920s and 1930s, but a group practice might. For the doctor who clung to individual business ownership, alternatives included outsourcing new diagnostic services to private laboratories or developing closer ties to large hospitals, where private patients could be referred for diagnostic services unavailable in the office. The conundrum for the modernizing doctor was that referring patients elsewhere meant losing billable services.

Besides affecting the structure of hospital and office practice, rising costs limited patient access to the benefits of modern medicine. By the 1910s, scholars, social reformers, and labor activists called attention to these problems. Their concern that sickness contributed to poverty and dependency inspired the first national movement to subsidize health care—the campaign for compulsory health insurance for industrial workers. Unlike similar campaigns in Europe, the American campaign ultimately failed due to ineffective leadership, growing opposition from the medical profession and some conservative labor leaders, and the increasingly persuasive claim by 1920 that compulsory health insurance was un-American.[3] The problems of rising costs and declining access only worsened with time, as revealed by the widely read reports of the Committee on the Costs of Medical Care from 1928 to 1933.[4] As the financial burdens of sickness and hospitalization increased, policy debates centered on ways to share risk, whether by new private insurance plans, public finance of health care through taxation, or some public-private scheme. Although bold legislative efforts to establish national health insurance failed repeatedly in the 1930s and 1940s, these efforts exposed the structural problems of health care such as the unequal distribution of health care services like doctor's offices. This chapter examines the changing geography of private medical practice in American cities during this turbulent period.

Contemporary analysis of the changing distribution of doctor's offices in the 1920s and 1930s primarily examined regional, state, and county patterns. These works compared the personal and professional traits of doctors with the locational characteristics of areas with low versus high doctor-to-population ratios. Personal and professional traits included the size of the doctor's hometown, the location of the doctor's alma mater, and other factors such as the doctor's specialization (if any) and experience (or years since graduation). Locational characteristics included the community's size, average or median income, number of hospitals, and percentage of residents living in urban areas. Generally, these early studies found that doctors favored practicing in urban and wealthy areas; in particular, specialists and young doctors were flocking to growing cities, and at a much greater pace than the population as a whole.[5] The incomes of doctors also increased with community size and wealth, which indicated to contemporaries that consumer demand shaped the geography of private practice to a much greater degree than community health needs.[6] As Assistant Surgeon General Joseph W. Mountin wondered in 1942, "Can the undirected forces in a free society be relied upon to effect an equitable distribution of physicians?" For Mountin, the answer was "no," at least "so long as there remain gross differences as well as deficiencies in individual and community resources."[7] Unevenly distributed doctor's offices were but one manifestation of growing inequality between the poor and the wealthy, the rural and the urban.

Yet precious few studies in the 1920s and 1930s examined health care distribution problems *within* American cities, where there were equally alarming disparities in the availability of doctor's offices.[8] For example, as sociologist James Bossard argued from his 1932 study of Philadelphia doctor's offices,

> There are, in Philadelphia, as in every large city, distinct areas, peopled by distinct social types, with their own distinctive needs for medical services. There are areas peopled exclusively or largely by racial groups. There are areas composed of poor people, with relatively high rates of sickness, and areas occupied by relatively rich people, with relatively low rates of sickness. What this means again is an inevitable conflict between medical demands, socially conceived, and medical services, conceived from the standpoint of a private profession. Socially speaking, medical service is most needed in the poorer areas; professionally, it is natural and inevitable for doctors to follow their paying patients.[9]

Professor Bossard's invective hit a nerve in the Philadelphia medical community, as did several fellow presenters at the conference on "The Medical Profession and the Public" sponsored by the College of Physicians of Philadelphia and the American Academy of Political and Social Science in 1934. In one scathing review of the conference published in *The Weekly Roster*, the official publication received by every member of the Philadelphia County Medical Society, Bossard was dismissed as a "comedian" who made "juvenile observations upon the location of the doctors of Philadelphia."[10] Such reactions were not unique to Philadelphia, as the AMA and its firebrand journal editor, Dr. Morris Fishbein, zealously defended the free market organization of American medicine against any and all perceived criticism, including even the timid recommendations of the final report of the Committee on the Costs of Medical Care.[11] In retrospect, though, patterns in the location of Philadelphia doctor's offices reveal significant and growing inequities in urban health care and American society, regardless of how early analysis by Dr. Bossard or the Committee on the Costs of Medical Care were received.

Doctors and Metropolitan Expansion

During the 1920s and 1930s, Philadelphia remained the third most populous American city, even though it had annexed little territory by comparison to New York and Chicago (see map 1).[12] The population of the city proper peaked in 1930, though metropolitan growth continued (figure 10). Despite ongoing restructuring and a decline in the blue-collar workforce after World War

I and again during the Great Depression, Philadelphia's industrial sector had rebounded by 1940 and still provided hundreds of thousands of jobs. Employment in other sectors expanded during this period, especially the white-collar, clerical workforce that staffed the growing number of offices and businesses in Center City. Thus, the Philadelphia region remained an attractive destination for job seekers, which partly explains the continued metropolitan growth.[13] Two developments in the social geography of Philadelphia affected the medical marketplace and opportunities for private practice therein: the shifting demographic profile of the city and the increasing pace of suburbanization.

With the first world war and the passage of restrictive immigration laws in the 1920s, foreign immigration declined precipitously as did the representation of foreign-born whites in Philadelphia (figure 11).[14] The foreign-born white residents who remained also began to be integrated into the social, political, and economic fabric of the city.[15] Although certain parts of town retained a distinct ethnic character, such as Little Italy in South Philadelphia, the days of vast segregated immigrant ghettoes had passed as immigrants dispersed residentially (map 6). By 1940, many foreign-born whites had simply

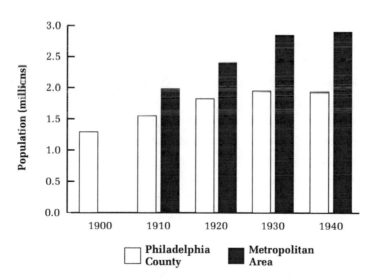

Figure 10. Population Growth in Philadelphia, 1900–1940

Sources: U.S. Bureau of the Census, *Thirteenth Census of the United States, 1910* (Washington, DC: U.S. G.P.O., 1913), vol. 3, *Population*, table 2, 527; U.S. Bureau of Census, *Fourteenth Census of the United States, 1920* (Washington, DC: U.S. G.P.O., 1921), vol. 1, *Population*, "Number and Distribution of Inhabitants," table 40, 64; U.S. Bureau of Census, *Sixteenth Census of the United States, 1940* (Washington, DC: U.S. G.P.O, 1942), *Population*, vol. 1, "Number of Inhabitants," 912 (table 3), 936 (table 7-F). Data on metropolitan districts were not collected before 1910.

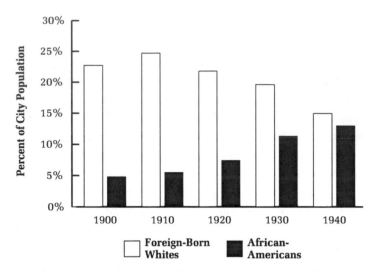

Figure 11.   The Changing Demography of Philadelphia, 1900–1940

Source: Data on the nativity and race of Philadelphia residents calculated from the Historical Census Browser at the University of Virginia, Geospatial and Statistical Data Center, http://mapserver.lib .virginia.edu.

capitalized on the opportunities available when they had arrived during the second wave of immigration (1885–1915) and had begun to prosper. For example, foreign-born whites were no longer as poor on average, and wards with high versus low immigrant residency rates had nearly indistinguishable average monthly rents in 1940, further suggesting residential integration (table 13). Greater economic prosperity enabled many foreign-born whites to leave the slum housing that had surrounded industrial and manufacturing sites where they worked, thereby weakening the former association of work and residence for immigrants.[16]

The experience of African Americans in Philadelphia differed considerably from that of foreign-born whites in 1940. Whether pushed out of the South by agricultural failure, the limited earning potential of tenant farming, and fear of racial violence, or pulled to northern industrial metropolises by the promise of a better job and a better life, the Great Migration of African Americans after the war changed cities like Philadelphia dramatically.[17] Although it already had a sizeable African American population for a northeastern city at the turn of the century, the number of African Americans in Philadelphia tripled between 1910 and 1940, and increased from 5.5 to 13.0 percent of the total population (figure 11).[18] Newly arrived African Americans settled mostly in South Philadelphia but also in sections of Western and inner Northwestern Philadelphia

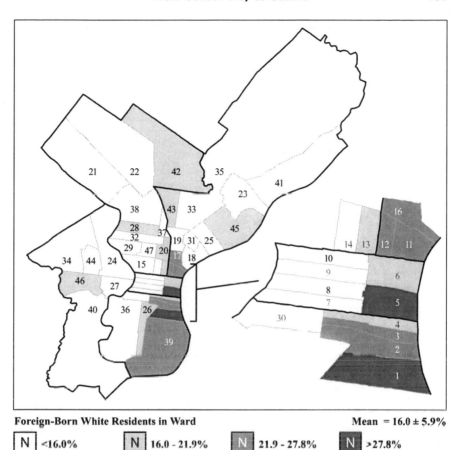

Foreign-Born White Residents in Ward   **Mean = 16.0 ± 5.9%**

| N | <16.0% | N | 16.0 - 21.9% | N | 21.9 - 27.8% | N | >27.8% |

Map 6. Residential Integration of Foreign-Born Whites in Philadelphia, 1940

Source: U.S. Bureau of the Census, *Sixteenth Census of the United States, 1940* (Washington, DC: U.S. G.P.O., 1942), *Population and Housing: Statistics for Census Tracts,* "Philadelphia, Pa." table 1, 4–5 and table 5, 140–163. Numbers indicate city wards. 15.0 percent of Philadelphia residents were immigrants. The map, however, compares immigrant residency rates in each ward to the mean of all city wards, which was 16.0 percent ± 5.9 percent. The city was then divided into four categories: wards below the mean rate, wards within one standard of deviation above the mean rate, wards one to two standards of deviation above the mean rate, and wards above two standards of deviation above the mean rate. No ward exceeded 31.0 percent.

(see map 4).[19] In general, African Americans were highly segregated residentially (map 7) and often lived in the poorest neighborhoods: wards with high African American residency rates had substantially lower rent than wards with low African American residency (see table 13). The causes of residential segregation included the clustering of available low-income housing, lending practices that reinforced racial segregation, and the ground-level enforcement of neighborhood boundaries by white residents.[20] The few areas where

Table 13.   **The Distribution of Residential Wealth in Philadelphia, 1940**

	Number of Wards	Average Rent
Wards with high foreign-born white residency rates	25	$30.95
Wards with low foreign-born white residency rates	22	$31.55
Wards with high African American residency rates	20	$27.28
Wards with low African American residency rates	27	$33.20
Wards with population gain from 1910–1940	21	$33.39
Wards with population loss from 1910–1940	26	$25.63
Wards losing PMPs from 1909–1940[†]	25	$29.08
Wards gaining PMPs from 1909–1940	22	$33.22
City of Philadelphia	47	$31.23

[†] The three wards having no gain or loss in PMPs from 1909 to 1940 are included with the "wards losing PMPs." See appendix for details.

Sources: U.S. Bureau of Census, *Thirteenth Census of the United States, 1910* (Washington, DC: U.S. G.P.O., 1913) vol. 3, *Population*, table 1, 549. U.S. Bureau of Census, *Sixteenth Census of the United States, 1940* (Washington, DC: U.S. G.P.O., 1942) *Population and Housing: Statistics for Census Tracts*, "Philadelphia, Pa." table 1, 4–5 and table 5, 140–63. *AMD* (1909) and *AMD* (1940) samples. The offices of each sample doctor in active practice were ward-coded. The total number of practices in each ward was extrapolated from the sample number in each ward by multiplying by five. Wards with residency rates above the citywide rate were classified as "high," and wards with residency rates below the citywide rate were classified as "low." Average monthly rent figures are per dwelling, and include estimated rent for owner-occupied dwellings. Data on average monthly rent per dwelling were therefore representative of the residential wealth of a census tract. Ward level data were tallied from census tracts, which were subdivisions of wards in 1940. "PMPs" are private medical practices.

African Americans could settle typically had declining industrial employment and were being vacated by older immigrant families. Hiring discrimination in unions and in industrial and manufacturing firms further restricted job opportunities for African Americans to unskilled manual labor for men and domestic service for women.[21] Although migrant African Americans generally had higher incomes in Philadelphia compared to jobs they held in the South, housing and employment conditions were not substantially better, and more than half of all migrants planned to return to the South.[22] In sum, African Americans arrived last among the major groups migrating to Philadelphia in the early twentieth century, but the opportunities that had sustained earlier immigrants were unavailable because of racial prejudice and declining social mobility.[23]

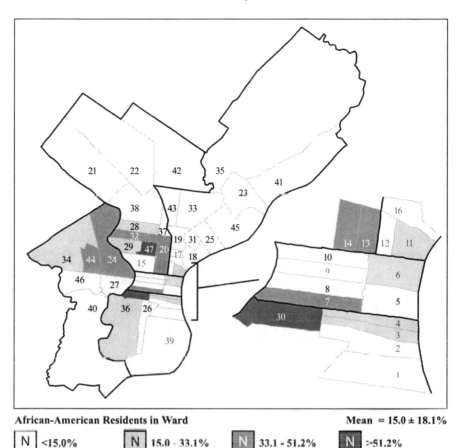

African-American Residents in Ward   Mean = 15.0 ± 18.1%

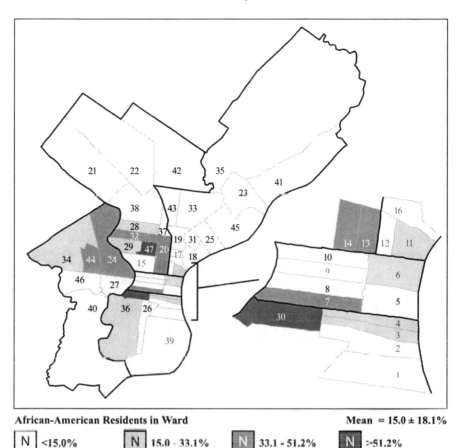 <15.0%   15.0 - 33.1%   33.1 - 51.2%   >51.2%

Map 7. Residential Segregation of African Americans in Philadelphia, 1940

Source: U.S. Bureau of the Census, *Sixteenth Census of the United States, 1940* (Washington, DC: U.S. G.P.O., 1942) *Population and Housing: Statistics for Census Tracts*, "Philadelphia, Pa." table 1, 4–5 and table 5, 140–163. 13.0 percent of Philadelphia residents were African Americans. The map, however, compares African American residency rates in each ward to the mean of all city wards, which was 15.0 percent ± 18.1 percent. The city was then divided into four categories: wards below the mean rate, wards within one standard of deviation above the mean rate, wards one to two standards of deviation above the mean rate, and wards above two standards of deviation above the mean rate. Wards 30 and 47 had rates of 80.4 percent and 57 percent, respectively. The high standard of deviation of the mean rate of African American residency when compared to foreign-born white residency indicates a higher level of segregation.

The social geography of the city also reflected economic stratification in the early twentieth century. From the workplace to entertainment and leisure to shopping, different social classes had distinct patterns of participation and consumption.[24] The same was true in housing: the poor and the working class lived mostly in South Philadelphia and in inner parts of the northern and western districts; the upper class resided in Rittenhouse Square downtown, in the suburbs of Chestnut Hill and Mount Airy to the northwest (ward 22), or else in more remote suburbs on the "Main Line" in Montgomery County; and the middle class lived in the outermost suburbs of the northern and western districts of the city (map 8).[25] Exceptions to this pattern could be found at the neighborhood level in any city ward, but by and large social class divided the residents of the city in 1940.

Suburbanization constituted the other significant influence upon the urban medical marketplace in 1940. Although well under way by the turn of

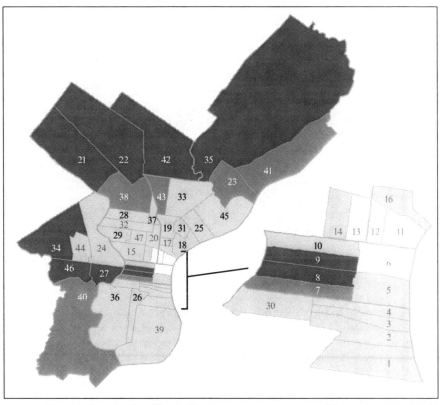

Average Monthly Rent Per Dwelling in Ward   **Mean = $27.95 ± $10.03**

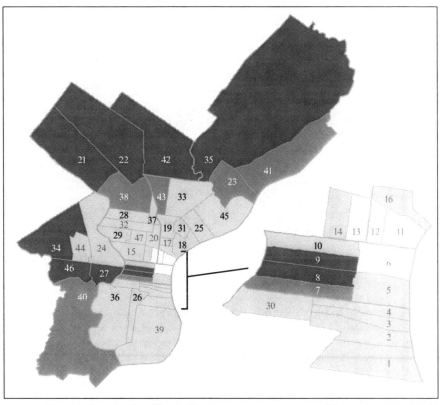 <$17.92 $17.92 - $27.95 $27.96 - $37.98   >$37.98

Map 8.   Average Monthly Rent in Philadelphia, 1940

Source: U.S. Bureau of the Census, *Sixteenth Census of the United States, 1940* (Washington, DC: U.S. G.P.O., 1942) *Population and Housing: Statistics for Census Tracts*, "Philadelphia, Pa." table 1, 4–5 and table 5, 140–163. The average monthly rent for all dwellings in the city was $31.21. The map, however, compares the average rent in each ward to the mean of average rents in all city wards, which was $27.95 ± $10.03. The city was then divided into quartiles: wards less than one standard of deviation above and below, and wards more than one standard above and below. Wards 22 and 8 had the highest rents, at $48.16 and $70.62, respectively.

the century, the pace of residential decentralization had increased dramatically by mid-century, transforming cities like Philadelphia in the process. As map 9 shows, the central wards of Philadelphia lost residents while the outer suburbs grew from 1910 to 1940. Suburbanization was distinctly wealth-based, as the wards that posted population gains from 1910 to 1940 had much higher average rent in 1940 than wards that posted population losses, or $33.39 to $25.63 (a 23 percent difference—table 13); likewise, wards with below median rent in 1940 had *lost* 76,299 residents since 1910, whereas wards with above median rent had gained 458,635 residents (table 14).

A variety of factors contributed to the increasing pace of suburbanization in Philadelphia from 1910–1940. Faster and cheaper public transportation, greater automobile ownership, more affordable housing, more available credit,

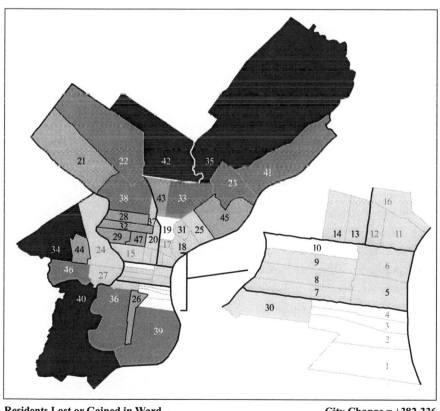

Residents Lost or Gained in Ward   City Change = +382,336

| N | < -10,000 | N | -10,000 to 0 | N | +1 to 10,000 | N | +10,000 to 50,000 | N | > +50,000 |

Map 9. Population Decentralization in Philadelphia, 1910–1940

Sources: See table 13.

Table 14.   **Comparison of Wards with Above and Below Median Monthly Rent in Philadelphia, 1940**

	Below Median Rent Wards	Above Median Rent Wards	City Combined
Number of wards	24	23	47
Total dwellings in 1940	183,410	342,487	525,897
Rent paid (actual and estimated)	$4,233,958	$12,192,241	$16,426,199
Average monthly rent	$23.08	$35.60	$31.23
Population	696,653	1,234,691	1,931,344
Foreign-born whites	119,045	171,280	290,325
African Americans	118,859	132,021	250,880
Share of city population (%)	36.1	63.9	100.0
Share of foreign-born whites (%)	41.0	59.0	100.0
Share of African Americans (%)	47.4	52.6	100.0
Foreign-born whites (%)	17.1	13.9	15.0
African Americans (%)	17.1	10.7	13.0
Population gain/loss, 1910–1940	-76,299	+458,635	+382,336
Private medical practice gain/ loss, 1909–1940	-295	+240	-55

Sources: See table 13.

and the growing purchasing power of middle- and even working-class incomes were all necessary for rapid suburban growth.[26] Also, as some large industrial and manufacturing firms relocated to the suburbs, so too did skilled workers who could now afford modest suburban homes. Besides being wealth-based, residential decentralization in Philadelphia conformed to the "white flight" trend in other cities as white residents vacated the lower-rent inner-city neighborhoods in which migrant African Americans settled.[27] Most white suburbanites still commuted to Center City for work and recreation, though dependence upon Center City for shopping declined as suburbs developed commercial centers of their own.[28]

The changing demographic profile of city residents and the increasing pace of suburbanization reinforced the specialization of different city districts (table 15).[29] Downtown Philadelphia remained the primary destination for work, shopping, and recreation for the middle class, and the central business district (CBD) at the heart of the district grew in size and prominence from 1910 to

1940. The expanding CBD even extended into the fifth and sixth wards, which had previously housed immigrant ghettoes and garment sweatshops, especially near the docks along the Delaware River (see map 1). Although peripheral business districts were developing, the CBD remained the largest (in terms of sales and employment) and it provided unique advantages to the firms located there.[30] Large companies and municipal government gained access to a regional pool of employees by having headquarters in the transportation hub. In addition, smaller and codependent manufacturing and distribution firms cut costs by clustering together downtown. Area retail stores and entertainment venues profited from their accessibility to the large number of middle-class commuters who lingered in the CBD after work; the CBD alone accounted for 37.4 percent of all retail sales in the city and for 71.5 and 63.2 percent of retail sales in general merchandise and apparel, respectively.[31] Finally, many professional firms, such as legal and accounting, chose downtown locations because of their accessibility to a metropolitan clientele; the growth of professional offices in turn sustained a host of secondary service industries and specialty stores that catered to the needs of office workers.[32] The few residents in this commercial district fell into two extremes: some of the wealthiest residents in the city lived around Rittenhouse Square (ward 8), while some of the poorest (African American) residents in the city lived but a few blocks south of Rittenhouse Square (ward 7—maps 7 and 8).

In stark contrast to the specialized functions of the downtown district as the metropolitan center of middle-class employment, recreation, and shopping, South Philadelphia remained quite poor and largely residential in 1940. South Philadelphia dwellings had the lowest average rent, and many residents began to leave the district once they could afford to do so (table 15). Contemporaries generally looked down on the district, and one travel guide described "the paralyzing poverty of South Philadelphia's Negro and foreign sections" with obvious disdain:

> The cobbled streets and uneven brick sidewalks, many reminiscent of Revolutionary days, are usually littered with dirt, rubbish, and torn newspapers. There are a few shopping districts, notably South Street, which sparkle with showy wares, but the prevailing note in the older quarters, is dull and depressingly minor in key. Slum areas splotch the scene like open sores. . . . Neglected children swarm about dingy alleyways. Ramshackle hovels, built without the benefit of bathtubs, huddle forlornly together . . . and society pays the usual price of its apathy in a high mortality, disease, and crime rate.[33]

Table 15. **District Summary of the Changing Social Geography of Philadel-phia, 1910–1940**

	DT	NE	NW	S	W	City
Population, 1910	89,267	392,740	482,939	336,134	247,928	1,549,008
Population, 1940	48,393	486,751	659,405	324,424	412,371	1,931,344
Pop. change, 1910–40	-40,874	+94,011	+176,466	-11,710	+164,443	+382,336
Share of city pop., 1910	5.8%	25.4%	31.2%	21.7%	16.0%	100.0%
Share of city pop., 1940	2.5%	25.2%	34.1%	16.8%	21.4%	100.0%
Percent of res. FBW, 1910	27.1%	26.4%	20.6%	34.6%	15.7%	24.7%
Percent of res. FBW, 1940	14.9%	14.9%	13.8%	19.8%	13.4%	15.0%
Percent of res. Afr-Am, 1910	17.5%	0.9%	5.4%	8.0%	4.9%	5.5%
Percent of res. Afr-Am, 1940	20.9%	1.8%	16.5%	17.8%	15.9%	13.0%
Avg. monthly rent, 1940	$42.26	$27.95	$33.86	$24.04	$34.00	$31.23

Sources: See map 2 and table 13. For abbreviations for the five districts of Philadelphia, see table 9. "Pop." is population, "Res." are residents, "FBW" are foreign-born whites, and "Afr-Am" are African Americans.

Many neighborhoods in the inner city areas of the northeast, northwest, and western districts began to resemble South Philadelphia by 1940: most were relatively poor and had lost residents from 1910 to 1940, though had a growing representation of African Americans (see maps 7–9 and table 15).[34] The exception was the inner northeast district, where a large factory district still thrived (especially in wards 16, 17, 18, 19, 25, and 31). The second- and third-generation immigrants who monopolized these skilled and semiskilled jobs still resided in the surrounding neighborhoods of Kensington and Fishtown, and they fought against perceived African American encroachment from the "Northern Liberties" neighborhood to the south (wards 11 and 12) and from central North Philadelphia to the west (wards 13, 14, and 20).[35] The outer portions of the western, northwestern, and northeastern districts, on the other hand, were fast-growing, white, middle-class suburbs by 1940, with few exceptions.

The ongoing social and spatial transformation of the city from 1910 to 1940 begs the question of how doctors adapted to new conditions in the medical marketplace. By 1940, there was only 1 doctor per 527 residents, and this less crowded marketplace was the cumulative result of licensing laws that had restricted the supply of medical graduates.[36] As in 1910, though, the demographic profile of doctors and city residents differed considerably: by comparison to all employed persons in Philadelphia, doctors were far more likely to have been white men (see table 11).[37] Moreover, growing professional income placed most Philadelphia doctors squarely in the upper middle class, having little in common with South Philadelphians or with the inner-city residents of Western, Northwestern, and Northeastern Philadelphia.[38] Whether and to what extent socioeconomic differences between doctors and the general population influenced location decisions in private practice are questions left to the next two sections. These sections also address the question of how larger developments in the social geography of Philadelphia shaped the career and business appeal of specialization.

The Changing Geography of Private Practice?

Private practices became more unevenly distributed from 1910 to 1940 (maps 5 and 10), although similar areas of the city had practice concentrations above or below the citywide average of 179 practices per 100,000 residents (PMP/100K). The eleventh ward still had nearly no doctor's offices, and the eighth and ninth retained their place as the most doctor-rich wards, even increasing their practice concentrations to 4,762 and 13,029, respectively. Similarly, 34 of the 47 wards had below average practice concentrations, and 13 of these wards had less than *half* the citywide rate of 179 PMP/100K. The handful of wards having twice the citywide practice concentration also remained roughly the same in 1940 as in 1909–1910—the fifth, sixth, seventh, eighth, ninth and twenty-seventh.[39] Again, factors other than population density must explain the location behavior of doctors; otherwise, there would not have been such variation in the concentration of private practices across the city. Although populous areas were certainly desirable, other factors were considered to be more important. As career and business advice author Dr. George D. Wolf explained in *The Physician's Business* (1938), "For obvious reasons, neighborhoods unable to support a physician should also be avoided, as should locations with inadequate transportation facilities, as inaccessibility is a serious handicap."[40] Philadelphia doctors followed this basic advice at mid-century much as their predecessors had followed similar advice decades earlier: they selected locations that were in central, accessible areas or in wealthy or growing suburbs, and avoided locations in the poorest neighborhoods of the city (maps 5 and 10). The uneven distribution of

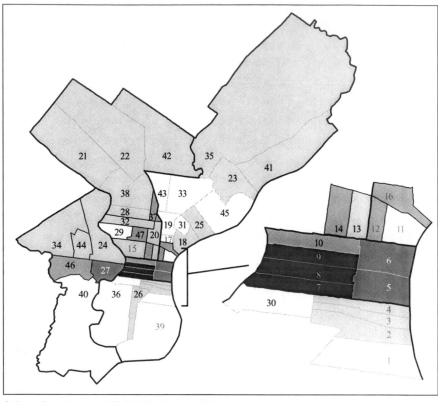

Private Practices per 100,000 Residents in Ward   **City Rate = 179**

| N | 0 - 89 | N | 90 - 179 | N | 180 - 358 | N | 359 - 1790 | N | >1790 |

Map 10.   The Distribution of Private Medical Practices in Philadelphia, 1940

Sources: See table 13. Doctors not in private practice in the *AMD* (1940) sample (184 of 879) were excluded. There were 700 practices addresses for 695 sample doctors in active practice. 690 practice addresses could be ward-coded. The total number of practices in each ward was extrapolated from the sample number in each ward by multiplying by five. See appendix for details.

doctor's offices at mid-century is explained by professional, social, and economic factors that continued to incentivize locating private practices in certain locations and not others.

Compared to the citywide rate of private practices per population in 1940, the downtown district contained the wards with the highest concentrations and no wards with rates below that of the city (table 16). To some degree, the high concentration of doctor's offices downtown can be explained as a mere mathematical artifact of the relatively small and shrinking population in this district. Nevertheless, the downtown had 32 percent of all Philadelphia

Table 16. **District Summary of the Changing Medical Marketplace in Philadelphia, 1909–1940**

	DT	NE	NW	S	W	City
Extrapolated PMP, 1909	1,090	310	1,295	280	530	3,505
Extrapolated PMP, 1940	1,100	475	960	275	640	3,450
PMP gain/loss, 1910–1940	+10	+165	-335	-5	+110	-55
PMP/100K, 1909–1910	1,221	79	268	83	214	226
PMP/100K, 1940	2,273	98	146	85	155	179
Share of all PMPs, 1909	31.1%	8.8%	37.0%	8.0%	15.1%	100.0%
Share of all PMPs, 1940	31.9%	13.8%	27.8%	8.0%	18.6%	100.0%
Avg. experience (yrs.), 1909	˙20.5	12.8	16.8	˙14.2	18.1	17.7
Avg. experience (yrs.), 1940	˙25.2	20.3	22.6	˙16.8	19.3	22.0
Specialization of PMPs, 1909	30.3%	3.2%	8.8%	7.1%	8.5%	14.8%
Specialization of PMPs, 1940	76.4%	32.6%	34.9%	21.8%	35.2%	46.8%
Share of specialty PMPs, 1909	63.5%	1.9%	22.1%	3.9%	8.7%	100.0%
Share of specialty PMPs, 1940	52.0%	9.6%	20.7%	3.7%	13.9%	100.0%
Full specialization of PMPs, 1940	68.2%	13.7%	18.8%	14.5%	22.7%	34.2%
Partial specialization of PMPs, 1940[†]	8.2%	18.9%	16.1%	7.3%	12.5%	12.6%
Share of full specialists, 1940	63.6%	5.5%	15.3%	3.4%	12.3%	100.0%
Share of partial specialists, 1940	20.7%	20.7%	35.6%	4.6%	18.4%	100.0%
Number of hospitals, 1940	10	12	24	8	15	69
Hospitals/100K, 1940	20.7	2.5	3.6	2.5	3.6	3.6
Share of hospitals, 1940	14.5%	17.4%	34.8%	11.6%	21.7%	100.0%

[†] The *AMD* (1909) did not recognize partial specialists.

˙ Difference in the mean experience level of downtown and South Philadelphia doctors differed significantly when measured by Student's t-test (p < .01). ANOVA indicated that the variation in the experience levels of doctors was significantly greater between districts than within a district (p < .01). Data not shown. See appendix for details.

Sources: See table 13 and maps 5 and 10. Data on Philadelphia hospitals in 1940 are from the *AMD* (1940), 1530–31. For abbreviations of the five districts of Philadelphia, see table 9. Percentages in the table are rounded to the nearest tenth of a percent, and therefore share percentages do not necessarily total 100.0 percent. "PMP" is private medical practice, and "PMP/100K" is the number of private medical practices per 100,000 residents in a district. "Avg. experience" is the average number of years since medical school graduation for the private practitioners in each district. Doctors not in private practice in the *AMD* (1909) and *AMD* (1940) samples were excluded, including interns and residents. "Specialization of PMPs" is the percentage of the total private practices in the district limited to a particular specialty, and the city rate is higher than reported elsewhere in this book because interns and residents are excluded.

practices despite having had less than 6 percent of its population. The share of doctor's offices located downtown nearly equaled the share located in Northwest Philadelphia, even though that district had ten times the population of the downtown and many growing suburbs (see map 9; tables 15 and 16).

The centralization of doctor's offices in Philadelphia became both possible and desirable for doctors for many of the same reasons as those identified for other cities in this period, such as San Francisco.[41] Center City doctors could recruit patients from throughout the region, as by 1940 the downtown had become even more accessible to the entire metropolitan area (including Camden, New Jersey, across the Delaware River) by automobile and by an extensive mass transit system that included buses, trolleys, subway and elevated trains, and commuter and regional trains.[42] As in other major cities, Philadelphians also made early use of new telephone networks, and it was common for doctors to include telephone connections on their business cards by the time of the first world war.[43] With the advent of telephony, doctors could locate centrally and still be reached in an instant for home visits and consultations, and colleagues throughout the city could more easily refer patients to centrally located doctors. The doctor's telephone became so fundamental to private practice, especially in central offices, that medical editorialists sung its praises and discussed the business etiquette of its use.[44]

Like other cities, downtown Philadelphia had also developed a vibrant real estate market for professional office buildings by 1920.[45] This market included buildings designed specifically for doctor's offices. For example, ads promising new buildings "devoted exclusively to offices for physicians" or "dedicated to the medical and dental professions" appeared in nearly every issue of the *Weekly Roster* from the late 1910s onward.[46] Rental prices for office suites in one of the first office buildings—the Medical Arts Building at Sixteenth and Walnut Streets (ward 8)—ranged from $500 to $1,500 per year in 1917, and prices in the overall medical office building market appear to have held in this range until the Great Depression.[47] But was the new supply of such buildings supported by demand? Was it even possible for the average doctor to afford these prices? As measured by a 1929 survey, the median gross income of Philadelphia doctors in private practice was $7,083, of which they spent, on average, $779 for office expenses and $2,833 for all expenses.[48] Thus the rental of a (low-end) downtown office was affordable to roughly half of Philadelphia doctors by 1929, a necessary condition for the sustained centralization of private practices.

In addition to factors that made centralization possible, such as better transportation, telephone networks, and a growing supply of medical offices, several factors made centralization *desirable*. First, new downtown offices better accommodated trends in private practice: technology-driven diagnosis, group practice, and specialization. With the growing technological complexity of diagnosis that followed in the wake of the "laboratory revolution" in medicine, doctors eventually needed on-site equipment to perform routine diagnoses, and real estate developers designed medical office suites with these needs in mind. A 1925 advertisement for the new Central Medial Building (1737 Chestnut Street in ward 9) lured doctors by noting that "this building offers you every convenience for the most effective practice of your profession," including "a gas line [that] feeds every office for laboratory work."[49] The Central Medical Building also housed commercial medical service firms, such as private laboratories like the Baker Biochemical Laboratories, which provided fee-for-service analyses of laboratory samples that included "biochemical research, blood chemistry, blood counts, serology, basal metabolism, food analyses, urinalysis, and smears."[50] Philadelphia doctors also coveted the spacious suites in new downtown office buildings. Larger offices satisfied the increased needs of group practices, which, as we have seen, had become more common by 1940.[51]

Downtown offices conferred another advantage overlooked by other studies of private practice location—namely the capacity to capture the business of a more lucrative client, the middle-class commuter.[52] Real estate advertisements for downtown offices celebrated their convenience to these potential customers. For example, the rendition of the Central Medical Building included a crowded street-level view that featured the heavy traffic of pedestrians, cars, and trolleys (figure 12). The lobby view depicted the well-heeled of Philadelphia society strolling to their doctor's offices along polished marble floors and beside handsome bronze railings (figure 13). Should the message of these two images have been lost on a dull reader of *The Weekly Roster*, the point was highlighted later in the five-page advertisement:

Why You Should Select the Central Medical Building

This building has an ideal location in the heart of the city, within a few minutes' walk of the railroad stations, the hotels and the central residential districts. Its main entrance is on the city's best street and its broadest frontage is on a select cross thorofare [sic]. The medical specialist who selects this location will add to his prestige, however notable it may be. His practice will not then be restricted to a single neighborhood. The entire city passes his door. He will work in an atmosphere that will be congenial, that will benefit his professional standing. Every opportunity of becoming better known and enhancing his reputation will be his. This

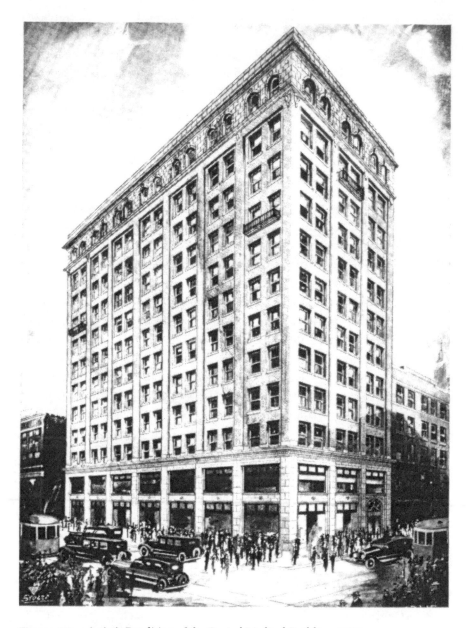

Figure 12. Artist's Rendition of the Central Medical Building, 1925

Source: "Central Medical Building," *WR* 20 (May 16, 1925): 25.

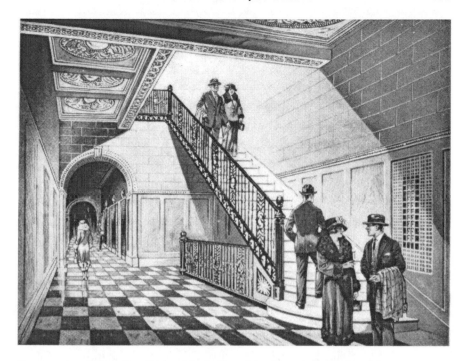

Figure 13. Artist's Rendition of the Lobby of the Central Medical Building, 1925
Source: "Central Medical Building," *WR* 20 (May 16, 1925): 27.

building offers a splendid opportunity to every professional practitioner
to broaden his work. It will be of real assistance in enabling him to find
his proper place in the professional and social life of the city.[53]

For most readers, though, the modern amenities and middle-class appeal were
obvious.

But the symbolic value of a downtown office mattered just as much. Early
twentieth-century bourgeois Philadelphians viewed suburbanization as a sign
of progress towards a rational and efficiently organized city in which residence,
work, commerce, and recreation were organized into discrete spaces.[54] Doctors with social aspirations could project a *public* image of success and status
attained simply by having a suburban home and a Center City office.[55] This
rhetorical link appeared in a 1917 advertisement for the Medical Arts Building:
"Tradition dies hard, but the instinct of self-preservation is driving doctors into
central buildings. The progressive physician realizes the necessity of divorcing
his practice from his home. Here is an opportunity to live in the suburbs and
get some enjoyment out of life. You will come to it eventually—why not now?
Offices are going fast."[56]

Doctors who located in the Medical Arts Building and other downtown offices also projected a particular *professional* image: that of a modern doctor who had achieved a certain level of success and status in private practice. At a time when numerous editorials heralded the demise of the "old-time doctor," or the GP who worked out of the home and made house calls, it became important for many Philadelphia doctors to appear modern. Although some editorialists lamented the disappearance of the old-time doctor as a sign of overspecialization or as evidence of over-reliance on knowledge gained at the laboratory bench rather than at the bedside, most cheered this trend as the inevitable march of medical progress.[57] In either case, being au courant had cultural purchase in the urban medical marketplace, and the location of a home or office was an integral part of crafting a modern professional image. For example, the advertisement for the Medical Arts Building targeted the "progressive physician" who appreciated the sensibility of "divorcing his practice from his home," the implied foil being the antiquated doctor for whom "tradition dies hard."[58]

This quest for a modern professional image also explains the appeal of early automobiles for wealthy city doctors. Early automobiles were not particularly useful for practicing medicine in a city because urban doctors relied more on income from seeing many patients in an office than on seeing fewer patients in house calls. After all, the whole purpose of renting an expensive downtown office was to have patients come to the doctor, not the other way around. Instead of facilitating patient care, early automobiles merely offered wealthy urban doctors another way to distinguish themselves from old-fashioned doctors, who still drove the proverbial horse and buggy.[59] Owning an automobile, like renting a downtown office or commuting to work from the suburbs, connoted professional success and status if only by virtue of the conspicuous wealth needed to purchase and maintain a car. The status of automobile ownership was not lost on the members of the Physicians' Motor Club in Philadelphia, which organized frequent weekend joyrides and countryside picnics. As the founders explained to potential members, the primary advantage of club membership was "the privilege of association with the better and most prosperous physicians of Philadelphia and vicinity."[60]

Doctors who located in expensive downtown offices enjoyed a luxury affordable to only half of their colleagues. In addition, downtown doctors had measurably higher professional status: three-quarters of the fellows of the elite College of Physicians of Philadelphia had downtown offices—a downtown rental rate twice that of all Philadelphia doctors combined.[61] Similarly, downtown offices were essentially out of reach for African American and immigrant doctors, who remained professionally and geographically marginalized in this period (see table 7). Given the social and professional composition of downtown officeholders, the very act of locating in the exclusive Center City signaled professional success—particularly for specialists, as we shall see. In a business where one's public and professional image provided the only legitimate forms of advertisement, renting a downtown office had great symbolic value.

The majority of doctors who could not afford a prime central office were nevertheless advised to find a "good" location elsewhere, in particular by avoiding "neighborhoods unable to support a physician."[62] The location behavior of Philadelphia doctors in 1940 indicates that they heeded such business advice: city wards with above-average rent had more than twice the practice concentration of wards with below-average rent (table 17). That doctors preferred wealthy over poor residential locations was not new.

In 1909–1910, immigrants were some of the poorest Philadelphians, and they tended to be segregated in the handful of city wards with cheap housing and a ready supply of unskilled or semiskilled jobs. It was therefore quite easy for doctors to avoid poverty-stricken immigrant ghettoes: the wards with high immigrant residency rates had one-third the concentration of private practices found in wards with low immigrant residency rates (table 17). In 1940, however, the

Table 17. The Changing Distribution of Private Medical Practices in Relation to the Nativity, Race, and Affluence of Residents in Philadelphia, 1909–1910 to 1940

	PMP/100K	
	1909–1910	*1940*
Wards with high immigrant residency rates	91.0	179.4
Wards with low immigrant residency rates	276.2	177.8
Wards with high African American residency rates	389.9	190.1
Wards with low African American residency rates	141.0	173.1
Wards with average monthly rent above median	N/A	280.5
Wards with average monthly rent below median	N/A	107.6
All city wards	226.3	178.6

Sources: See table 13 and maps 5 and 10. *AMD* (1909) and *AMD* (1940) samples. Wards with residency rates above the city rate were defined as "high," and wards with residency rates below the city rate were classified as "low." Average monthly rent figures are per dwelling. Data on average monthly rent per dwelling were not collected in the 1910 census. "PMP/100K" is the number of private medical practices per 100,000 residents in these wards. See appendix for details.

geography of private practice did not correspond as closely with immigrant resi-dency patterns, even though doctors still preferred wealthy over poor residential locations (table 17). As foreign-born whites became more integrated socially and economically in the city (see map 6, tables 13 and 15), it was no longer possible for doctors to avoid foreign-born white residents as had been the case earlier in the century, even had most doctors so desired. Moreover, as foreign-born whites gained social acceptance and enjoyed greater prosperity, doctors no longer viewed locations near immigrant neighborhoods as bad for business.

The spatial relationship between African American residency and doctor's offices was more complex in the early twentieth century. Like most working-class Philadelphians, African Americans tended to live close to work, which meant living near the wealthy neighborhoods that supplied domestic ser-vice and manual labor jobs. Because doctors were eager to locate in wealthy neighborhoods, there was a false positive association between wards with high African American residency rates and wards with high concentrations of private practices in 1909–1910, and the same was true in 1940 (table 17). African Americans may have had more diverse occupations by mid-century, but African American men still depended upon lower-status jobs, especially as janitors and low-wage workers, and African American women still worked pre-dominantly in domestic service.[63] Although a middle-class African American community had developed in Philadelphia by 1940, this social and occupa-tional group was relatively small, and most African American neighborhoods remained quite poor (see table 13), especially those where recent migrants from the South had settled.[64] Given this occupational profile, many African Ameri-cans still lived on the outskirts of Center City because it had the best supply of jobs in the many office buildings of the CBD and in the wealthy homes near Rittenhouse Square.

Proximity to downtown doctor's offices did not mean, however, that Afri-can Americans could afford the many choices for private medical care avail-able nearby. Even when correcting for the lower occupational status of African Americans by comparison to whites, African American families still earned less and spent less on medical care. One Philadelphia-based study of wage earners and low salary clerical workers in 1933–1935 found that African American households only earned an average of $1,203 per year and spent an average of only $32.17 on medical care, whereas white households had average incomes of $1,601 and spent an average of $51.66 on medical care. Although the two groups spent an equal amount on care from GPs, white families were able to afford far more on care from specialists.[65] Racial prejudice and the legacy of slavery and sharecropping resulted in persistent economic hardship, social immobility, and poor health for African Americans in Philadelphia, even for those living in the shadows of downtown medical office buildings.

In addition to residential clusters on the outskirts of Center City, the newest areas of African American settlement in the city were found in the inner northwestern and inner western districts, both of which had been affluent streetcar suburbs earlier in the century. As African Americans began to settle in these areas, white middle-class residents began to leave for more remote suburbs, and doctors followed suit.[66] For example, as the number of African American residents increased nearly fivefold in the forty-seventh ward, the center of African American settlement in North Philadelphia, the number of white residents declined by half, as did the number of doctor's offices (see table 7).[67] Because suburban white flight was still under way in 1940, some African American neighborhoods like the forty-seventh ward still had above-average concentrations of private practices (see map 10), but only because a number of white doctors in these areas had not yet relocated their offices. Thus the even distribution of private practices among wards with high and low African American residency rates in 1940 should not be interpreted as evidence that the white majority of Philadelphia doctors solicited or even welcomed African American clientele. On the contrary, it was common for white doctors to harbor contemporary racial and class prejudices and therefore to avoid practicing medicine amid the poverty that disproportionately affected African American neighborhoods at this time. Only African American doctors were on the increase in places like the forty-seventh ward, which had once been one of the most desirable office locations in Philadelphia (see map 5).[68]

As judged by their location behavior, doctors were keenly aware of shifting patterns of residential wealth in Philadelphia. Not only did they tend to practice in the wealthiest wards of the city (see table 17), many also followed the middle class to the fastest growing or the wealthiest suburbs (map 11). For doctors unable to afford "convenient offices in the central section" from which they could "hold onto their clientele," it made good business sense to follow the people and the money to the outer suburbs.[69] Classified advertisements in *The Weekly Roster* commonly referred to an "unusual opportunity in fast growing northeast community" or appealed to doctors "wishing to locate in fast growing N.E. section."[70] As George Wolf explained in *The Physician's Business* (1938), "Naturally, with the development of rapid means of transportation and good roads, the suburban sections of large cities have grown and so have become increasingly popular for medical practice."[71] Indeed, Philadelphia wards that gained population from 1910 to 1940 gained a total of 210 private practices over the same period, while the wards that lost population actually *lost* 265 practices altogether.[72] Philadelphia doctors followed the money as well: wards with above median rent in 1940 had gained a total of 240 private practices since 1909, while wards with below median rent had *lost* 295 practices altogether (see table 14); similarly, wards that gained private practices after 1909 had higher average rent in 1940 than wards that lost (or did not gain) practices over the same period, or $33.22 versus $29.08 (see table 13). Contemporary observers, such as the aforementioned James Bossard, noticed the appeal of suburban offices to doctors.[73] Although some doctors denied the financial incentives behind the uneven distribution of private practices, their location behavior tells a different story.

The New Suburban Market Niche for Private Practice

As we have seen, most Philadelphia doctors followed normative location advice in 1940, much as they had earlier in the century. Some doctors nevertheless adapted to locations that did not conform to the received wisdom of the day; otherwise there would have been no practices at all in the poorest neighborhoods. To a large degree, whether by choice or by lack of opportunity, immigrant and African American doctors continued to locate their offices in some of the poorest neighborhoods in the city (see map 8 and table 7). In other words, social background still distinguished doctors in different corners of the medical marketplace. But evidence demonstrates that specialization and experience also distinguished doctors who located in different market niches for private medical practice. Two of these niches—the downtown district and South Philadelphia—retained many of their respective market characteristics from earlier in the century, and the same kinds of doctors could be found in both areas. Historians have ignored, however, the niche that developed last in the twentieth century: the suburbs. By focusing on the suburbs, which attracted an altogether different kind of doctor, a more dynamic and previously unrecognized picture of the changing urban marketplace emerges.

    The downtown district still functioned primarily as a niche for specialists, particularly "full specialists," or doctors who had limited their practices to a particular medical or surgical specialty such as obstetrics and gynecology. With two-thirds of downtown private practices having been fully specialized in 1940, the district had the highest specialization rate in the city and three times the rate of any other district. Moreover, the downtown district retained its majority share of the fully specialized practices in the city, or 64 percent,

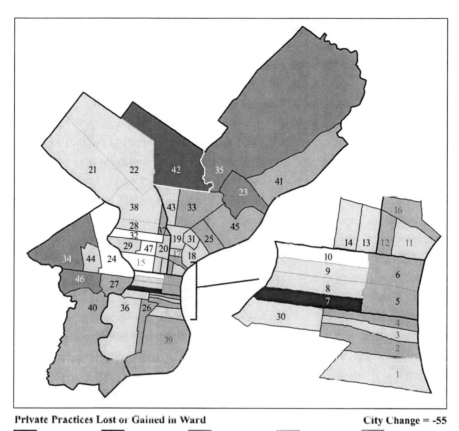

Private Practices Lost or Gained in Ward　　　　　　　　　**City Change = -55**

| N | < -50 | N | -50 to 0 | N | +1 to 50 | N | +50 to 100 | N | > +100 |

Map 11.　The Emerging Suburban Niche for Private Practice in Philadelphia, 1909–1940

Sources: See table 13 and maps 5 and 10. *AMD* (1909) and *AMD* (1940) samples. "Practices Gained or Lost in Ward" refers to the number of private medical practices (PMPs). Wards 3, 11, and 43 had no net change in the number of PMPs.

which was well above its share of all private practices combined, or 31 percent (see table 16).

Professional as well as economic factors explain why full specialists flocked to the downtown district. Full specialists depended upon business from referrals and consultations. Because of its centrality and accessibility, the downtown niche provided an ideal location for the full specialist to treat patients who had been referred from throughout the metropolitan area and to consult with other doctors who solicited diagnostic and therapeutic advice from the specialist. Full specialists also depended upon part-time teaching and clinical positions in hospitals for career development and advancement. Although the downtown district no longer possessed the greatest share of the city's hospitals, it still had the highest concentration of hospitals per area or population (see table 16), including many of the largest and most reputable hospitals, such as Jefferson Medical College Hospital, Hahnemann Hospital, and Pennsylvania Hospital. In addition, the new hospital complex around the University of Pennsylvania School of Medicine in West Philadelphia was but a short distance away by car, bus, trolley, or elevated subway. By locating their offices near downtown medical institutions, full specialists cut the time (and money) lost in transit between various worksites: from private practice in an office, to lectures at a medical school, to clinical or surgical staff duties at a hospital or clinic. Because the downtown functioned as the center of a vast metropolitan referral network, full specialists in downtown offices were unaffected by close proximity to other specialists, as there were more than enough patients referred to downtown specialists from GPs in the metropolitan area. On the other hand, GPs were very sensitive to professional overcrowding because they still depended upon unscheduled walk-by business and upon business cultivated in the immediate neighborhood, at least at first. As such, the sparsely populated and professionally overcrowded downtown district held more limited appeal. The downtown district also attracted the middle-class clientele who could afford specialty care. Because the central business district in downtown Philadelphia remained the primary destination for work, recreation, shopping, and entertainment for the middle class in 1940, specialists found it an ideal location to provide medical services for their target customer. Finally, and of most significance, because the average gross income of full specialists in Philadelphia doubled that of GPs and far exceeded that of partial specialists, full specialists were best able to afford the higher rent of the larger, more modern, and more prestigious downtown offices.[74]

Besides specialists, the downtown market niche also continued to select for experienced doctors in 1940 (see table 16). In part, the greater experience of downtown doctors (25.2 years on average) merely reflected the association between experience and specialization, but professional and economic factors also made it especially difficult for young doctors to succeed there. They first needed to build up collegial and institutional networks before relocating to a downtown office where income depended upon referrals and consultations rather than upon unscheduled walk-by business in a sea of office buildings and placards. Experienced doctors were more likely to have established these networks. Downtown doctors also needed a good reputation from satisfied patients or from impressed colleagues in order to attract clientele, who would have been disinclined to pay downtown prices for private medical care from an unknown doctor. Finally, young doctors earned less income, on average, than experienced doctors, and typically could not afford the expense of renting a prestigious downtown office.[75] Thus for most young doctors, it would have been premature, even foolhardy, to rent a downtown office immediately following internship and licensure. Young doctors who aspired to work downtown usually had to start elsewhere.

In stark contrast to the prestigious specialty market in downtown Philadelphia, very few doctors were interested in opening private practices in South Philadelphia: the district had the lowest concentration of practices in the city, or less than 1 practice per thousand residents (see table 16). Not only was the district neither centrally located nor easily accessible, it also had the poorest residents in the city, with average rent per dwelling at $24.04 per month, or $7.21 less than the citywide average (see table 15). Although gone were the days of vast immigrant ghettoes in South Philadelphia, the area still had some neighborhoods like South Street, which had lingering ethnic stigma, even if a less coherent ethnic self-identity. Of the few doctors who remained in the second and third wards, for example, over half were immigrants and another third were second-generation immigrants (see table 7). There were, however, growing African American ghettoes in South Philadelphia: the thirtieth ward, for example, had the highest rate of African American residency in the city, at more than 80 percent, and the ward, like the rest of the district, was also quite poor, with average rent at $24.78 (see maps 7 and 8). Doctors avoided the thirtieth ward, which had only 1 practice per 1,380 residents (see map 10).[76] In a place like the thirtieth ward, contemporary class and racial prejudices contributed to the doctor shortage. For example, young interns commonly dismissed all of South Philadelphia as nothing more than "slums" populated by "the scum of the city."[77] Even if some doctors harbored no prejudices against South Philadelphia, most believed they could make more money elsewhere and therefore avoided the district as a matter of business.

Besides a handful of immigrant and African American doctors, there were two kinds of doctors willing to open practices in the less crowded marketplace of South Philadelphia—young doctors and GPs. South Philadelphia had the youngest doctors in the city, on average, and more than three in four doctors in the district were GPs (see table 16). The lower overhead for office space in South Philadelphia appealed to some young doctors, who needed time to build a practice slowly without being bankrupted by fixed costs. Advertisements for the rental of office space or for the sale of a practice in South Philadelphia often promised a "rare opportunity for a young doctor" or an "ideal place for young man just starting," and typically featured "moderate rent to responsible tenant."[78] Lower overhead compensated for the lower fees earned in the poverty-stricken district, as did higher patient volume due to the minimal competition from other doctors or from medical institutions (see table 16). For example, as Dr. Lee Winston Silver noted of her first practice after finishing her residency in the late 1930s, "I enjoyed a colorful pediatric practice in South Philadelphia." Of her income from her practice at 1321 South Sixth Street (ward 1), she later recalled, "Fees were small but the large number of patients helped."[79] Finally, young doctors and GPs could further cut overhead in South Philadelphia by combining home and office—an arrangement that was impossible and undesirable for most downtown doctors, given the expensive real estate market in the CBD and the status gained by separating home and office. In contrast, advertisements for "physician's office and residence" in South Philadelphia were common, which suggests that older business models for private practice prevailed there.[80]

Other than the distinct market niches in downtown and South Philadelphia, the suburbs comprised the newest niche for private medical practice in 1940: the outer wards of the west, northwest, and northeast districts had the largest gains from 1909 to 1940 (see table 16 and map 11). The population growth and affluence of the suburbs appealed to many Philadelphia doctors, especially white doctors leaving inner-city neighborhoods like the forty-seventh ward. For example, in the suburbs of Germantown, Mount Airy, and Chestnut Hill (ward 22), only 4.9 and 2.4 percent of doctors were immigrants or African Americans, respectively (see table 7). But the typical suburban doctor differed in other ways from those who practiced downtown or in South Philadelphia: the suburbs attracted doctors with intermediate experience, and suburban doctors had only modest specialization rates (see table 16). When it came to *partial* specialism, though, the suburbs had the highest rates in the city: three-quarters of all partial (or part-time) specialists could be found in the suburbs (see table 16).

The intermediate levels of experience and specialization in the new suburban niche can be explained by the unique professional and economic factors that created market conditions favorable to a wide range of doctors. Young doctors and GPs could economize by combining home and office in the more residential sections of the suburbs, much as they did in the working-class district of South Philadelphia. Classified ads, such as one 1937 listing for a "suburban office and home ideally combined," indicate that this arrangement appealed to many suburban doctors.[81] Newly built homes in the suburbs were also larger and better suited for combining home and office than the cramped, outdated dwellings of South Philadelphia, which may explain the continued appeal of this arrangement. For example, the above ad for a suburban home/ office featured a "modern, newly painted" home with a "double garage" in "desirable surroundings," while still boasting "waiting, consultation, and treatment rooms," and a "separate entrance and exit" for patients.[82] In addition, the relatively low concentration of private practices in suburbs, particularly in residential neighborhoods, attracted many young doctors and GPs who could not compete in the crowded, referral- and consultation-based market downtown.

The suburbs also appealed to specialists and to more experienced doctors who were drawn not to residential areas but rather to business districts that were beginning to form in the suburbs.[83] Even if suburban business districts were relatively small, they nonetheless provided certain goods and services to local residents and therefore promoted commerce of all kinds, including private medical practice. For example, in 1935, the business district in Germantown (the southernmost portion of ward 22, plus nearby sections of wards 38, 42, and 43) had 358 stores, and ranked as the second largest business district outside Center City, which had 2,715 stores.[84] Small suburban business districts like the one in Germantown were typically located in or near important transportation nodes, and thus had the accessibility that specialists and more experienced doctors found important for referrals and consultations. Some suburban business districts even began to develop professional office buildings, such as the Germantown Professional Building (located one block off the main traffic artery of Germantown Avenue), where specialists and more experienced doctors could rent a separate office from their home, not unlike their Center City counterparts.[85] The doctors in suburban business districts further benefited from their proximity to the residences of the affluent clientele they hoped to cultivate. The hybrid market features of the suburbs made it ideal for those beginning to specialize in Philadelphia's medical marketplace.

As in 1909–1910, many Philadelphia doctors relocated one or more times in mid- to late career as circumstances warranted and income permitted. In addition, a few doctors maintained a general practice in a first location while opening a second office in a different location, typically one better suited for specialty practice. Although advice literature still cautioned young doctors about premature relocation and against opening too many "branch offices," it was common to change locations once a doctor had become established and could count on retaining loyal clients during the move.[86] Mid-career specialization was the most common motivation for relocation. After becoming established and deciding to specialize, doctors in mid-career had attained the income needed to rent a central and accessible office and had cultivated the kind of practice and networks that both demanded and benefited from such an office location. Phrases such as "present owner going to specialize" or "reason for selling—specializing" appeared in many classified ads for combined home and office space.[87]

Besides seeking new accommodations and office space, doctors who relocated in mid-career often changed market niches altogether: young doctors in South Philadelphia left the district once they could afford to practice in a wealthier residential neighborhood; doctors who became partial specialists began to think about renting a more central office location, perhaps separate from the home; and doctors who fully specialized their practices began to think about renting the most central and accessible office space they could afford, ideally an office in Center City. But as the following example illustrates, mid-career transitions did not necessarily lead doctors to relocate to Center City, as had been the case in the early century. Instead, the suburbs had become a viable alternative by mid-century.

After graduating from Hahnemann Medical College in 1928 and completing his internship and state board examinations in 1929, Dr. Carl C. Fischer developed an interest in pediatrics that ultimately led him to become a board-certified, full specialist in pediatrics by 1940. In the intervening years, Dr. Fischer underwent a series of moves. As mentioned in chapter 4, he secured his first opportunity for private practice through family connections, settling for a preceptorship in the office of Dr. C. S. Raue. At the time, Dr. Raue was an eminent pediatrician in Philadelphia who had offices at 1530 Locust Street (ward 8), near fashionable Rittenhouse Square in Center City. As Dr. Fischer explained, Dr. Raue, "like most leading [Philadelphia] specialists at that time, had his office in center city."[88] In exchange for a small salary, Dr. Fischer assisted Dr. Raue during the morning office hours at the Locust Street office, where he helped examine patients, took patient histories, performed routine laboratory analyses, and discussed patient cases with Dr. Raue. On occasion, at Dr. Raue's behest, Dr. Fischer would make house calls to patients. Several afternoons a week, Dr. Fischer also worked in a nearby pediatric outpatient department, which he regarded as "a rare privilege and for which no compensation was either expected or given."[89]

It was not uncommon for recent medical licentiates to assist the practice of older doctors, and Dr. Fischer intended to continue in this capacity for two years, as had his predecessor, Dr. J. H. Reading Jr. In 1931, however, Dr. Fischer decided to leave the Center City practice of Dr. Raue and to establish his own pediatric practice in the suburb of Germantown. He explained, "The trend away from center city to the suburbs was rapidly increasing. More and more families were seeking pediatricians in their home neighborhoods, and central city practices declined. After about a year and a half or so it became apparent that I was no longer truly needed in Dr. Raue's private office, and that it was time for me to set out on my own. I had become engaged in 1930 and married in 1931 (March 7), and had settled shortly thereafter in a semi-detached home on Glen Echo Road, Mount Airy. Therefore an office location in the Germantown area seemed logical."[90] Starting a first practice meant finding a good location, and as his unpublished memoirs reveal, Dr. Fischer considered the new opportunities in the changing medical marketplace at that time. For young pediatricians, relocating to the suburbs made good sense not only because of the aforementioned market benefits of the suburbs for young specialists but because the suburbs had young families with children.[91]

In 1931, Dr. Fischer found office space to share in the Germantown Professional Building, which was located at Greene Lane and Coulter Street and was a short commute from his home in Mount Airy. For the first several months, Dr. Fischer remembered that he "spent many an afternoon in [his] office eagerly awaiting his practice to grow."[92] In the meantime, he established collegial relations with other eminent pediatricians who had offices in the same building, such as Dr. J. J. Stokes Jr., who later became a professor of pediatrics at the University of Pennsylvania and physician-in-chief of the renowned Children's Hospital of Philadelphia.[93] Eventually, Dr. Fischer's practice grew, and "in response to local demand," he even opened a branch office near his family's new home in the suburb of Bala Cynwyd in Montgomery County, a short drive across the Schuylkill River from his Germantown office. As his practice expanded, Dr. Fischer first took on a pediatric resident as an assistant; he later added two partners in what had become a small group practice by 1941. By that point, Dr. Fischer had become fully established, and he began to enjoy his private practice a bit more. In particular, he liked that group practice enabled him and his partners "to provide continuous service to our patients and still have occasional nights and weekends to ourselves and our families. Thus ended the long period of 60-hour weeks with little or no relief, found in solo practice."[94]

Dr. Fischer's decision calculus for leaving downtown for suburban practice combined personal goals (such as wanting to get married, buy a house, and start a family) with professional goals (such as wanting independence and a private practice). To achieve these goals, Dr. Fischer made explicit and calculated assessments of market opportunities for private pediatric practice that led him to the suburbs. There he stayed for the rest of his career, until he left private practice in 1958 for salaried position as the director of medical services at Girard College (ward 47). Dr. Fischer's career illustrates the new appeal of the suburbs for many doctors at mid-century. The suburbs formed a distinct niche from downtown and South Philadelphia, with each of these niches selecting for different kinds of doctors. Thus, in 1940, private practice continued to be divided into different strata of doctors on the basis of specialization, experience, and social background. Each stratum had distinct career paths, distinct business practices, and, as I have argued here, distinct location behaviors in the urban medical marketplace.

Mandatory Internships and the Selection of an Office Location

From an analytical perspective, the different niches for private medical practice that were emerging at the turn of the century had become more pronounced by mid-century. But these niches were more than an interesting pattern identified from historical hindsight; contemporary doctors were also keenly aware of them and had opinions about the kinds of doctors and the types of private practices that were best adapted to different parts of the city. Even though contemporary doctors may have understood these market niches in different terms from historians, contemporary doctors both cultivated and used their understanding of the city, however inaccurate, incomplete, or prejudiced it may have been, to guide their career paths and business decisions. In this respect, then, mid-century doctors were no different from their forbears, who had also taken an interest in the social geography of the city when considering the important question of where to locate a practice.

But the workplace in which young doctors first developed their understanding of the urban medical marketplace had changed drastically from the early twentieth century, moving from the office to the hospital. At the beginning of the twentieth century, the majority of doctors entered private practice directly from medical school, including many doctors who had specialty aspirations. This career path began to change in 1914, when Pennsylvania became the first state to require one year of hospital internship for licensure; by 1940, the hospital internship year had become universally required across America (see figure 1). At the same time, medical reformers succeeded in placing the hospital at the center of both undergraduate and graduate medical education. Hospital instruction, in other words, had become the training ground for all young doctors, regardless of their career or business plans. Under these new circumstances, young doctors first practiced medicine as interns, which meant that the first postgraduate, professional exposure of young doctors to the social geography of cities no longer came in a neighborhood office with a newly hung shingle but rather in the confines of an urban hospital ward while on a rotating internship. This significant structural change begs the question of whether and to what extent the advent of the hospital internship changed the lens through which young doctors first viewed the city and their own place in the urban medical marketplace. Did young hospital interns reach different conclusions about the urban medical marketplace than had young doctors in private practice at the turn of the century?

Historians have debated whether the rise of "hospital medicine" in late eighteenth-century Europe transformed medical knowledge and doctor-patient relations thereafter.[95] This question does not pertain to America until much later, as very few hospitals existed in the United States before the Civil War and as the majority of doctors never undertook internship until the first world war.[96] Although some of the epistemic priorities of hospital medicine and the professional worldview it inspired no doubt diffused outward from large American cities and downward from hospital-trained elites by the late nineteenth century, the process was slow and uneven.[97] I would suggest that discussion of "hospital medicine" and its diffusion should refocus on where and when hospital internships became universal, as mandatory rather than voluntary internships had greater potential to inculcate young doctors with these professional values and bedside manners. We might begin by determining whether the advent of the universal internship in early twentieth-century America fundamentally changed how urban doctors developed their views of the social geography of the city and the opportunities available in the medical marketplace. These questions defy quantification, so I offer the following evidence of how one young doctor crafted his self-image as a modern physician during his internship year, a self-image molded by new patterns in medical careers, business practices, and office locations in the 1930s.

After earning his M.D. from the University of Minnesota in 1936, Dr. Harold Scheie came to Philadelphia for what became five years of graduate medical education at the University of Pennsylvania Hospital, by the end of which he had established himself as a full specialist. Besides providing important insight into the factors that led him to specialize and into his experiences during his first year as a hospital intern, his second year as the assistant chief medical officer, and his subsequent three years as a resident and budding ophthalmologist, Dr. Scheie's correspondence reveals his developing perception of the city's social geography and what he regarded to be the problems and promises for private practice in various parts of Philadelphia. Of particular interest in the letters are the ways in which Dr. Scheie's early views of patients and place were shaped by the structure of hospital practice.

Several important features distinguished hospital practice as a young intern from private practice as a young doctor earlier in the century: a larger caseload, a wider variety of cases, and geographical isolation from patients. Unlike young private practice doctors earlier in the century who typically had been accustomed to "wait for patients" while they struggled to make ends meet, hospital interns handled a much heavier caseload.[98] To be sure, interns also struggled financially, but they at least had a regular stipend, even if small, and often room and board in the hospital. As young Harold Scheie noted of his arrangement, "I gain weight steadily. . . . This is the first time I have eaten so well and regularly since leaving home. That is my only luxury so I take full advantage of it. They feed us remarkably well. We earn it though for I haven't had a night off for two weeks."[99] Interns generally viewed their meager earnings and hard work as fair trade for the experience that they gained in their challenging year. Scheie expressed this sentiment in no uncertain terms: "My internship is still very satisfactory. We are very well taught and medicine is really practiced right in this hospital. What is more they keep us on our toes. I don't believe I could have chosen or been accepted at a better place."[100] As interns rotated from service to service in the hospital over the course of a year, they gained experience treating a wide range of patients suffering from diseases and injuries of different severity and progression. Obviously, the variety of cases depended on the size and purpose of the hospital; as a large teaching hospital, the University of Pennsylvania Hospital no doubt gave young Dr. Scheie one of the most diverse caseloads available in the United States. By contrast, young doctors earlier in the century were so desperate for patients that they gladly accepted whoever walked into their fledgling practices. Even though private practitioners had treated the occasional emergency patient or rare disease, their typical patients were ambulatory and presented with a limited range of complaints.

The size and diversity of intern caseloads necessarily limited the relationships they could establish with their hospital patients. Whereas the business success of private practice depended upon trust and the careful cultivation of loyal and satisfied patients, hospital practice, especially during an internship, did not place great emphasis on bedside manner. Although interns had other incentives for doing a good job, their contact with patients was often impersonal or short in duration in part because such contact had no immediate business goal in mind.

Indeed, these structural features of hospital internship diminished Dr. Scheie's ability to empathize with his patients. From the very first days, he described how busy he was with his large caseload at the University Hospital. During the first rotation of his internship, he wrote to his parents, with apparent nervous agitation, about his overwhelming schedule:

> My behavior [in not writing more often] is quite shameful but I have been terribly busy. Since arriving at this hospital I haven't even slept. We are all on call 24 hours a day and work like troopers. . . . To show you how busy I am I take care of all the eye patients, X ray patients, and those with skin diseases in addition to taking care of all emergencies every third night and giving all the anesthetics every third night. Last evening I was on and gave anesthetics for two babies, had a baby come in with insect bites, a boy with a broken leg, a lady with a severe headache and one other. You can see I didn't sleep—oh yes a baby came in which had been vomiting for 2 days. Taking care of those kept me interested. Tonite [sic] I have a man who is dying so again I won't sleep.[101]

His large caseload and busy schedule not only made life difficult for Dr. Scheie on a physical level, but they also led him to see his patients more as interesting cases than as people who needed compassion alongside good medical care. For example, he recorded during his first rotation: "Right now my patients keep me interested. I help on all the eye operations. Afterwards must follow them through to recovery. Then on X ray I have all the cancer patients etc. that we treat by X ray and radium. My skin patients are the prize collection. You would hardly know they are human. One is nearly ready to die. . . . How he has lasted till now is miraculous. One thing about this hospital is that we can do anything for our patients no matter how expensive. All that is asked is that we do everything possible."[102] Whereas the financial incentives of private medical practice had forced young doctors to cultivate their bedside manner and to empathize with their patients, hospital interns simply did not have the same practical considerations during their first postgraduate exposure to patients.

The final distinct feature of hospital practice, one that also constrained doctor-patient relations, was the geographical isolation of interns from the city that surrounded the hospital. After several nights on call, interns mostly spent their free time sleeping in their hospital quarters. For example, Harold Scheie left the hospital for the first time only after a month of internship. When he was finally outside of the walls, his two-hour walk took him from the hospital (at Thirty-fourth and Spruce Streets in West Philadelphia—ward 27) to Fairmount

Park, then to the Franklin Museum, and the zoo—the kinds of destinations that a tourist might visit. His first walk was not one that a local West Philadelphian might take on a daily basis, nor was it a route which could have generated a greater appreciation for the social and spatial realities of ordinary city life.[103] In contrast, young doctors at the turn of the century not only got their start in private practice rather than hospital internship, but they often located their offices in the interstices of city neighborhoods, even residing on the same blocks as their patients, at least at first. Their smaller caseload and closer proximity to the neighborhoods of their patients connected them, even if but a little, with the social geography of the city. Young interns at mid-century typically lacked this connection. In a moment of reflection, Dr. Scheie reached this very conclusion: "In this hospital, I seem to be isolated from the world, eating, sleeping, and working in the same building."[104] While this isolation intensified homesickness, it also changed the lens through which Dr. Scheie perceived the social and spatial organization of the city. Specifically, firsthand knowledge of the relationship between patient and place had become abstracted by the hospital internship.

At large teaching hospitals, patients came not only from the surrounding neighborhood but from all over the city, and often from the poorest city wards in search of charity medical care. Young interns therefore treated patients from whom they were isolated socially, economically, and also spatially. This additional geographic isolation further inhibited empathy. The effects of his isolation surfaced when Dr. Scheie described one of his rotations to his parents: "On emergencies I have sewed up more broken open heads and what not than you can imagine. You get to see everything here [in emergencies], mostly niggers. The police brought in a couple of them one night—not married—but they had been having a battle royal. He socked her with his fists a few times—she picked up a club and walloped him over the head cutting it open about 5 inches right down to the skull. She was built like Mrs. Larson but taller. I fixed them both up—from there they both went to jail. They come in drunk, sober, crazy, and what not."[105] For his parents back in a small farming town in North Dakota, this must have been a shocking story indeed, perhaps even one that confirmed their misgivings about "big city" life and their son's safety. For Dr. Scheie, this experience also left an indelible impression at this early stage in his internship, but this impression did little to spark interest into the everyday lives of these charity patients. His snap judgments about his charity patients and his inability to relate to their material circumstances came not only from his latent racism and social class prejudice but from a geographical ignorance of the city bred by his isolation in the hospital. He did not bother to ask about the material and social circumstances that might have led to this and other violent episodes. Nor did Dr. Scheie appreciate that the clinical experience he gained in a large urban teaching hospital depended to a large degree upon the poor health of inner-city residents.

Isolation could breed not only callousness and prejudice in young interns but outright resentment of charity patients, whom interns not infrequently dismissed as unworthy ingrates tolerated only for their value as interesting "clinical material." At the University of Pennsylvania Hospital, Dr. Scheie did get to treat private-ward patients (middle or upper class) in addition to charity patients (poor or working class), an arrangement which he liked because at least then, in his estimation, he could have a few patients "of the better and more appreciative sort."[106] In stark contrast to his disinterest in his poorer patients, Dr. Scheie made an effort to get acquainted with his private-ward patients. In one letter to his parents, he rattled off the distinctions of some of these patients: "One is a doctor, quite famous, from Korea, an island next to Japan. He is here for an unusual operation. Also a professor from the Philippine Islands, and a doctor from Cleveland, a newspaper man from Montgomery, Alabama." He summarized his other hospital patients with telling brevity: "the rest are charity."[107]

For only a brief, three-week period during his internship, Dr. Scheie practiced medicine outside the hospital. During their obstetric rotation at the University Hospital, Dr. Scheie and other interns were sent to the Southeastern Dispensary, which was located at 736 South Tenth Street, on the border of the third and fourth wards in South Philadelphia (see map 1). As discussed earlier, very few doctors located private practices in this part of the city (see map 10), partly because it lacked a commercial or transportation hub but also because of its long-lived notoriety as a poor, overcrowded, insalubrious ghetto. Before beginning his new obstetric rotation, Dr. Scheie dreaded going to the Southeastern Dispensary, mostly because of what he had heard from other doctors. In one update to his parents, he noted, "I am now on my last week of Pediatrics. Next Friday I start on obstetrics on which I stay till January 1st. While on that [rotation] we have some interesting work. For three weeks I will be at a dispensary up town from where we go out to these homes in the slums to deliver babies. The people are mostly Italian and Negroes. And from all that I can gather [from what other interns have said] we see some fine messes."[108] Dr. Scheie later elaborated on his meaning of "fine messes" by characterizing the homes where he would go as "not so much homes as slums, for there I will care for the scum of the city." He was quick to note, however, that the rotation in the Southeastern Dispensary was "a great experience from all that the fellows say."[109] Just as Harold Scheie often valued his charity patients in the hospital only for their

value as "clinical material," it should be no surprise that he valued the delivery of babies in the poorest homes of South Philadelphia only for the experience he gained, not for the moral imperative and ethical value of treating poor
patients for free. Had Dr. Scheie bothered to consult a map, he might also have
learned that the Southeast Dispensary was *crosstown*, and not "up town," from
his internship quarters.

Although geographical isolation hindered the ability to empathize with
charity patients, this isolation did not prevent young interns from developing
their own views about the social organization of the city, however misguided,
judgmental, or prejudiced these views may have been. In the social and spatial
logic of Dr. Scheie and like-minded pre-specialist interns, the city was a collection of discrete market niches with varying degrees of career and business
utility: the wealthiest or most accessible neighborhoods were ripe for locating a
private medical practice after internship, whereas the rest of Philadelphia was
valued only to the extent that it provided "a great experience" during charity
home visits or interesting "clinical material" in the form of charity patients
who sought treatment in free outpatient clinics and charity wards of teaching
hospitals. Along with this calculated view of the city came distinct preferences
(or prejudices) that directed the career decisions of young doctors as they finished their internships—decisions that included whether or not to specialize,
where to locate a private practice in the city, and what kind of patients to seek.

The preferences that Dr. Scheie developed during his internship directed
his later career decisions, professional ambitions, and social aspirations. Given
Dr. Scheie's revulsion to many aspects of city life and to urban medical practice, and given his concerns about the difficulty of starting a specialty practice
in the city, it is no wonder that he daydreamed about ditching his residency
for general practice in a small town. Dr. Scheie ultimately decided to follow
the advice of his mentors and persevered as a budding specialist in the city,
where he believed his future to be "more promising" despite short-term financial sacrifices during his prolonged postgraduate education.[110] His patience,
hard work, and loyalty paid career dividends in the long run, for he became
the junior partner and heir to the private ophthalmology practice of his mentor,
Dr. Adler. By joining this specialty private practice, Dr. Scheie secured a bright
financial future and situated himself in the social and professional niches to
which he aspired and in which he felt the most comfortable. The success of the
practice enabled Dr. Adler and Dr. Scheie to locate their offices in prime space
at 313 South Seventeenth Street (ward 7), only two blocks from the affluent
neighborhood of Rittenhouse Square, close to the heart of the commercial and

transportation hub of Center City and in the most popular niche for private specialty practice (see map 10). As a result of these career and business decisions, Dr. Scheie could afford to live in an upscale bedroom community in West Philadelphia and hire a private cook.[111]

The preferences that Dr. Scheie developed in his internship also found expression in the kind of patients he sought. From early on, when Dr. Scheie treated both private and charity patients in the hospital, he articulated his preference for more affluent patients, a preference that shaped his vision of future practice. As he put it, "Private patients also teach you how to get along with and handle people of the type you will later have. You tend to become high handed with the charity cases alone."[112] Given Dr. Scheie's preference for affluent clientele and his prejudices towards charity patients, especially poor foreign-born whites and African Americans, it is no surprise that he treated charity cases only in his hospital clinic work as a resident. In his private specialty practice, Dr. Scheie treated the patients who could afford Dr. Adler's fees, whom Scheie described as "wealthy Easterners," one of whom paid Dr. Adler $1,000 for an interstate house call to Charleston, South Carolina.[113]

Thus, Dr. Scheie's understanding of the social geography of the city and the preferences he developed as a hospital intern later informed his decisions to specialize, to locate his practice in an elite section of the city, and to cater to affluent patients. These career choices, moreover, only further distanced him from his charity patients—socially, economically, and spatially—as his only exposure to the poorest Philadelphians came during the few hours that he practiced or taught in the eye clinic at University Hospital. Because hospital practice separated patient and place, this formative training was unlikely to create greater familiarity with or sympathy for charity patients. As Dr. Scheie's career progressed, his social identification with Philadelphia's elites strengthened at pace with his professional success. By 1939, Dr. Scheie's social calendar indicates that he had begun to be embraced by the upper echelons of society. After a weekend visit to the Du Pont family on their vast estate outside of Philadelphia, Dr. Scheie defended the lavish lifestyle of his high-society patrons: "all wealthy people aren't snobbish. They [the Du Ponts] have a simply beautiful home, servants, racehorses, and all you usually see in the movies but never experience."[114] Dr. Scheie had come a long way indeed from North Dakota, from the daydreams of a country doctor to those of the modern urban specialist.

From this close reading of one doctor's correspondence, I do not mean to imply that hospital internships completely determined how doctors understood the social geography of the city and developed their preferences in relation to the medical marketplace. Unlike Scheie, some young interns nevertheless became GPs and even practiced medicine in poor neighborhoods throughout their careers. Nor do I wish to suggest that doctors before mandatory hospital internship somehow had more noble aims or greater commitment to social justice when they opened their first private practice, or even that earlier generations had truer or less prejudiced understanding of the social geography of the city. Professional ambition and pecuniary motives restrained humanitarian impulses before as well as after the advent of universal internship. Instead, I merely wish to demonstrate that hospital training added another lens through which doctors viewed the social geography of the city, and which therefore influenced how doctors interpreted their relation to patients, to the medical marketplace, even to modern medicine. The influence of the internship on the career paths and business practices of young doctors, in other words, extended far beyond the supplemental medical and surgical training received inside the hospital. The views of Philadelphia and of the medical marketplace from inside the hospital led many interns, like Dr. Scheie, to avoid general practice in a neighborhood office altogether.

As has been argued, there continued to be distinct patterns to the location behavior of Philadelphia doctors in the 1920s and 1930s. In general, Philadelphia doctors continued to prefer office locations in central and accessible areas or else in affluent suburbs, and practices were therefore unevenly distributed with respect to the population. Philadelphia also had distinct niches for private practice in the medical marketplace: first, in the prestigious and expensive downtown niche, especially in the CBD and around Rittenhouse Square, where specialists and experienced doctors based office practices upon consultations and referrals and sought to attract middle-class clientele; second, in the poverty-stricken and undesired South Philadelphia niche, where some GPs and young doctors were sheltered by the low level of competition and by lower fixed costs; and third, in the hybrid suburban niche, where many kinds of doctors could make a living but where doctors with intermediate levels of experience found it convenient to begin to specialize. These market niches were defined in relation not only to medical institutions but also to larger social and economic change in the city. The changing geography of private medical practice was bound to the changing social geography of Philadelphia: the decline of foreign immigration, the "Great Migration" of African Americans from the South, and the increasing pace of suburbanization all reconfigured market niches for private practice during the interwar years.

Using evidence from advice literature, classified advertisements, doctors' memoirs, and the actual office locations of Philadelphia doctors, I have also argued that individual doctors deliberately cultivated and deployed their own knowledge about opportunities in the medical marketplace when deciding where to locate their private practices, as had their predecessors earlier in the century. The worksite in which doctors first developed their understanding of the social geography of the city and its influence upon niches for private medical practice had changed, however, from the office to the hospital ward. Because the hospital separated patient and place, the city and the doctor, the advent of universal hospital internships changed the environment in which doctors developed their self-image and their roles in the city. It is impossible to quantify the extent to which the hospital internships alienated young doctors socially, economically, and spatially from their patients and from the city outside of the hospital, just as it is impossible to quantify the extent to which such alienation explains the demise of community-based, general medical practice in the interstices of inner-city neighborhoods. What can be argued, however, is that doctors' perceptions of the medical marketplace shaped their location behavior as much as the reality of social and economic change at the ground level.

Conclusion

The Business of Private Medical Practice analyzes the urban origins of one of our nation's most intractable health care access problems: the uneven distribution of doctor's offices, or private medical practices. Unlike early studies of the location of doctor's offices published from the 1920s to the 1940s, which focused on rural-urban divisions at the county, state, and regional level, this book examines distribution problems within American cities, using the example of Philadelphia, Pennsylvania, from 1900 to 1940. Although a spate of *intra*-urban studies were published from the late 1960s through the early 1980s, very few analyzed office locations before mid-century. This oversight matters, for as *The Business of Private Medical Practice* demonstrates, we can trace the beginnings of unevenly distributed private practices to early twentieth-century urban growth. In other words, the hallmark features of the "urban health crisis" identified by health care economists and geographers from the late 1960s through the early 1980s—especially doctor shortages in impoverished inner-city neighborhoods—formed much earlier than previous work has suggested.[1]

There were several objectives in this historical geography of private practice: determining where doctors were *advised* to locate their offices ("normative location advice"), where doctors *actually* located their offices ("location behavior"), and *why* doctors collectively preferred certain locations and avoided others ("location decisions" or "location calculus"). In general, whether in the aphorisms of career guides, in editorials of medical journals, or in lectures to medical students and young doctors, normative location advice remained consistent throughout the early twentieth century. Urban doctors were advised to locate their private practices on busy streets or else near wealthy neighborhoods.

   Doctors conformed their location behavior to this advice. Depending on
the particular city, though, adherence to such advice resulted in different patterns of office location, as cities had distinctive relationships between central
areas, transportation arteries, commercial activity, and residential affluence,
let alone different stages of development and change in these relationships. In
early twentieth-century Philadelphia, doctors clustered in the central business
district (CBD) and in growing middle-class suburbs to the west and north of
Center City. Over time, ever fewer doctors worked in poor inner-city neighborhoods, especially South Philadelphia. Although other historical geographies of
private practice have identified similar trends, *The Business of Private Medical Practice* places the development of a distinct suburban market niche much
earlier in the twentieth century than previously thought. In part, this early suburban niche reflected new patterns of work and housing in Philadelphia and
their influence on the medical marketplace. Unlike the changing distribution of
doctor's offices in other early twentieth-century cities that have been studied,
which exhibited strong centralization (San Francisco and Toronto), decentralization (Brooklyn), or initial centralization followed by rapid decentralization
after mid-century (Bloomington-Normal, Illinois), Philadelphia exhibited contemporaneous centralization and decentralization, yielding doctor shortages in
the inner-city slums that ringed the CBD.[2] This pattern reflected the enduring vitality of the CBD as the heart of middle-class employment, recreation,
and (health care) consumption even though middle-class residential clusters
shifted to the suburban and later metropolitan periphery.

   It should not be surprising that different cities exhibited distinctive patterns of office location. After all, as more recent urban historiography notes,
there was no monolithic or unidirectional urban transformation in the early
twentieth century.[3] The purpose of *intra*-urban analysis of doctor's offices is
to understand how trends in the medical marketplace, and in the geography
of private practice specifically, were linked to broader changes in the social
and spatial order of American cities. Health care services like doctor's offices
became but another unevenly distributed resource alongside quality education,
affordable housing, and gainful employment as cities like Philadelphia became
specialized, postindustrial metropolises by mid-century.[4]

   In order to explain the modern pattern of unevenly distributed doctor's
offices that first emerged in early twentieth-century cities, it is essential to
understand not only how broader urban change (or "ecological factors") shaped
the opportunity structure for private practice but *why* doctors selected certain
office locations over others within the medical marketplace. The first step to
answering this question is to uncover the career and business significance of

private practice. As we have seen, despite the rise of medical institutions, especially hospitals, as sites for career development and income supplementation for American doctors, private practice remained the ultimate goal, even for specialists who had strong institutional ties throughout their careers. In fact, career and business goals were inseparable in private practice, and decisions about whether to undertake an internship or residency, whether to specialize, or whether to seek institutional positions reflected the financial aspirations of doctors in private practice as much or more than their intellectual affinities or technical abilities. Given the significance of private practice, it is not surprising that career and business advice focused to a great degree on the selection of an appropriate and profitable office location.

In addition to knowing the significance of private practice, we must also understand the different interests of doctors in private practice. Like other works that have come to revise the standard historical narrative of professionalization, *The Business of Private Medical Practice* uncovers a divided and rapidly changing profession in which Philadelphia doctors were adopting a variety of new careers paths and business practices in the early twentieth century. Much of the "new" historiography of medical professionalization has identified income or social background as enduring sources of such professional division and conflict.[5] Income and social background also divided Philadelphia doctors, particularly as discrimination restricted the ability of women, African American, and working-class doctors to gain access to graduate medical education, to institutional positions, and thereby to lucrative private practice in medical specialties. In addition, experience and specialization themselves were equally fundamental sources of stratification, as experienced and young doctors had very different career and business interests, as did specialists and GPs. Although doctors reached consensus on broad professional matters such as licensing reform and enforcement, these different interest groups often clashed on business issues, especially with regard to the proper relationship between hospitals, private practices, and the medical marketplace in the early twentieth century.

Upon closer examination of the social and professional lives of an entire community of urban doctors, then, we can begin to understand why doctors selected certain locations and not others for their offices. Different market niches for private practice mapped onto different social and spatial niches in the city. In Philadelphia, many doctors aspired to locate their offices in the CBD, but the niche was best suited to doctors who could afford the high cost of rent and whose business was based upon patient referrals from throughout the metropolitan region. As such, specialists and established doctors flourished downtown. By contrast, doctors generally avoided working-class neighborhoods, like those in South Philadelphia, yet the area proved acceptable to doctors who needed low overhead and a less competitive market. As such, some GPs spent their early years in these densely populated neighborhoods, though many relocated in mid-career. Finally, the "suburban niche" constituted the newest corner of the marketplace. It was a hybrid niche, with some residential locations suited for general practice and some satellite business districts suited for partial specialists. The geography of early twentieth-century private practice therefore highlights the connection between the career, business, and location decisions of individual doctors.

That economic self-interest motivated career, business, and office location decisions is the premise, not the conclusion, of this book. Instead, *The Business of Private Medical Practice* reveals how a constellation of interests yielded the characteristic pattern of office locations that emerged in cities like Philadelphia in the early twentieth century, and that emerged in other cities by mid-century. Professional factors remained relevant, of course, but so too did the changing environment in which doctors practiced. When we look at particular cities such as Philadelphia, not only do we find the obvious link between cities and the medical marketplaces but also how changes in opportunity structures limited the career, business, and location choices available to urban doctors in different professional strata.

Furthermore, because the growth of medical specialties and hospital-based medical care were centered in American cities, the historical processes we think of as "the specialization of American medicine" or "the institutionalization of American medicine" took their particular shape as a result of the career and business imperatives of doctors who practiced medicine in the urban medical marketplace. That is to say, specialization and institutionalization were neither externally produced structural changes in medical practice nor internally generated strategies for acquiring status or legitimacy, but rather the organizational choices of a modern medical workforce that emerged under the influence of market pressures in urban private medical practice.[6] Although professional values discouraged crass commercialism in the conduct of private practice, doctors nonetheless pursued economic self-interest and competitive advantage in the urban marketplace, which yielded the particular maldistribution of private practices that scholars first began to notice in the late 1960s.

The maldistribution of doctor's offices that developed in some early twentieth-century American cities like Philadelphia emerged in other cities by mid-century. In general, among academic and policy circles since the 1960s, there has been rough agreement on two trends since mid-century: urban doctors have been moving from low-income areas to high-income areas, and from inner-city neighborhoods to the suburbs, with the exception of hospital-based (rather than office-based) specialists, who have tended to remain centrally located and near to hospitals.[7] Closer examination of particular cities, though, has identified distinctive patterns of office location that reflect slightly different developments in the social and spatial organization of each city, such as the timing and extent of suburbanization.[8] The uneven distribution of urban private medical practices relative to the population matters because numerous studies have found that a greater distance to the doctor predicts lower patient access to and utilization of health care.[9] Furthermore, hospital outpatient departments and emergency rooms have not filled the void left by inner-city doctors as they retired or relocated. This sad reality inspired the community health center movement in the 1960s and 1970s, though such centers have never secured steady funding to address the health care needs of people living in areas with limited access to doctors.[10]

Although there has been rough agreement on trends in intra-urban location of doctor's offices, scholars and policy analysts have disagreed considerably on the causes of and solutions to unevenly distributed health care services like private practices. On one end of the spectrum, advocates for national health insurance or (in more modern parlance) universal health care have alleged that unevenly distributed health care signals the failure of the free market to address the nation's health care needs.[11] In this school of thought, maldistributed doctor's offices are but one symptom of the for-profit U.S. health care system that has resulted in exorbitant costs and growing ranks of uninsured. In the absence of universal, publicly financed health insurance, the economic self-interest of health care providers, insurance companies, the pharmaceutical industry, and the hospital industry will always lead to inequitably distributed health care goods and services. The only solution is to pass comprehensive health care reform, thereby eliminating some of the economic disincentives to provide primary health care to the poor or to the remotely located. There is some evidence to suggest that this approach works: for example, studies of English industrial practices before and after the National Insurance Act of 1911 have found more evenly distributed primary care doctors after subsidies became available.[12] However, after the establishment of the National Health Service in 1948, many scholars in the 1970s and 1980s still found unevenly distributed doctor's offices, suggesting that government subsidy alone cannot completely eliminate perverse market incentives and location behaviors.[13]

At the other end of the ideological spectrum, advocates for free market solutions to health care problems deny the existence of distribution problems, instead arguing that doctor-to-population ratios are poor measures of health care efficiency by comparison to health care utilization or health maximization. In a classic series of essays published in conjunction with the RAND Corporation in the early 1980s, health policy contrarian Joseph P. Newhouse made exactly these arguments, even asserting that the distribution of specialists was becoming *more* equitable over time as the oversupply of specialists in urban areas began to push specialists from large cities to midsize towns, where demand was rising in response to the decline of rural GPs. Such studies roundly criticized even limited government intervention, claiming that incentives for rural medical practice could never overcome the market forces that shaped the distribution of health care.[14] Furthermore, Newhouse and others alleged that incentives rarely achieved their objectives, as doctors in the National Health Service Corps, for example, typically relocated to cities after fulfilling their contractual obligations to the program.[15] Like-minded English scholars also contended that the failure of the NHS to eliminate the pooling of health care personnel and resources in areas where they were least needed—what a generation termed the "inverse care law"—signaled the failure of nationalized medicine to address problems fundamental to the marketplace.[16] Rather than interfere with the laws of supply and demand, free market enthusiasts advised investment in better transportation and infrastructure, thereby shortening the travel time from rural areas to city doctors and hospitals.[17]

With the repeated failure of national health insurance in Congress, the tactics of American health care reformers shifted to the pursuit of incremental policies after mid-century.[18] Despite the dramatic expansion of the medical welfare state with Medicare and Medicaid in 1965, these programs did little to redistribute health care. Because of restrictive eligibility for Medicaid, only the very poorest could enroll, and many states were slow to fully implement programs. As Medicaid did little to alter the incentive for doctors to maximize profit in a private provider marketplace, and as reimbursements from Medicaid struggled to match reimbursements from private third parties, there was little incentive for doctors to relocate their private practices to rural or poor areas, at least from the perspective of economic self-interest. This was as true for solo practices as it was for the corporate-owned managed care practices that emerged in the 1980s. With the limited redistributive effect of Medicaid, more limited subsidy programs were established to right the perceived wrongs of the market on a case-by-case basis. From the NHSC (established in 1970) to the many experimental programs in the

Patient Protection and Affordable Care Act of 2010, pilot programs to incentivize rural medical practice have been fairly small in scope and have been subjected to continual and highly politicized reauthorization by Congress.

Related to policy debates about whether we have unevenly distributed doctor's offices, let alone what can be done about it, are two more fundamental questions. How many doctors are needed to provide adequate medical care? What is the ideal distribution of doctors? The answers to these questions have also been ideologically charged. Generally speaking, health policy analysts in the 1960s found too few doctors and a looming doctor shortage.[19] In response, the federal government began to subsidize medical education to increase supply. As a result of such programs, between 1965 and 1980, the number of medical schools grew from 88 to 126 and the number of medical graduates doubled, from roughly 7,500 to 15,000 annually. So successful were these programs that health policy analysts in the 1980s began to predict a doctor surplus by the year 2000. As a result, Congress eliminated some subsidies. Finally, since beginning of the twenty-first century, the doctor supply debate has shifted back to predictions of doctor shortages by 2020, especially as demand increases due to the retirement of the baby boom generation.[20] Determining the truth-value of these predictions is not of primary concern here. It is important to note, though, that these debates have informed (or misinformed) contemporaneous discussions of health care distribution.

Generally speaking, calls to subsidize medical education and training assume that increasing the supply of doctors will produce more equitable distribution as doctors leave oversupplied cities for underserved areas.[21] Critics of federal subsidies to increase the supply of doctors rightly note that these programs are expensive and overlook many important causes of rising cost and declining access. Instead, policy should incentivize medical students to enter primary care rather than medical specialties and subspecialties, as specialists tend to cluster in cities and specialty care is one of the drivers of health care cost inflation.[22] Furthermore, critics argue that increasing the supply of doctors artificially increases demand in the medical marketplace, especially in wealthy areas, thereby diminishing any redistributive pressure toward medically underserved areas. Finally, critics rightly note that subsidizing medical education and training is expensive, and the more immediate goal of improving health care access could be achieved more directly by subsidizing public health insurance for the millions of Americans who lack health insurance (who are disproportionately poor and rural).[23] Furthermore, why not subsidize the training of allied health professionals, such as advanced nurse practitioners and physician-assistants, who are quickly becoming more affordable providers of primary care?

Even if consensus could be reached on the ideal supply of doctors, how should these doctors be distributed? Should we expect even distribution of doctors across regions, states, counties, and even cities? Or is there a way to have efficiently clustered medical goods and services while maximizing health care access and outcomes? What should be the measure of equitable and just health care organization? These questions remain hotly debated among health care geographers, economists, and policy analysts.[24]

To some extent, it is beyond the scope of historical scholarship to resolve questions about the ideal supply or distribution of health care goods and services. Instead, it is the duty of historians to call attention to the fact that the structure of our current health care system did not arise by accident nor was it the inevitable, essentialist destiny for the United States. Instead, our current health care system resulted from health care policy choices over the past century, choices that invariably privileged the private sector and individual rights—in private practice as in so many other areas of health care provision—over collective sacrifice to finance universal health care. In the absence of comprehensive health care reform, the peculiar influences of the free market directed the reorganization of our health care system.

Although this author's sympathies lie with the proponents of universal health care, that is the subject of a different book. Instead, this concluding analysis of intra-urban doctor's office locations since mid-century is intended to highlight the following points about the business of private medical practice and specialization. First, the inequitable patterns that emerged in some early twentieth-century cities like Philadelphia spread to other cities and worsened after mid-century. Second, the debate about distribution problems misses the point to a degree. The expensive, unevenly distributed, unequally accessible, highly specialized care that we receive today took its present shape during the urban transformation of the United States in the early twentieth century, when early specialists and hospital-trained doctors forged new career paths, business practices, and office locations in the rapidly changing medical marketplaces of cities. This means that in order to fully address today's health care problems, especially through subsidy for more equitably distributed or accessible health care, policymakers must address more fundamental structural causes of our inefficient system: poverty, discrimination, and economic self-interest all generate or exacerbate health care inequities. Without attention to economic and social injustice in modern urban society, greater subsidy for the purchase of health care can only go so far in solving our present health care crisis.

Appendix

Notes on Sources and Methods

This appendix provides interested readers a detailed account of the sources and methods used in this book to measure changes in the careers and office locations of Philadelphia doctors from 1900 to 1940. At the evidentiary core of this quantitative analysis are samples of Philadelphia doctors listed in the second and sixteenth editions of the *American Medical Directory* compiled by the American Medical Association—hereafter referred to as the *AMD* (1909) and *AMD* (1940) samples. I will explain the samples, their promises and challenges, and how the following were defined and counted: private practitioners; the specialization, experience, and position-holding patterns of doctors; the office addresses of private practices; and hospitals. The majority of these data were collected from the *AMD* (1909) and *AMD* (1940) samples, however, additional sources were used, as noted.

The *AMD* (1909) and *AMD* (1940) Samples

To answer quantitative questions about Philadelphia doctors, quantitative sources must to be used. There are two main quantitative sources for diachronic data on American doctors from 1900 to 1940—the federal census and national or local medical directories. For Philadelphia, the decennial censuses were only useful for data on the total number of "physicians and surgeons" in the city (though not at the ward or census tract level) and for comparative data on the gender, race, and nativity of persons in the city. The census did not further subdivide "physicians and surgeons," and identifying particular "physicians and surgeons" in the manuscript census enumerator sheets proved too laborious, though not altogether impossible for select neighborhoods of interest (see discussion below). In order to answer quantitative questions about the characteristics of individual doctors, one must turn to a combination of national and local medical directories.[1]

In Philadelphia, there were several for-profit local medical directories, the best of which was *The Professional Directory of Doctors and Druggists of Philadelphia, Including Camden and Atlantic City and Eighty Nearby Towns.* Although *The Professional Directory* contained a variety of useful data, including the names and office addresses of Philadelphia doctors, a listing of the Philadelphia medical school faculty, and the most comprehensive listing of hospital staff positions, it lacked data on the specialization of individual doctors. In addition, there was no single local medical directory that spanned the years 1900 to 1940 that could provide consistent listing procedures from which to draw samples at two time points. Thus, while *The Professional Directory* (1910) was useful for enhancing the *AMD* (1909) sample, it could not serve as the basis for a diachronic study of the career and office locations of Philadelphia doctors.

Instead, it was necessary to use a national medical directory. Fortunately for the purposes of this study, the AMA began compiling and publishing the *AMD* in 1906, with new editions every two to three years into the 1940s. It boasted a complete alphabetical list of "legally qualified physicians of the United States and Canada" arranged by state and city. The AMA made every effort update their index files by enlisting the help of state licensing boards, medical school registrars, and local medical societies. The AMA also circulated questionnaire forms in *The Journal of the American Medical Association* asking doctors, especially ones not previously listed in the *AMD*, to send in their information.[2] Over the years, little changed in the basic information the *AMD* provided about doctors: birth year, medical society membership, medical school attended, graduation year, state licensure year, specialization (with the 1909 edition), high-level faculty positions held (though *The Professional Directory* was superior), and, of great importance for this book, the office addresses for doctors. I selected the 1909 and 1940 editions for my diachronic study for two reasons. First, these editions were close to decennial federal census years, making cross-referencing with census data more meaningful. The *AMD* (1909) had to be used, as the third edition was not published until 1912. Second, unlike the 1906 edition of the *AMD*, subsequent editions listed specializations. Although the number of AMA-recognized specialties expanded over time, the *AMD* nonetheless had thorough listings of specialists that used consistent and well-defined criteria.

Using 20 percent skip-interval samples of Philadelphia doctors listed in the *AMD* (1909) and *AMD* (1940), the biographical data for every fifth doctor were key-entered into a searchable card index that was created using widely available database software. The *AMD* (1909) listed 3,316 Philadelphia doctors, yielding 664 in the sample. The *AMD* (1940) listed 4,392 Philadelphia doctors, yielding 879 in the sample. The addresses listed for every doctor in the samples were coded by city ward using street atlases and a city ward genealogy.[3]

The data listed for doctors in the *AMD* (1909) and *AMD* (1940) samples were not always complete. Many had missing birth dates in the *AMD* (1909) sample. Nearly all, however, had graduation dates listed, which is why years since graduation was used as a measure of experience rather than age. Gender had to be inferred from the first names (and occasionally alma maters) of sample doctors. A handful of doctors, however, had names of indeterminate gender, especially those listing only initials or those with names of ambiguous gender, like Macy, Hilary, or Francis. In addition, some doctors listed addresses which could not be located on city atlases, or which were too general to be located in a specific ward. For example, an address at "Eighteenth and Chestnut" could be in either of two neighboring city wards, depending on which corner the doctor was located. In instances where analysis used incomplete data in the book, detailed numbers are given in the endnotes so that the reader can find a complete accounting of what and how much was missing. Missing data never exceeded 5 percent of the doctors or practitioners studied in any descriptive statistics or measures of variance, which meant that any preservation bias would have had little, if any, effect on data interpretation. This is a rare achievement in social science history. For example, although incomplete data were available on graduation date and gender in the *AMD* (1909) sample, 636 of 664 doctors in the sample had both graduation date listed and a name of discernable gender (table 18).

Table 18.   **Characteristics of Data Collected on Philadelphia Doctors in the 1909 and 1940 Samples of the *American Medical Directory***

	1909		1940	
	N	%	N	%
Total Philadelphia doctors listed in *AMD*	3,316	N/A	4,392	N/A
Total doctors in 20 percent skip interval sample	664	100.0	879	100.0
Year of birth given	333	50.2	858	97.6
Year of medical school graduation given	650	97.9	879	100.0
Gender discernable from name or alma mater	647	97.4	868	98.7

Sources: See appendix for discussion.

Unfortunately, the *AMD* did not collect data on nativity or social class of Philadelphia doctors, and only incomplete data on race. For doctors in select city neighborhoods in the *AMD* (1909) and *AMD* (1940) samples, individual data on race and nativity were retrieved from the manuscript census in the 1910 and 1940 (see table 7). Nativity and race were also studied at the city level for "physicians and surgeons" versus other occupied persons using data from the federal census (see tables 5 and 11). The social class of Philadelphia doctors as a whole or for individual doctors could not be studied using existing sources.

Private Practitioners

In chapters 1, 2, and 4, I refer to doctors who were "private practitioners" in the *AMD* (1909) and *AMD* (1940) samples. I defined practitioners as any doctor in the *AMD* who had a private practice address listed (see definition of private practice address below). I therefore excluded any doctor who had only an institutional address listed, such as a hospital, medical school, or government agency. Many of the doctors having only a hospital address were interns or residents and well on their way to private practice, though not actively practicing in a private office. Many interns and residents were labeled as such in the *AMD*, but others were not. I defined interns and residents as any doctor who graduated from medical school less than five years prior to the publication date of the *AMD*, and whose only listed address was a hospital. Also excluded from the tally of private practitioners were doctors listed as "retired" or "not in practice." Table 19 summarizes the number of private practitioners versus other categories of doctors in the *AMD* (1909) and *AMD* (1940) samples.

Table 19. **The Relative Proportion of Private Practitioners versus Other Doctors in the 1909 and 1940 Samples of the *American Medical Directory***

	1909		1940	
	N	%	N	%
Philadelphia doctors in sample	664	100.0	879	100.0
Private practitioners in sample	632	95.2	695	79.1
Interns/residents in sample	16	2.4	110	12.5
Doctors only in institutional practice in sample	5	0.8	44	5.0
Doctors retired or not in practice in sample	11	1.7	29	3.3

Note: Percentage totals are round to the nearest tenth of a percent, and therefore do not necessarily total 100 percent. The doctor missing from the 1940 sample did not fall into these four categories because he lived in Philadelphia but had his office outside of the city.

Sources: See appendix for discussion.

Specialization, Experience, and Position Holding

The AMA first recognized specialties in the *AMD* (1909), wherein it listed full specialists in one of eight specialties. The AMA did not recognize partial specialists until the *AMD* (1914), and so partial specialists could not be quantified in the *AMD* (1909) sample. By 1921, the *AMD* had recognized more than a dozen additional specialties. From the beginning, however, the AMA restricted who could be listed as a specialist in the *AMD* to those "who are members of a national or local specialty society or one of the special sections of the AMA, or who hold teaching positions, either didactic or clinical, on the faculty of some medical school."[4] As a result of its strict definition, the rate of specialization calculated using the *AMD* was likely less than the actual rate in practice. For instance, 14 and 20 percent of Philadelphia doctors were partial and full specialists, respectively, in the *AMD* (1929), whereas a questionnaire-based study of Philadelphia doctors conducted that same year found that 33 and 37 percent were partial and full specialists.[5] In the absence of more complete diachronic data on specialists, the *AMD* was used in spite of its known limitations. Because the *AMD* provided a stable definition of specialists, it permits an internally consistent measure of the growth of specialization from 1909 to 1940, even if the list of AMA-recognized specialties grew somewhat.

A doctor's "experience" was defined as the number of years since medical school graduation. The term "experience" was used instead of "years since graduation" for word economy, and does not presume a positive association between seniority and clinical abilities. Experience instead measures the relative opportunity to have become established in private practice and as a medical professional. In this respect, age would have been an equivalent measure. However, the experience of sample doctors was measured instead of age due to the incomplete data for birth dates in the *AMD* (1909) sample (table 18).

Two directories were used in order to determine patterns in position holding among doctors in 1909. Although the *AMD* (1909) listed some medical school faculty positions, these tended to be at the professor level only. Furthermore, the *AMD* (1909) did not list hospital or other institutional positions held. As a result, it was necessary to supplement position-holding data on doctors in the *AMD* (1909) sample using *The Professional Directory* (1910), which listed every medical school faculty position at Philadelphia medical schools, from full professor to assistant demonstrator.[6] *The Professional Directory* (1910) also had the most comprehensive hospital staff list available, with every position from superintendent to intern listed in 51 Philadelphia hospitals.[7] These hospitals were the largest and most significant, though a few smaller ones were not counted in *The Professional Directory* (1910). Thus the count of hospital positions was incomplete, though fairly comprehensive given source limitations.

For the *AMD* (1940) sample, no sources had comprehensive listings of medical school and hospital positions held by Philadelphia doctors. A handful of hospital staff lists were able to be located, though too few to warrant counting the number of positions held by doctors in the 1940 sample. As a result, the relationship between position holding and the specialization and experience of Philadelphia doctors could not be studied directly in the *AMD* (1940) sample. As described in chapter 4, there were a number of contemporary studies of Philadelphia or American doctors that provided general information on position holding, specialization, and experience from 1929 to 1940.

Several methods were used to determine the relationship between specialization, experience, and position holding for Philadelphia doctors in the *AMD* (1909) sample. First, descriptive statistics were used to tabulate totals and percentages for each variable, and bar charts compared variables. In addition, various means were calculated: average experience of specialists versus GPs, average positions held by specialists versus GPs, and average experience levels of position holders and non-position holders. In order to determine if two groups were different—say the average experience of GPs and specialists—means were compared for significant differences in variance using Student's t-test.[8] Student's t-tests were performed using an algorithm for two samples of different sizes, assuming unequal variance in each sample.[9] These algorithms are available in all major spreadsheet and statistical software packages. Significance levels (p-values) were reported in endnotes. Similar methods were used to establish the relationship between specialization and experience among Philadelphia doctors in the *AMD* (1940) sample, though position-holding data were unavailable.

Private Practices

In order to track patterns in the distribution of private medical practices in Philadelphia in the *AMD* (1909) and *AMD* (1940) samples, it was necessary to determine which of the addresses listed for sample doctors were private practices. I defined a "private practice" as any non-institutional location at which a doctor practiced medicine. At times in the book, I refer to private practices as "offices" and to private practice addresses as "office addresses" or "office locations." Before the turn of the century, doctors, especially in small towns, practiced medicine in their residence rather than in a separate rented office space. By my definition, these home offices addresses ought to be counted as private practice addresses. However, given that urban doctors in this period increasingly separated home and office, it was important to determine the meaning of the addresses listed in the *AMD* (1909) and *AMD* (1940).[10] Which non-institutional addresses were private practices, and which were non-work residences?

I developed inclusion criteria in order to eliminate non-work residences from my count of private practices in the *AMD* (1909) and *AMD* (1940) samples. Descriptions of early editions, including the *AMD* (1909), stated that the purpose of the directory, among other things, was to list the "office addresses and office hours" for all American doctors.[11] For the Philadelphia doctors in the sample who had only one address listed (85 percent), I tallied their sole address as a private practice so long as it was non-institutional and so long as the doctor was in active practice (defined above). It is likely that many of these addresses doubled as residences, but these would have been work addresses given the stated meaning of the addresses for early editions. For the few Philadelphia doctors having two addresses listed in *AMD* (1909), all non-institutional addresses were counted as practices so long as the doctor was in active practice. For doctors having two practice addresses, the practices were enumerated separately. By these inclusion criteria, there were 724 practice addresses among the 632 private practitioners in the 1909 sample. 713 of these practices were located in city limits, and 701 of these Philadelphia practices could be located on a street atlas and ward-coded (table 20). The number of practices in the city was extrapolated from the 20 percent sample by multiplying by five. By this method, there were an estimated 3,505 practices in the city in 1909.

Between publication of the *AMD* (1909) and *AMD* (1940), the editors changed their listing conventions for addresses. For doctors having two or three addresses listed in the *AMD* (1940), the first was identified as a residence and the second (and third) as an office.[12] This change in listing conventions, combined with evidence that few doctors worked from home in 1941, meant that different inclusion criteria were needed for the *AMD* (1940) sample. Residences had to be eliminated because most residences were non-working addresses in 1940. For doctors having only one address listed in the 1940 sample, I counted their sole address as a practice so long as the sole address was non-institutional and so long as the doctor was in active practice (defined above). A few of these sole addresses may have doubled as residences, but these would have been work addresses. The assumption was that in a professional directory, single address doctors would have listed the address at which they worked (whether a home or separate office) rather than a non-work residence. For doctors having two or three addresses listed, I did not count first addresses as private practices, as these were designated "residences" in the key to the 1940 edition.[13] This marked a significant

Table 20. **The Number of Private Practices in the 1909 and 1940 Samples of the _American Medical Directory_, with Non-Private-Practice Addresses Sorted by Exclusion Criteria**

	1909	1940
Philadelphia doctors in sample	664	879
Single-address doctors:	564	610
Total first addresses of single-address doctors	564	610
First addresses excluded because		
Non-work residence	N/A	N/A
Institutional address	-21	-130
Doctor not in practice or retired	-4	-29
Address not found or could not be ward-coded	-6	-4
Address not in city limits	0	0
Total first addresses of counted as private practices	533	447
Two-address doctors:	93	263
Total first addresses of two-address doctors	93	263
First addresses excluded because		
Non-work residence	N/A	-263
Institutional address	-1	N/A
Doctor not in practice or retired	0	N/A
Address not found or could not be ward-coded	-2	N/A
Address not in city limits	-10	N/A
Total first addresses of counted as private practices	80	0
Total second addresses of two-address doctors	93	263
Second addresses excluded because		
Non-work residence	N/A	N/A
Institutional address	0	-15
Doctor not in practice or retired	0	-9
Address not found or could not be ward-coded	-4	-5
Address not in city limits	-1	-1
Total second addresses of counted as private practices	88	233
Three-address doctors:	0	6
Total addresses of three-address doctors	0	18

(_continued_)

Table 20. **The Number of Private Practices in the 1909 and 1940 Samples of the *American Medical Directory*, with Non-Private-Practice Addresses Sorted by Exclusion Criteria (*continued*)**

	1909	1940
Addresses excluded because		
Non-work residence	N/A	-6
Institutional address	0	0
Doctor not in practice or retired	0	0
Address not found or could not be ward-coded	0	-1
Address not in city limits	0	-1
Total addresses of counted as private practices	0	10
Total addresses listed for all doctors in sample	750	1,154
Total addresses counted as private practices	701	690

Sources: See appendix for discussion.

departure from the inclusion criteria used for counting private practices in the *AMD* (1909) sample. The second and third addresses of multi-address doctors were counted as private practices so long as the second and third addresses were non-institutional and so long as the doctor was in active practice (defined above). By these inclusion criteria, there were 797 private practice addresses among the 695 private practitioners in the 1940 sample. 709 of these practices were located in city limits, and 690 of these practices could be located on a Philadelphia street atlas and ward-coded (table 20). The estimated number of practices in the city was extrapolated from the 20 percent sample by multiplying by five. By this method, there were an estimated 3,450 practices in the city in 1940.

Hospitals and Dispensaries

Counting the number of hospitals and dispensaries for the purposes of analyzing the *AMD* (1909) sample proved challenging. The definition of a hospital, in particular, was changing in the early twentieth century. Therefore it is not surprising that different sources yielded different counts for Philadelphia hospitals (and dispensaries). There were 135 "Hospitals, Sanitaria, and Charitable Institutions" in the *AMD* (1909), 53 "Hospitals and Sanitariums" and 49 "Dispensaries" in the federal census of *Benevolent Institutions* (1910), and 283 "Hospitals, Asylums, Dispensaries, and Homes" listed in the *Philadelphia City Register* (1910).[14] These lists had many overlapping institutions, and yielded a total of 294 institutions. This combined list was sorted into institutions having medical functions, social functions (or any institution having no obvious medical care functions from the name or from the staff list), both medical and social functions (or any institution with obvious social functions but having a doctor on staff), or unknown functions. Of these, 113 institutions had medical functions or both medical and social functions, and were counted as Philadelphia hospitals and dispensaries in 1909–1910. Of these 113 institutions, 111 could be ward-coded and used in geographical analysis. It is important to reiterate that a different hospital count was used for enumerating staff positions in 1909–1910. *The Professional Directory* (1910) had the most complete listing of hospital staff positions available, but these covered just the 51 largest and most significant hospitals (and their dispensaries). *The Professional Directory* did not include the other sixty or so small hospitals and homes. In the absence of a more complete source, *The Professional Directory* was used to measure hospital position-holding patterns in 1910.

By 1940, the definition and functions of a hospital had become more standardized. As a result, it was only necessary to use the *AMD* (1940), which counted 69 different "Hospitals, Sanatoriums, and Related Institutions."[15] The decreasing number of hospitals from 1909 to 1940 reflected the closures of small, neighborhood hospitals and dispensaries or mergers with larger hospitals. All 69 listed hospitals in 1940 were ward-coded and used in geographical analysis.

Notes

Introduction

1. National health expenditure (NHE) is the sum of all money, public and private, spent on health care in a given nation in a given year. Anne B. Martin, David Lassman, Benjamin Washington, Aaron Catlin, and the National Health Expenditure Accounts Team, "Growth in U.S. Health Spending Remained Slow in 2010; Health Share of Gross Domestic Product Was Unchanged from 2009," *Health Affairs* 31, no. 1 (2012), doi:10.1377/hlthaff.2011.1135. Organization for Economic Cooperation and Development, "OECD Health Data 2012," http://www.oecd.org/health/healthdata.

2. For recent overviews, see Sven Steinmo and Jon Watts, "It's the Institutions, Stupid! Why Comprehensive National Health Insurance Always Fails in America," *Journal of Health Politics, Policy, and Law* 20, no. 2 (1995): 329–72; Beatrix Hoffman, "Health Care Reform and Social Movements in the United States," *American Journal Public Health* 93, no. 1 (2003): 75–85; Colin Gordon, *Dead on Arrival: The Politics of Health Care in Twentieth-Century America* (Princeton, NJ: Princeton University Press, 2003); Jill Quadagno, "Why the United States Has No Health Insurance: Stakeholder Mobilization against the Welfare State, 1945–1996," in "Health and Health Care in the United States: Origins and Dynamics," ed. Donald W. Light and Ivy Bourgeault, extra issue, *Journal of Health and Social Behavior* 45 (2004): 25–44; and Rosemary A. Stevens, "History and Health Policy in the United States: The Making of a Health Care Industry, 1948–2008," *Social History of Medicine* 21, no. 3 (2008): 461–83. The Patient Protection and Affordable Care Act of 2010 did nothing to change this hybrid system.

3. U.S. Bureau of Labor Statistics, "Labor Force Statistics from the Current Population Survey," Household Data Historical table A-1, 2012, http://www.bls.gov/web/empsit/cpseea01.htm. Carmen DeNavas-Walt, Bernadette D. Proctor, and Jessica C. Smith, U.S. Census Bureau, Current Population Reports, P60–243, *Income, Poverty, and Health Insurance Coverage in the United States: 2011* (Washington, DC: U.S. Government Printing Office, 2012), 23, 65, http://www.census.gov/prod/2012pubs/p60–243.pdf.

4. U.S. Congressional Budget Office, "Estimates for the Insurance Coverage Provisions of the Affordable Care Act Updated for the Recent Supreme Court Decision" (July 2012), table 3, http://www.cbo.gov/publication/43472.

5. Michael E. Martinez and Robin A. Cohen, "Health Insurance Coverage: Early Release of Estimates from the National Health Interview Survey, January–June 2011" (National Center for Health Statistics, December 2011), http://www.cdc.gov/nchs/nhis/releases.htm. Other methods place this figure closer to 1 in 3 adults: Commonwealth Fund Commission on a High Performance Health System, *Why Not the Best? Results from the National Scorecard on U.S. Health System Performance, 2011* (Commonwealth Fund, October 2011), 43, exhibit 18, "Access Problems Because of Costs, 2010."

6. Michael Halpern et al., "Association of Insurance Status and Ethnicity with Cancer Stage at Diagnosis for Twelve Cancer Sites: A Retrospective Analysis," *Lancet Oncology* 9, no. 3 (2008): 222–31.

7. Institute of Medicine, Committee on the Consequences of Uninsurance, *Insuring America's Health: Principles and Recommendations* (Washington, DC: National Academies Press, 2004), 46.

8. Andrew P. Wilper et al., "Health Insurance and Mortality in U.S. Adults," *American Journal of Public Health* 99, no. 12 (2009): 2289–95. Mortality differences between the insured and uninsured persisted even after controlling for age, gender, race, ethnicity, income, education, and variables related to lifestyle and health. For 2005 mortality data, see Hsiang-Ching Kung et al., "Deaths: Final Data for 2005," *National Vital Statistics Reports* 56, no. 10 (Hyattsville, MD: National Center for Health Statistics, 2008), 5, table B.

9. For expenditure rankings, see I. S. Falk, C. Rufus Rorem, and Martha D. Ring, *The Costs of Medical Care: A Summary of Investigations on the Economic Aspects of the Prevention and Care of Illness*, Publications of the Committee on the Costs of Medical Care, 27 (Chicago: University of Chicago Press, 1933), 9, and Martin et al., "Growth in U.S. Health Spending," 209, exhibit 1.

10. George Rosen, *The Structure of American Medical Practice, 1875–1941*, ed. Charles E. Rosenberg (Philadelphia: University of Pennsylvania Press, 1983). Neil Larry Shumsky, James Bohland, and Paul Knox, "Separating Doctors' Homes and Doctors' Offices: San Francisco, 1881–1941," *Social Science and Medicine* 23, no. 10 (1986): 1051–57. Donald L. Madison and Thomas R. Konrad, "Large Medical Group-Practice Organizations and Employed Physicians: A Relationship in Transition," *Milbank Quarterly* 66, no. 2 (1988): 240–82.

11. For comparison of administrative costs, see the Commonwealth Fund, *Why Not the Best?* 49.

12. Lawrence P. Casalino, "Physicians and Corporations: A Corporate Transformation of American Medicine?" in "Transforming American Medicine: A Twenty-Year Retrospective on The Social Transformation of American Medicine," special issue of *Journal of Health Politics, Policy, and Law* 29, no. 4–5 (2004): 869–84. Gardener Harris, "More Doctors Giving Up Private Practices," *New York Times*, March 25, 2010. Timothy Hoff, *Practice Under Pressure: Primary Care Physicians and Their Medicine in the Twenty-First Century* (New Brunswick, NJ: Rutgers University Press, 2010).

13. U.S. Bureau of the Census, *1990 Census of Population and Housing: Population and Housing Unit Counts, United States*, Publication CPH-2-1 (Washington, DC: United States Census Office, 1990), 5, "Table 4: United States Urban and Rural," http://www.census.gov/population/censusdata/table-4.pdf.

14. The primary literature on this topic is too vast to cite in a single footnote. For major overviews published from the 1920s to the 1960s, see Lewis Mayers and Leonard V. Harrison, *The Distribution of Physicians in the United States* (New York: General Education Board, 1924); R. G. Leland and the AMA Bureau of Medical Economic Research, *Distribution of Physicians in the United States* (Chicago: AMA Press, 1935); Joseph W. Mountin, Elliott H. Pennell, and Georgie S. Brockett, "Location and Movement of Physicians, 1923 and 1938: Changes in Urban and Rural Totals for Established Physicians," *Public Health Reports* 60, no. 7 (1945): 173–85; Frank Greene Dickinson, *Distribution of Physicians by Medical Service Areas* (Chicago: AMA, 1954); H. G. Weiskotten et al., "Trends in Medical Practice: An Analysis of the Distribution and Characteristics of Medical College Graduates, 1915–1950," *Journal of Medical Education* 35, no. 12 (1960): 1071–1121; and Rashi Fein, *The Doctor Shortage: An Economic Diagnosis* (Washington, DC: Brookings Institution, 1967).

15. Daniel M. Fox, *Health Policies, Health Politics: The British and American Experience, 1911–1965* (Princeton, NJ: Princeton University Press, 1986), 123–31. Rosemary Stevens, *In Sickness and In Wealth: American Hospitals in the Twentieth Century*, updated ed. (Baltimore: Johns Hopkins University Press, 1999), 216–26. Fitzhugh Mullan, "The National Health Service Corps," *Lancet* 313, no. 8125 (1979): 1071–73.

16. David C. Goodman, "Twenty-Year Trends in Regional Variations in the U.S. Physician Workforce," *Health Affairs* 23 (2004): 90–97. David C. Goodman, Elliott S. Fisher, and Kristen K. Bronner, "Hospital and Physician Capacity Update," Dartmouth Institute for Health Policy and Clinical Practice, March 30, 2009, http://www.dartmouthatlas.org/downloads/reports/Capacity_Report_2009.pdf.

17. Donald Dewey, *Where the Doctors Have Gone: The Changing Distribution of Private Practice Physicians in the Chicago Metropolitan Area, 1950–1970*, Chicago Regional Hospital Study (Chicago: Illinois Regional Medical Program, 1973). Pierre de Vise, *Misused and Misplaced Hospitals and Doctors: A Locational Analysis of the Urban Health Care Crisis* (Washington, DC: Association of American Geographers, Commission on College Geography, 1973). See also John C. Norman and Beverly Bennett, eds., *Medicine in the Ghetto* (New York: Appleton-Century-Crofts, 1969), and Pierre de Vise, ed., *Slum Medicine: Chicago's Apartheid Health System* (Chicago: Community and Family Study Center, University of Chicago, 1969). Only a couple of intra-urban studies were conducted before the late 1960s: Rollo H. Britten, "The National Health Survey: Receipt of Medical Services in Different Urban Population Groups," *Public Health Reports* 55, no. 48 (1940): 2199–2224, and Stanley Lieberson, "Ethnic Groups and the Practice of Medicine," *American Sociological Review* 23, no. 5 (1958): 542–49.

18. For example, see Sheila Joroff and Vicente Navarro, "Medical Manpower: A Multivariate Analysis of the Distribution of Physicians in Urban United States," *Medical Care* 9, no. 5 (1971): 428–38, and Stephen C. Guptill, "The Spatial Availability of Physicians," *Proceedings of the Association of American Geographers* 7 (1975): 80–84.

19. This argument was first made by Paul Knox, James Bohland, and Neil Larry Shumsky, "The Urban Transition and the Evolution of the Medical Care Delivery System in America," *Social Science and Medicine* 17 (1983): 37–43.

20. Notable exceptions include David Rosner, *A Once Charitable Enterprise: Hospitals and Health Care in Brooklyn and New York, 1885–1915* (Princeton, NJ: Princeton University Press, 1982); Shumsky et al., "Separating Doctors' Homes and Doctors' Offices"; Paul F. Mattingly, "The Changing Location of Physician Offices in Bloomington-Normal, Illinois: 1870–1988," *Professional Geographer* 43, no. 4 (1991): 465–74; and Anne-Marie Adams and Stacie Burke, "A Doctor in the House: The Architecture of Home-Offices for Physicians in Toronto, 1885–1930," *Medical History* 52, no. 2 (2008): 163–94.

21. For the best definition of "the medical marketplace," see Mark S. R. Jenner and Patrick Wallis, "The Medical Marketplace," in *Medicine and the Market in England and Its Colonies, c. 1450–1850*, ed. Mark S. R. Jenner and Patrick Wallis (New York: Palgrave, 2007), 1–23.

22. Lisa Rosner, "Thistle on the Delaware: Edinburgh Medical Education and Philadelphia Practice, 1800–1825," *Social History of Medicine* 5, no. 1 (1992): 19–42. Leo J. O'Hara, *An Emerging Profession: Philadelphia Doctors 1860–1900* (New York: Garland Publishing, Inc., 1989). On the relationship of medical institutions to early American cities, see Simon P. Newman, *Embodied History: The Lives of the Poor in Early Philadelphia* (Philadelphia: University of Pennsylvania Press, 2003), Billy G. Smith, ed., *Down and Out in Early America* (University Park: Pennsylvania State

University Press, 2004), and Simon Finger, The Contagious City: The Politics of Public Health in Early Philadelphia (Ithaca, NY: Cornell University Press, 2012).

23. Rosner, A Once Charitable Enterprise. Thomas Bonner, Medicine in Chicago, 1850–1950: A Chapter in the Social and Scientific Development of a City (Madison: American History Research Center, 1957). Christopher Crenner, Private Practice: In the Early Twentieth Century Medical Office of Dr. Richard Cabot (Baltimore: Johns Hopkins University Press, 2005). Charles E. Rosenberg, "Making It in Urban Medicine: A Career in the Age of Scientific Medicine," BHM 64 (1990): 163–86.

24. H. G. Weiskotten and Marion E. Altenderfer, "Trends in Medical Practice," Journal of Medical Education 27, no. 5 (1952): 3–41, esp. tables 9 and 10.

25. David P. Adams, "Community and Professionalization: General Practitioners and Ear, Nose, and Throat Specialists in Cincinnati, 1945–1947," BHM 68 (1994): 664–84. See also Oswald Hall, "The Informal Organization of Medical Practice in an American City" (PhD diss., University of Chicago, 1944).

26. For an excellent theoretical framework, see Patricia Gober and Rena J. Gordon, "Intraurban Physician Location: A Case Study of Phoenix," Social Science and Medicine 14D (1980): 407–17.

27. For overviews, see Sam Bass Warner Jr., Streetcar Suburbs: The Process of Growth in Boston, 1870–1900, 2nd ed. (Cambridge, MA: Harvard University Press, 1978); Theodore Hershberg, ed., Philadelphia: Work, Space, Family, and Group Experience in the Nineteenth Century (New York: Oxford University Press, 1981); Kenneth T. Jackson, Crabgrass Frontier: The Suburbanization of the United States (New York: Oxford University Press, 1985); Robert Fishman, Bourgeois Utopias: The Rise and Fall of Suburbia (New York: Basic Books, 1987); Sam Bass Warner Jr., The Private City: Philadelphia in Three Periods of Its Growth, 2nd ed. (Philadelphia: University of Pennsylvania Press, 1987); and Colin Gordon Mapping Decline: St. Louis and the Fate of the American City (Philadelphia: University of Pennsylvania Press, 2008). Medical care has so rarely been put in the context of urban change: Paul Knox, James Bohland, and Neil Larry Shumsky, "Urban Development and the Geography of Personal Services: The Example of Medical Care in the United States," in Public Service Provision and Urban Development, ed. Andrew Kirby, Paul Knox, and Steven Pinch (New York: St. Martin's Press, 1984), 152–75.

28. The historiography of the professionalization of American medicine is both too familiar and too vast to cite in a single footnote. For overviews, see Joseph Kett, The Formation of the American Medical Profession: The Role of Institutions 1760–1860 (New Haven: Yale University Press, 1968); James G. Burrow, Organized Medicine in the Progressive Era: The Move toward Monopoly (Baltimore: Johns Hopkins University Press, 1977); Gerald E. Markowitz and David Rosner, "Doctors in Crisis: Medical Education and Medical Reform during the Progressive Era, 1895–1915," in Health Care in America: Essays in Social History, ed. Susan Reverby and David Rosner (Philadelphia: Temple University Press, 1979), 185–205; Paul Starr, The Social Transformation of American Medicine (New York: Basic Books, 1982); Rosen, The Structure of American Medical Practice; Barbara G. Rosenkrantz, "The Search for Professional Order in Nineteenth-Century American Medicine," in Sickness and Health in America: Readings in the History of Medicine and Public Health, ed. Judith W. Leavitt and Ronald Numbers, 2nd ed. (Madison: University of Wisconsin Press, 1985), 219–32; William G. Rothstein, American Medical Schools and the Practice of Medicine: A History (New York: Oxford University Press, 1987); Ronald Numbers, "The Fall and Rise of the American Medical Profession," in Sickness and Health in America: Readings

in the History of Medicine and Public Health, ed. Judith Walzer Leavitt and Ronald Numbers, 3rd ed. (Madison: University of Wisconsin Press, 1997), 225–36.

29. See, for example: Thomas Goebel, "American Medicine and the 'Organizational Synthesis': Chicago Physicians and the Business of Medicine, 1900–1920," *BHM* 68 (1994): 639–63; Goebel, "The Uneven Rewards of Professional Labor: Wealth and Income in the Chicago Professions, 1870–1920," *Journal of Social History* 29, no. 4 (1996): 749–77; Donald L. Madison, "Preserving Individualism in the Organizational Society: 'Cooperation' and American Medical Practice, 1900–1920," *BHM* 70 (1996): 442–83; Christopher Crenner, "Organizational Reform and Professional Dissent in the Careers of Richard Cabot and Ernest Amory Codman, 1900–1920," *Journal of the History of Medicine and Allied Sciences* 56 (2001): 211–37; John Harley Warner, "Grand Narrative and Its Discontents: Medical History and the Social Transformation of American Medicine," in "Transforming American Medicine" (see note 12), 757–80.

30. Norman Gevitz, ed., *Other Healers: Unorthodox Medicine in America* (Baltimore: Johns Hopkins University Press, 1988). Charlotte G. Borst, *Catching Babies: The Professionalization of Childbirth, 1870–1920* (Cambridge, MA: Harvard University Press, 1995).

31. One notable exception is Rosenberg, "Making It in Urban Medicine." Nineteenth-century studies of rank-and-file doctors abound: Judith W. Leavitt, "'A Worrying Profession': The Domestic Environment of Medical Practice in Mid-Nineteenth Century America," *BHM* 69, no. 1 (1995): 1–29; Steven M. Stowe, "Seeing Themselves at Work: Physicians and Case Narrative in the Mid-Nineteenth-Century American South," *American Historical Review* 101 (1996): 41–79; Stowe, *Doctoring the South: Southern Physicians and Everyday Medicine in the Mid-Nineteenth Century* (Chapel Hill: University of North Carolina Press, 2004).

32. For biographies detailing career paths and occupational activities, see Rosenberg, "Making It in Urban Medicine"; Bonnie E. Blustein, *Preserve Your Love for Science: Life of William A. Hammond, American Neurologist* (Cambridge: Cambridge University Press, 1991), and Crenner, *Private Practice*. Notable studies of private practice as an urban occupational system include Rosner, *A Once Charitable Enterprise*, 13–35; Hall, "The Informal Organization of Medical Practice"; and Shumsky et al., "Separating Doctors' Homes and Doctors' Offices." By comparison, histories of medical practice in Britain abound: Rosemary Stevens, *Medical Practice in Modern England: The Impact of Specialization and State Medicine* (New Haven: Yale University Press, 1966); Irvine Loudon, *Medical Care and the General Practitioner, 1750–1850* (New York: Oxford University Press, 1986); Anne Digby, *Making a Medical Living: Doctors and Patients in the English Market for Medicine, 1720–1911* (Cambridge: Cambridge University Press, 1994); Irvine Loudon, John Horder, and Charles Webster, eds., *General Practice Under the National Health Service, 1948–1997* (London: Clarendon Press, 1998); and Anne Digby, *The Evolution of British General Practice, 1850–1948* (New York: Oxford University Press, 1999).

33. Women doctors are an exception. Because they worked in a male-dominated profession and faced frequent gender discrimination, women doctors viewed their careers as extraordinary, even if they did not achieve great fame. As a result of their worldview, and of the effort of Woman's Medical College of Pennsylvania to keep track of their alumnae, a more representative corpus of papers from Philadelphia's women doctors survives than that of their medical brethren.

34. For background, see George Weisz, "Medical Directories and Medical Specialization in France, Britain, and the United States," *BHM* 71, no. 1 (1997): 23–68.

35. There are, however, quantitative histories of medical practice in Britain: Digby, *Making a Medical Living* and *The Evolution of British General Practice.*

36. George Weisz, "Mapping Medical Specialization in Paris in the Nineteenth and Twentieth Centuries," *Social History of Medicine* 7, no. 2 (1994): 177–211; Weisz, "The Emergence of Medical Specialization in the Nineteenth Century," *BHM* 77 (2003): 536–75. By "specialists," I am referring only to orthodox doctors and not to the large cast of alternative healers, such as bonesetters or herbalists, who flourished in early modern medical marketplaces.

37. George Weisz, *Divide and Conquer: A Comparative History of Medical Specialization* (New York: Oxford University Press, 2006), 68–76.

38. U.S. Department of Health, Education, and Welfare, *Health Manpower Source Book*, Sec. 14, "Medical Specialties" (Washington, DC: U.S.G.P.O., 1962), esp. 3, 7, and 9. See also George Rosen, "Changing Attitudes of the Medical Profession to Specialization," *BHM* 12 (1942): 343–54; Rosen, "Whither Specialization," *Medicine and Society: Contemporary Medical Problems in Historical Perspective*, vol. 4 (Philadelphia: American Philosophical Society, 1971), 196–219; and Rosen, *The Structure of American Medical Practice*, 85–94.

39. For a recent review, see Weisz, *Divide and Conquer* (2006), xii–xv. One rare example of a local study is Weisz, "Mapping Medical Specialization in Paris."

40. George Rosen, *The Specialization of Medicine with Particular Reference to Ophthalmology* (New York: Froben Press, 1944).

41. Weisz, "The Emergence of Medical Specialization"; Weisz, *Divide and Conquer*. Rosemary Stevens, *American Medicine and the Public Interest*, updated ed. (Berkeley: University of California Press, 1998). Stevens, *Medical Practice in Modern England.*

42. See, for example: Sydney Halpern, *American Pediatrics: The Social Dynamics of Professionalism, 1880–1980* (Berkeley: University of California Press, 1988); Glenn Gritzer and Arnold Arluke, *The Making of Rehabilitation: A Political Economy of Medical Specialization, 1890–1980* (Berkeley: University of California Press, 1985); and Russell C. Maulitz and Diana E. Long, eds., *Grand Rounds: One Hundred Years of Internal Medicine* (Philadelphia: University of Pennsylvania Press, 1988).

1. The Primacy of Private Practice

1. Samuel L. Baker, "Physician Licensure Laws in the United States, 1865–1915," *Journal of the History of Medicine and Allied Sciences* 39 (1984): 174. Richard H. Shryock, *Medical Licensing in America, 1650–1965* (Baltimore: Johns Hopkins University Press, 1967), 3–42. Joseph Kett, *The Formation of the American Medical Profession: The Role of Institutions 1760–1860* (New Haven: Yale University Press, 1968), 14–30.

2. Harold F. Alderfer, "Legislative History of Medical Licensure in Pennsylvania," *PMJ* 64 (1961): 1605–9, and Shryock, *Medical Licensing in America*, 23, 48.

3. For an overview, see Kett, *The Formation of the American Medical Profession;* James G. Burrow, *Organized Medicine in the Progressive Era: The Move toward Monopoly* (Baltimore: Johns Hopkins University Press, 1977); Gerald E. Markowitz and David Rosner, "Doctors in Crisis: Medical Education and Medical Reform during the Progressive Era, 1895–1915," in *Health Care in America: Essays in Social History*, ed. Susan Reverby and David Rosner (Philadelphia: Temple University Press, 1979), 185–205; Paul Starr, *The Social Transformation of American Medicine* (New York: Basic Books, 1982); George Rosen, *The Structure of American Medical Practice, 1875–1941*, ed. Charles E. Rosenberg (Philadelphia: University of

Pennsylvania Press, 1983); Barbara G. Rosenkrantz, "The Search for Professional Order in Nineteenth-Century American Medicine," in *Sickness and Health in America: Readings in the History of Medicine and Public Health*, ed. Judith W. Leavitt and Ronald Numbers, 2nd ed. (Madison: University of Wisconsin Press, 1985), 219–32; and Ronald Numbers, "The Fall and Rise of the American Medical Profession," in *Sickness and Health in America: Readings in the History of Medicine and Public Health*, ed. Judith Walzer Leavitt and Ronald Numbers, 3rd ed. (Madison: University of Wisconsin Press, 1997), 225–36.

4. William G. Rothstein, *American Medical Schools and the Practice of Medicine: A History* (New York: Oxford University Press, 1987)), esp. tables 3.1 and 7.2.

5. Leo J. O'Hara, *An Emerging Profession: Philadelphia Doctors, 1860–1900* (New York: Garland Publishing, 1989), esp. 111–61. Steven J. Peitzman, *A New and Untried Course: Woman's Medical College and the Medical College of Pennsylvania, 1850–1998* (New Brunswick, NJ: Rutgers University Press, 2000), 74–81. Naomi Rogers, *An Alternative Path: The Making and Remaking of Hahnemann Medical College and Hospital of Philadelphia* (New Brunswick, NJ: Rutgers University Press, 1998), 50–53, 84–95. Janet Tighe, "'Never Knowing One's Place': Temple University School of Medicine and the Medical Education Hierarchy," *Transactions of the College of Physicians of Philadelphia*, 5th ser., 12, no. 3 (1990): 311–34.

6. Alderfer, "Legislative History of Medical Licensure in Pennsylvania," 1605–9.

7. Baker, "Physician Licensure Laws in the United States," 173–97. L. E. Miller and R. M. Weiss, "Medical Education Reform Efforts and Failures of U.S. Medical Schools, 1870–1930," *Journal of the History of Medicine and Allied Sciences* 63, no. 3 (2008): 348–87.

8. "Report the Medical Newcomers in Your Neighborhood" *WR* 2, no. 16 (1906): 7.

9. Charles E. Rosenberg, "Community and Communities: The Evolution of the American Hospital," in *The American General Hospital: Communities and Social Contexts*, ed. Diana E. Long and Janet Golden (Ithaca, NY: Cornell University Press, 1989), 3–17.

10. Kenneth M. Ludmerer, *Learning to Heal: The Development of American Medical Education* (Baltimore: Johns Hopkins University Press, 1985), 47–71.

11. O'Hara, *An Emerging Profession*, 174–178. Peitzman, *A New and Untried Course*, 77–81, 125–30.

12. Rosenberg, "Community and Communities," 8–15.

13. George W. Norris, "Medical Memories: An account of events and personalities that I saw and heard as a medical student at the University of Pennsylvania, 1895–1899," George W. Norris Papers, 1898–1962, Collection 1826, HSP.

14. Alderfer, "Legislative History of Medical Licensure in Pennsylvania," 1605–9. Stevens, *American Medicine and the Public Interest*, 116–20. O'Hara, *An Emerging Profession*. For overviews of American hospitals, see Morris J. Vogel, *The Invention of the Modern Hospital, Boston, 1870–1930* (Chicago: University of Chicago Press, 1980); David Rosner, *A Once Charitable Enterprise: Hospitals and Health Care in Brooklyn and New York, 1885–1915* (Cambridge: Cambridge University Press, 1982); Charles E. Rosenberg, *The Care of Strangers: The Rise of America's Hospital System* (Baltimore: Johns Hopkins University Press, 1987); Diana E. Long and Janet Golden, eds., *The American General Hospital: Communities and Social Contexts* (Ithaca, NY: Cornell University Press, 1989); and Rosemary Stevens, *In Sickness and In Wealth: American Hospitals in the Twentieth Century*, paperback ed. (Baltimore: Johns Hopkins University Press, 1999). On graduate medical education and Philadelphia hospitals, see Steven J. Peitzman, "'Thoroughly Practical': America's

Polyclinic Medical Schools," *BHM* 54 (1980): 166–87; Charles E. Rosenberg, "From Almshouse to Hospital: The Shaping of Philadelphia General Hospital," *Milbank Memorial Fund Quarterly/Health and Society* 60, no. 1 (1982): 108–54; Rosemary Stevens, "Sweet Charity: State Aid to Hospitals in Pennsylvania, 1870–1910," *BHM* 58 (1984): 287–314; Edward T. Morman, "Clinical Pathology in America, 1865–1915: Philadelphia as a Test Case," *BHM* 58 (1984): 198–214; David McBride, *Integrating the City of Medicine: Blacks in Philadelphia Health Care, 1910–1965* (Philadelphia: Temple University Press, 1989); and O'Hara, *An Emerging Profession.*

15. J. A. Curran, "Internships and Residencies: Historical Backgrounds and Current Trends," *Journal of Medical Education* 34, no. 9 (1959): 873–84.

16. "Editorial" *The Jeffersonian* 12, no. 95 (1911): 10–11. The term "intern" was often used synonymously with "resident" until standardization in the 1910s and 1920s, when "internship" referred to the first year of general hospital work and "residency" referred to any education in a specialty beyond internship. See Curran, "Internships and Residencies," 873–84.

17. "Editorial" *The Jeffersonian* 12, no. 95 (1911): 10–11.

18. "The Education of the Interne," *JAMA* 43, no. 7 (1904): 469–70, and "The Hospital Intern Year," *JAMA* 60, no. 25 (1913): 2017. The authors of the 1913 article acknowledged that the cited ratio of interns to graduates was likely artificially high, because some graduates occupied internships for more than one year. The sample was also biased toward graduates of elite schools, which likely had higher internship rates for their graduates.

19. "The Hospital Intern Year," 2017.

20. Data based on a 20 percent skip-interval sample of all listed doctors for Philadelphia, Pennsylvania in the *AMD* (Chicago: AMA Press, 1909). See the appendix of this book for details on the sample. Of the 664 doctors in the 1909 sample, graduation dates were listed for 650 doctors (97.8 percent). Of these, 10 of 22 who graduated in 1908 had internships in 1909 (45.5 percent).

21. Rosen, *The Structure of American Medical Practice*, 21–32, 53–60. Neil Larry Shumsky, James Bohland, and Paul Knox, "Separating Doctors' Homes and Doctors' Offices: San Francisco, 1881–1941," *Social Science and Medicine* 23, no. 10 (1986): 1051–57. Anne Marie Adams and Stacie Burke, "A Doctor in the House: The Architecture of Home-Offices for Physicians in Toronto, 1885–1930," *Medical History* 52, no. 2 (2008): 163–94.

22. For numbers for 1880 faculty, see O'Hara, *An Emerging Profession* (1989), 145–54. Numbers for 1910 faculty were gathered from *The Professional Directory of Philadelphia, Including Camden and Atlantic City and Eighty Near-by Towns* (Philadelphia: Edward Trust, 1910), 163–75. See the appendix of this book for more details.

23. This transformation is discussed, at length, in chapter 4 of this book.

24. All hospital staff positions in 1910 were enumerated from the fifty-one Philadelphia hospitals listed in *The Professional Directory*, 209–66. See the appendix of this book for details.

25. O'Hara, *Emerging Profession*, 145–54. On the later movement for full-time faculty (who had no private medical practice on the side), see Rothstein, *American Medical Schools*, 160–78, and Ludmerer, *Learning to Heal*, 207–18.

26. See the appendix of this book and table 19 for details.

27. Thomas Goebel, "The Uneven Rewards of Professional Labor: Wealth and Income in the Chicago Professions, 1870–1920," *Journal of Social History* 29, no. 4 (1996): 749–77. On earlier patterns of institutional tenure in Philadelphia, see O'Hara, *An Emerging Profession*, 295–327.

28. George Weisz, "Medical Directories and Medical Specialization in France, Britain, and the United States," *BHM* 71 (1997): 23–68. Weisz, *Divide and Conquer: A Comparative History of Medical Specialization* (New York: Oxford University Press, 2006), esp. 87–92. George Rosen, *The Specialization of Medicine, with Particular Reference to Ophthalmology* (New York: Froben Press, 1944), esp. 30–49.

29. Measured another way, the average experience of specialists exceeded that of GPs in Philadelphia in 1909–1910: specialists had been out of medical school for an average of 21.4 years by comparison to 17.7 years for GPs. Differences were significant when measured by Student's t-test (p < .01). Data not shown. See the appendix of this book for details.

30. Dr. DeForest Porter Willard is listed as a partial specialist in orthopaedic surgery in 1914 and a full specialist of orthopaedic surgery in the 1916—see *AMD*, 4th ed. (Chicago: AMA Press, 1914), 1297, and *AMD*, 5th ed. (Chicago: AMA Press, 1916), 1368. The AMA did not recognize partial specialists until the fourth edition in 1914, thus it is possible that Dr. Willard had partially specialized his practice earlier than 1914, especially given his many hospital appointments immediately after his internship ended in 1910. See the appendix of this book for discussion.

31. Elizabeth L. Peck, "The President's Address," *Transactions of the Alumnae Association of the Woman's Medical College of Pennsylvania*, Twenty-sixth Annual Meeting (1901): 42–46.

32. Edwin B. Cragin, "Specialism in Medicine," *The Jeffersonian* 13, no. 100 (1911): 2–9.

33. Joseph McDowell Matthews, *How to Succeed in the Practice of Medicine* (Philadelphia: W. B. Saunders, 1905), 99.

34. Weisz, "Medical Directories and Medical Specialization," 23–68. Weisz, *Divide and Conquer*, 127–46. Rosemary Stevens, *American Medicine and the Public Interest*, updated ed. (Berkeley: University of California Press, 1998). Rothstein, *American Medical Schools*, 314–24.

35. Peitzman, "'Thoroughly Practical,'" 166–87. Stevens, *American Medicine and the Public Interest*, 113–31. Jennifer L. Gunn, "Science and Skill: Educating the Medical Practitioner at the Graduate School of Medicine of the University of Pennsylvania," (PhD diss., University of Pennsylvania, 1997).

36. See chapter 2 in this book for further discussion.

37. Private specialty practice had begun to depend upon hospital position holding by 1900: O'Hara, *An Emerging Profession*, 174–78. Salaried positions in health departments and laboratories were still very rare, and salaried doctors often relied upon private practice for income: Charles E. Rosenberg, "Making It in Urban Medicine: A Career in the Age of Scientific Medicine," *BHM* 64 (1990): 163–86.

38. According to cross-references of the *AMD* (1909) and *The Professional Directory* (1910) there were 3,155 faculty and hospital positions combined (excluding internships) for 3,316 doctors in Philadelphia, or enough for 95 percent of doctors to hold one position apiece. Multiple office holders, though, limited positions to just 41 percent of Philadelphia doctors. My data for 1909–1910 are consistent with O'Hara's for 1900: *An Emerging Profession*, 312n31.

39. Of non–position holders in the *AMD* 1909 sample, 13 of 375 (4 percent) were specialized; of position holders, 72 of 257 were specialized (28 percent). Differences in the mean number of positions held by specialists and general practitioners were significant when measured by Student's t-test (p < .0001). Data not shown. See the appendix of this book for details.

40. See chapter 2 in this book for further discussion.

41. The same was also true for lawyers and engineers: Goebel, "The Uneven Rewards of Professional Labor," 749–77.

42. Arthur B. Emmons, *The Profession of Medicine: A Collection of Letters from Graduates of the Harvard Medical School* (Cambridge, MA: Harvard University Press, c.1914), 60, 105.

43. Goebel, "The Uneven Rewards of Professional Labor." Emmons, *The Profession of Medicine*, 60, 105. David W. Galenson, "Economic Opportunity on the Urban Frontier: Nativity, Work, and Wealth in Early Chicago," *Journal of Economic History* 51, no. 3 (1991): 581–603.

44. Rothstein, *American Medical Schools*, 96, table 5.3.

45. For later income data, see R. G. Leland, "Income from Medical Practice" *JAMA* 96, no. 20 (1931): 1683–91; I. S. Falk, C. Rufus Rorem, and Martha D. Ring, *The Costs of Medical Care: A Summary of Investigations on the Economic Aspects of the Prevention and Care of Illness*, Publications of the Committee on the Costs of Medical Care, no. 27 (Chicago: University of Chicago Press, 1933), 205–7; Maurice Leven, *The Income of Physicians: An Economic and Statistical Analysis*, Publications of the Committee on the Costs of Medical Care, no. 24 (Chicago: University of Chicago Press, 1932); and Nathan Sinai and Alden B. Mills, *A Survey of the Medical Facilities of the City of Philadelphia: 1929*, Publications of the Committee on the Costs of Medical Care, no. 9A (Washington, DC: Committee on the Costs of Medical Care, 1931).

46. Dr. DeForest Porter Willard Jr. finished third in his class at the University of Pennsylvania in 1908, and presented or published many papers in just his first few years after graduation (see table 3). Clearly, he was no slouch.

47. Matthews, *How to Succeed in the Practice of Medicine*, 93. See chapter 5 for discussion of the tarnishing image of the "old-time" or "country" doctor in professional discourse by the mid-twentieth century.

48. John Harley Warner, *The Therapeutic Perspective: Medical Practice, Knowledge, and Identity in America, 1820–1885*, paperback ed. (Princeton, NJ: Princeton University Press, 1997), 11–36. E. B. Ketcherside, "The Old-Time Doctor" *The Jeffersonian* 9, no. 76 (1908): 7–9.

49. *How to Be Successful as a Physician: Heart-to-Heart Talks of a Successful Physician with His Brother Practitioners* (Meriden, CT: Church Publishing, 1902), 122–23.

50. Newspaper clippings of "The New Medical Professor," *The Press*, April 12, 1910 in "Scrapbook 1909–1912," Charles K. Mills Papers, 1864–1941, Collection 424, HSP.

51. George Rosen, "Changing Attitudes of the Medical Profession to Specialization," *BHM* 12 (1942): 343–54.

52. This story of Dr. William Fisher Norris, recounted to his son by Dr. George E. de Schweinitz, appeared in George William Norris, "Medical Memories," HSP.

53. Matthews, *How to Succeed in the Practice of Medicine*, 96.

54. Abraham Flexner, *Medical Education in the United States and Canada*, bulletin no. 4 (New York: Carnegie Foundation for the Advancement of Teaching, 1910), 42–51, 178–81.

55. Tighe, "Never Knowing One's Place," 311–34. Flexner, *Medical Education in the United States and Canada*, esp. 42–51. Todd L. Savitt, *Race and Medicine in Nineteenth- and Early-Twentieth-Century America* (Kent, OH: Kent State University Press, 2007), 252–66, 269–94.

56. U.S. Bureau of the Census, *Thirteenth Census of Population: 1910*, vol. 4, "Occupation Statistics" (Washington, DC: U.S. G.P.O., 1914), 192–193. Women had higher

representation in the Philadelphia medical profession (9.1 percent) than in the American medical profession, as a whole (6 percent) in 1910. See Regina Morantz-Sanchez, *Sympathy and Science: Women Physicians in American Medicine*, new ed. (Chapel Hill: University of North Carolina Press, 2000), esp. 232–65. On early support for women's medical education in Philadelphia, see Steven J. Peitzman, "Why Support a Women's Medical College? Philadelphia's Early Male Medical Pro-Feminists," *BHM* 77 (2003): 576–99.

57. O'Hara, *An Emerging Profession*, 295–327. Douglas M. Haynes, "Policing the Social Boundaries of the American Medical Association," *Journal of the History of Medicine and the Allied Sciences* 60, no. 2 (2005): 170–95.

58. Peitzman, *A New and Untried Course*, 66. Morantz-Sanchez, *Sympathy and Science*, 90–202, 232–311.

59. Peck, "The President's Address," 45.

60. Morantz-Sanchez, *Sympathy and Science*, 184–202. On the "maternalist" influence upon social welfare reform in the Progressive Era, see Theda Skocpol, *Protecting Soldiers and Mothers: The Political Origins of Social Policy in the United States* (Cambridge, MA: Harvard University Press, 1992).

61. See, for example, essentialist advice given in Louise G. Rabinovitch, "The Woman Physician, and a Vast Field of Usefulness Unrecognized by Her," *Transactions of the Alumnae Association of the Woman's Medical College of Pennsylvania*, 28th Annual Meeting (1903): 72–81, and in V. A. Latham, "Special Lines of Research Work for Women," *Transactions of the Alumnae Association of the Woman's Medical College of Pennsylvania*, 31st Annual Meeting (1906): 76–78. On rhetoric leading many women doctors into restricted specialties, see Morantz-Sanchez, *Sympathy and Science*, 182–83, 266–311; Carla S. Bittel, *Mary Putnam Jacobi and the Politics of Medicine in Nineteenth Century America* (Chapel Hill: University of North Carolina Press, 2009); Ann K. Boulis and Jerry A. Jacobs, *The Changing Face of Medicine: Women Doctors and the Evolution of Health Care in America* (Ithaca, NY: ILR Press, 2008); and Ellen S. More, Elizabeth Fee, and Manon Parry, eds., *Women Physicians and the Cultures of Medicine* (Baltimore: Johns Hopkins University Press, 2009).

62. Helen Murphy, "The City of Philadelphia," *Transactions of the Alumnae Association of the Woman's Medical College of Pennsylvania*, Twenty-fifth Annual Meeting (1900): 147–49.

63. The mean number of positions held by women doctors and men doctors were 1.13 and 0.95 per doctor, respectively. When compared by Student's t-test, these means were statistically indistinguishable ($p > .05$). Data not shown. See the appendix of this book for details. Similar percentages of women and men doctors held positions—47 percent and 41 percent respectively (see table 4).

64. See chapters 2 and 3 in this book for further discussion. For comparisons to women doctors today, see Boulis and Jacobs, *The Changing Face of Medicine*.

65. McBride, *Integrating the City of Medicine*. Isabella Vandervall, "Some Problems of the Colored Woman Physician" *Woman's Medical Journal* 27 (1917): 156–58. Lauran Kerr-Healy, "Race, Gender, and African American Women Doctors in the Twentieth Century" (PhD diss., University of Houston, 2010). University of Houston Center for Public History and the Houston Medical Forum, "To Bear Fruit for Our Race: A History of African-Americans in Houston," http://www.history.uh.edu/cph/tobearfruit/index.htm.

66. McBride, *Integrating the City of Medicine*.

67. Ibid. W.E.B. Du Bois, *The Philadelphia Negro: A Social Study* (1899; repr. Philadelphia: University of Pennsylvania Press, 1996). Joel D. Howell and Catherine G. McLaughlin, "Race, Income, and the Purchase of Medical Care by Selected 1917 Working-Class Urban Families," *Journal of the History of Medicine and Allied Sciences* 47 (1992): 439–61.

68. Edward H. Beardsley, "Making Separate, Equal: Black Physicians and the Problems of Medical Segregation in the Pre–World War II South," *BHM* (1983) 57: 382–96. Beardsley, *A History of Neglect: Health Care for Blacks and Mill Workers in the Twentieth-Century South* (Knoxville: University of Tennessee Press, 1987). Savitt, *Race and Medicine*, 269–94. Lynn Marie Pohl, "Long Waits, Small Spaces, and Compassionate Care: Memories of Race and Medicine in a Mid-Twentieth-Century Southern Community," *BHM* 74, no. 1 (2000): 107–37. Thomas J. Ward Jr., *Black Physicians in the Jim Crow South* (Fayetteville: University of Arkansas Press, 2003), 239–64. Kerr-Healy, "Race, Gender, and African American Women Doctors."

69. McBride, *Integrating the City of Medicine*, esp. 3–55. Samuel K. Roberts, *Infectious Fear: Politics, Disease, and the Health Effects of Segregation* (Chapel Hill: University of North Carolina Press, 2009). Savitt, *Race and Medicine*, 252–66.

70. J. Torrance Rugh, "The Resident Physician and the Hospital," *The Jeffersonian* 8, no. 58 (1906): 158–66. O'Hara, *An Emerging Profession*, 295–327.

71. See chapter 2 in this book for further discussion.

2. The Doctor as Business Owner

1. John B. Roberts, "The Doctor's Fee—A Plea for Honorable Dealing," *Proceedings of the Philadelphia County Medical Society* 22 (1901): 168–69.

2. Samuel Hopkins Adams, "The Vanishing Country Doctor," *Ladies' Home Journal* 40, no. 10 (1923): 23, 178, 180; Adams, "Why the Doctor Left," *Ladies' Home Journal* 40, no. 11 (1923): 26, 218–19; Theodore Dreiser, "The Country Doctor," *Harper's Monthly Magazine* 137 (July 1918): 193–202.

3. "The Physicians' Home—the First Medical Hearthstone in America," *Medical Journal and Record* 122 (August 4, 1925): 171. See also John A. Lapp, "David A. Mountain Home for Aged Physicians: A Project for the Care of Those Grown Old in the Service of Their Fellowmen," *The Nation's Health* 4, no. 6 (1922): 380–81. On the Philadelphia home, see "Aged Physicians' Home to Come" *WR* 8, no. 20 (1913): 8; "Planning for the 'Home,'" *WR* 8, no. 21 (1913): 1; "Home for Aged Doctors in Prospect," *WR* 8, no. 22 (1913): 7; Meyer Solis-Cohen, "The Work of the Aid Association of the Philadelphia County Medical Society," *WR* 27, no. 41 (1932): 23–24; and Charles Sinker, "A Different Picture of Doctor," *WR* 27, no. 41 (1932): 19, 21.

4. D. W. Cathell, *Book on the Physician Himself and Things That Concern His Reputation and Success*, twentieth century ed. (Philadelphia: F. A. Davis Company, 1911), 1.

5. For an overview, see Mark S. R. Jenner and P. Wallis, "The Medical Marketplace," in *Medicine and the Market in England and Its Colonies, c. 1450–1850*, ed. Mark S. R. Jenner and Patrick Wallis (New York: Palgrave Macmillan, 2007), 1–23.

6. On early modern Europe, see Harold Cook in *The Decline of the Old Medical Regime in Stuart London* (Ithaca, NY: Cornell University Press, 1986); Margaret Pelling, "Medical Practice in Early Modern England: Trade or Profession?" in *The Professions in Early Modern England*, ed. Wilfrid Prest (London: Croom Helm, 1987), 90–128; Dorothy Porter and Roy Porter, *Patient's Progress: Doctors and Doctoring in Eighteenth-Century England* (Stanford, CA: Stanford University Press, 1989). On early America, see Edward C. Atwater, "The Medical Profession in a New Society,

Rochester, New York (1811–60)," *BHM* 47, no. 3 (1973): 221–35; Lisa Rosner, "Thistle on the Delaware: Edinburgh Medical Education and Philadelphia Practice, 1800–
1825," *Social History of Medicine* 5 (1992): 19–42; and George Rosen, *The Structure
of American Medical Practice, 1875–1941*, ed. Charles E. Rosenberg (Philadelphia:
University of Pennsylvania Press, 1983), 19–25.

7. Jenner and Wallis, "The Medical Marketplace," 7–16.

8. Paul Starr, *The Social Transformation of American Medicine* (New York: Basic
Books, 1982). Rosen, *The Structure of American Medical Practice.*

9. James G. Burrow, *Organized Medicine in the Progressive Era: The Move towards
Monopoly* (Baltimore: Johns Hopkins University Press, 1977). Gerald E. Markowitz
and David Rosner, "Doctors in Crisis: Medical Education and Medical Reform dur-
ing the Progressive Era, 1895–1915," in *Health Care in America: Essays in Social
History*, ed. Susan Reverby and David Rosner (Philadelphia: Temple University
Press, 1979), 185–205.

10. Two studies of individual doctors have answered these questions: Charles E. Rosenberg, "Making It in Urban Medicine: A Career in the Age of Scientific Medicine,"
BHM 64 (1990): 163–86, and Christopher Crenner, *Private Practice: In the Early
Twentieth-Century Medical Office of Doctor Richard Cabot* (Baltimore: Johns Hopkins University Press, 2005), 30–70.

11. Hans Ulrich Deppe, "The Nature of Health Care: Commodification versus Solidar-
ity," in "Morbid Symptoms: Health Under Capitalism," ed. Leo Panitch and Colin
Leys, *Socialist Register* 46 (2010): 29–38.

12. David J. Rothman, *Strangers at the Bedside: A History of How Law and Bioethics Transformed Medical Decision Making* (New York: Basic Books, 1991), 101–47. Christopher
Crenner, "Professional Measurement: Quantifying Health and Disease in American
Medical Practice, 1880–1920" (PhD diss., Harvard University, 1993). Olga Amsterdam-
ska and Anja Hiddinga, "The Analyzed Body," in *Medicine in the Twentieth Century*,
ed. Roger Cooter and John V. Pickstone (Amsterdam: Harwood Academic Publishers,
2000), 417–33. Nancy Tomes and Beatrix Hoffman, "Introduction: Patients as Policy
Actors," in *Patients as Policy Actors*, ed. Beatrix Hoffman, Nancy Tomes, Rachel Grob,
and Mark Schlesinger (New Brunswick, NJ: Rutgers University Press, 2011), 1–16.

13. Christopher Crenner, "Diagnosis and Authority in the Early Twentieth-Century
Medical Practice of Richard C. Cabot," *BHM* 76, no. 1 (2002): 30–55.

14. Nancy Tomes, "Patients or Health-Care Consumers? Why the History of a Contested
Term Matters," in *History and Health Policy in the United States: Putting the Past
Back In*, ed. Rosemary A. Stevens, Charles E. Rosenberg, and Lawton R. Burns (New
Brunswick, NJ: Rutgers University Press, 2006), 83–110. Einer Elhauge, "The Irrel-
evance of the Broccoli Argument against the Insurance Mandate," *New England
Journal of Medicine* 366, no. 1 (2012): e1. James B. Stewart, "How Broccoli Landed
on the Supreme Court Menu," *New York Times*, June 13, 2012. *National Federation
of Independent Business v. Sebelius*, 567 U.S. ___ (2012).

15. Alfred D. Chandler Jr., *The Visible Hand: The Managerial Revolution in American
Business* (Cambridge, MA: Belknap Press, 1977). Marc Levinson, *The Great A&P
and the Struggle for Small Business in America* (New York: Hill and Wang, 2011).

16. Arthur B. Emmons, *The Profession of Medicine: A Collection of Letters from Graduates of the Harvard Medical School* (Cambridge, MA: Harvard University Press,
1914), 81, 108.

17. See, for example, Thomas Reilly, *Building a Profitable Practice: Being a Text-Book
on Medical Economics* (Philadelphia: J. B. Lippincott, 1912), 1–7.

18. See discussion in chapter 1 of this book on the growth of hospital internships in Philadelphia. On internships nationwide, see "The Education of the Interne," *JAMA* 43, no. 7 (1904): 469–70 and "The Hospital Intern Year," *JAMA* 60, no. 25 (1913): 2017.

19. J. A. Curran, "Internships and Residencies: Historical Backgrounds and Current Trends," *Journal of Medical Education* 34, no. 9 (1959): 873–84.

20. Edith Flower Wheeler, "She Saunters Off Into Her Past," 116–17, 128, Edith Flower Wheeler Papers, Acc x.2002.1–5, box 1, DUCOM Archives. The dollar value of room and board was estimated from what Dr. Wheeler paid to a local boarding house after she left her internship.

21. "Register of Employees, 1892 Oct. 1–1940 Jan. 1," Philadelphia Orthopaedic Hospital and Infirmary for Nervous Diseases, MS 6/0009–01, Box 7, LCPP.

22. Emmons, *The Profession of Medicine*, 71. There were no comprehensive studies of the incomes of young doctors in Philadelphia, let alone the United States as a whole, at this time.

23. Ibid.

24. Catherine MacFarlane, [Autobiography], 3, Catherine MacFarlane Papers, Acc 195, box 1, DUCOM Archives. Ellen Culver Potter, "The Slow Development of Income from Practice," Ellen Culver Potter Papers, Acc 40, box 1, folder 16—Miscellaneous, DUCOM Archives.

25. On rising tuition, see William G. Rothstein, *American Medical Schools and the Practice of Medicine* (New York: Oxford University Press, 1987), 150–52.

26. George W. Norris, "Medical Memories: An account of events and personalities that I saw and heard as a medical student at the University of Pennsylvania, 1895–1899," George W. Norris Papers, 1898–1962, collection 1826, HSP.

27. Harriet L. Hartley, "The Woman in Medicine," *The Esculapian* 2, no. 6 (1911): 4–6.

28. Philip H. Moore, "Beginning a Medical Career," *The Jeffersonian* 9, no. 74 (1908): 2–4.

29. Reilly, *Building a Profitable Practice*, 3.

30. Ibid., 7.

31. Emmons, *The Profession of Medicine*, 71.

32. MacFarlane, [Autobiography], 52. Potter, "The Slow Development of Income from Practice."

33. Reilly, *Building a Profitable Practice*, 1–2.

34. Medical Staff, "Minutes of regular and special meetings," January 13, 1901, Saint Christopher's Hospital Collection, MSS 6/0007–01, LCPP.

35. Letter to Interns, June 8, 1898, Philadelphia General Hospital Collection, MSS 6/0005–05, box 2, folder 20, LCPP.

36. Reilly, *Building a Profitable Practice*, 8.

37. An estimated 15,000 American doctors undertook postgraduate education between 1870 and 1914 in Germany alone, or 341 doctors per year: Thomas N. Bonner, *American Doctors and German Universities: A Chapter in International Intellectual Relations* (Lincoln: University of Nebraska Press, 1963). By comparison, about 13,000 doctors undertook postgraduate education in the three largest American "polyclinic" medical schools combined between 1882 and 1899, or 722 doctors per year: Steven J. Peitzman, "'Thoroughly Practical': America's Polyclinic Medical Schools," *BHM* 54 (1980): 166–87.

38. Peitzman, "'Thoroughly Practical,'" 166–87. Kenneth Ludmerer, *Learning to Heal: The Development of American Medical Education* (Baltimore: Johns Hopkins

University Press, 1985). Rothstein, *American Medical Schools and the Practice of Medicine*. George Weisz, *Divide and Conquer: A Comparative History of Specialization* (New York: Oxford University Press, 2006).

39. Reilly, *Building a Profitable Practice*, 8–9.
40. Harold F. Alderfer, "Legislative History of Medical Licensure in Pennsylvania," *PMJ* 64 (1961): 1605–09.
41. Martin E. Rehfuss, "Your First Patient," 1–2, Martin E. Rehfuss Collection, MS 30, box 2, [Speech Transcripts], TJU Archives.
42. D. W. Cathell, *Book on the Physician Himself and Things That Concern His Reputation and Success* (Philadelphia: F. A. Davis Company, 1913), 3.
43. C. R. Mabee, *The Physician's Business and Financial Adviser*, 4th ed. (Cleveland: Continental Publishing Company, 1900), 93.
44. Reilly *Building a Profitable Practice*, 30.
45. Moore, "Beginning a Medical Career," 2.
46. Reilly *Building a Profitable Practice*, 26–27. See also Joseph McDowell Matthews, *How to Succeed in the Practice of Medicine* (Philadelphia: W. B. Saunders, 1905), 28–31, and Cathell, *Book on the Physician Himself* (1913), 4–7.
47. Mabee, *The Physician's Business*, 79.
48. Of the 664 Philadelphia doctors in the *AMD* (1909) sample, the educational backgrounds of 650 were ascertainable. Of these, 588 were alumni of Philadelphia medical schools (90.5 percent). See the appendix of this book for details. Some Philadelphia medical school faculty advised graduates to leave the city: Ella B. Everitt, "Timely Suggestions to the Recent Graduate," *The Iatrian* 3, no. 8 (1912): 3–6.
49. Rosen, *The Structure of American Medical Practice*. Irvine Loudon, "The Concept of the Family Doctor," *BHM* 58 (1984): 347–62. Crenner, *Private Practice*, 30–70. Neil Larry Shumsky, James Bohland, and Paul Knox, "Separating Doctors' Homes and Doctors' Offices: San Francisco, 1881–1941," *Social Science and Medicine* 23, no. 10 (1986): 1051–57.
50. Rosen, *The Structure of American Medical Practice*, 25–32.
51. Reilly, *Building a Profitable Practice*, 32.
52. Ibid., 33–34.
53. Howard A. Kelley, "Success in Life," *The Jeffersonian* 8, no. 64 (1907): 86–98.
54. "Doctor's Office for Rent," *WR* 10, no. 25 (1915): 19.
55. Reilly *Building a Profitable Practice*, 68.
56. Listed under the section for "Practices for Sale" in *WR* 10, no. 7 (1914): 23.
57. Reilly *Building a Profitable Practice*, 68–69.
58. Rita S. Finkler, "Good Morning Doctor!" 90–93, R154.F5, DUCOM Archives.
59. Reilly *Building a Profitable Practice*, 32. "A List of Practical Instruments and Necessary Medicines Selected for the Young Practitioner by Professors of Jefferson Medical College," *The Jeffersonian* 5, no. 33 (1903): 3–5.
60. Moore, "Beginning a Medical Career," 2.
61. Excerpted as "Saving Doctors," in *The Jeffersonian* 16, no. 124 (1914): 17.
62. Hartley, "The Woman in Medicine," 4.
63. Ibid., 4–5.
64. MacFarlane, [Autobiography], 36.
65. Ibid., 36.
66. Ibid.
67. Ibid., 37–38.
68. Ibid., 52.

69. This text quoted from the 1903 AMA Code of Ethics, but was contained, nearly verbatim, in the 1912 version as well. Reprinted in Robert B. Baker et al., eds., *The American Medical Ethics Revolution: How the AMA's Code of Ethics Has Transformed Physicians' Relationships to Patients, Professionals, and Society* (Baltimore: Johns Hopkins University Press, 1999), 335–54. See also John Harley Warner, "Ideals of Science and Their Discontents in Late Nineteenth-Century American Medicine," *Isis* 82 (1991): 454–78.

70. Albert V, Harmon, *Large Fees and How to Get Them: A Book for the Private Use of Physicians* (Chicago: W. J. Jackman, 1911), 61–71.

71. Ibid., 67.

72. Reilly *Building a Profitable Practice*, 70. Steven M. Stowe, *Doctoring the South: Southern Physicians and Everyday Medicine in the Nineteenth Century* (Chapel Hill: University of North Carolina Press, 2004), 88–90. On the market value of laboratory diagnosis skills for young doctors in the early twentieth century, see Crenner, *Private Practice.*

73. MacFarlane, [Autobiography], 37.

74. Rehfuss, "Your First Patient," 2.

75. Reilly, *Building a Profitable Practice*, 49.

76. Ibid., 49–67.

77. Rosenberg, "Making It in Urban Medicine," 164.

78. MacFarlane, [Autobiography], 37–38.

79. See, for example: Rehfuss, "Your First Patient," 2; Moore, "Beginning a Medical Career," 2–4; Hartley, "The Woman in Medicine," 4–6; Kelley, "Success in Life," 86–98; and John B. Roberts, "Some Causes of Inefficiency in Medical Practice," *PMJ* 10, no. 2 (1906): 91–93. See also Crenner, "Diagnosis and Authority."

80. MacFarlane, [Autobiography], 37–59.

81. Ibid., 52.

82. Mabee, *The Physician's Business*, 93.

83. Hartley, "The Woman in Medicine," 4–6.

84. Edwin B. Cragin, "Specialism in Medicine," *The Jeffersonian* 13, no. 100 (1911): 2–9.

85. Crenner, *Private Practice*, 49–62.

86. MacFarlane, [Autobiography], 52.

87. Data compiled by Rothstein, *American Medical Schools and the Practice of Medicine*, 143.

88. U.S. Bureau of the Census, *Twelfth Census of Population: 1900*, Special Reports, "Occupations" (Washington, DC: U.S. G.P.O., 1904), 672, 676. U.S. Bureau of the Census, *Fourteenth Census of Population: 1920*, vol. 4, "Occupations" (Washington, DC: U.S. G.P.O., 1923), 218. U.S. Bureau of the Census, *Fourteenth Census: 1920*, vol. 1, "Population" (Washington, DC: U.S. G.P.O., 1921), 69. U.S. Bureau of the Census, *Twelfth Census: 1900*, vol. 1, part 1, "Population" (Washington, DC: U.S. Census Office, 1901), lxix.

89. Norman Gevitz, ed., *Other Healers: Unorthodox Medicine in America* (Baltimore: Johns Hopkins University Press, 1988). James C. Wharton, *Nature Cures: The History of Alternative Medicine in America* (New York: Oxford University Press, 2002), 1–130.

90. Robert H. Wiebe, *The Search for Order, 1877–1920* (New York: Hill and Wang, 1967). Burrow, *Organized Medicine in the Progressive Era.* Starr, *The Social Transformation of American Medicine.* Barbara G. Rosenkrantz, "The Search for Professional Order in Nineteenth-Century American Medicine," in *Sickness and Health in America: Readings in the History of Medicine and Public Health*, ed. Judith W. Leavitt and Ronald Numbers, 2nd ed. (Madison: University of Wisconsin Press, 1985), 219–32.

91. Samuel Baker, "Physician Licensure Laws in the United States, 1865–1915," *Journal of the History of Medicine and Allied Sciences* 39 (1984): 173–97. Pennsylvania had separate boards for homeopaths and for Eclectic doctors until 1911: Alderfer, "Legislative History of Medical Licensure in Pennsylvania," 1605–09.

92. Naomi Rogers, *An Alternative Path: The Making and Remaking of Hahnemann Medical College and Hospital of Philadelphia* (New Brunswick, NJ: Rutgers University Press, 1998). Norman Gevitz, *The D.O.'s: Osteopathic Medicine in America* (Baltimore: Johns Hopkins University Press, 1982).

93. I thank Christopher Crenner for this insight.

94. Mabee, *The Physician's Business*, 188.

95. Ibid., 188–218; Harmon, *Large Fees and How to Get Them*, 141–78; Matthews, *How to Succeed in the Practice of Medicine*, 109–29; Reilly, *Building a Profitable Practice*, 138–62; and Cathell, *Book on the Physician Himself* (1913), 327–64.

96. Reilly, *Building a Profitable Practice*, 146–49.

97. Thomas R. Neilson to patient, July 22, 1901, Thomas R. Neilson Papers, closed stacks (Phi) Amp 5885, Ledger and Correspondence, 1901–1908, "Correspondence and Notes found in Ledger," HSP.

98. Thomas R. Neilson to patient, November 14, 1906, Neilson Papers, HSP.

99. Thomas R. Neilson to patient, March 19, 1912, Neilson Papers, HSP.

100. "Northeastern Physicians Unite for Protection," *WR* 3, no. 4 (1907): 4.

101. Thomas Goebel, "American Medicine and the 'Organizational Synthesis': Chicago Physicians and the Business of Medicine, 1900–1920," *BHM* 68 (1994): 655. On corporatism and efficiency in American business, see: Chandler, *The Visible Hand*; Louis Galambos, "The Emerging Organizational Synthesis in Modern American History," *Business History Review* 44 (1970): 279–90; Galambos, "Technology, Political Economy, and Professionalization: Central Themes of the Organizational Synthesis," *Business History Review* 57 (1983): 473–91; Galambos, "Recasting the Organizational Synthesis: Structure and Process in the Twentieth and Twenty-First Centuries," *Business History Review* 79 (2005): 1–38; and Brian Balogh, "Reorganizing the Organizational Synthesis: Federal-Professional Relations in Modern America," *Studies in American Political Development* 5 (1991): 119–72.

102. Goebel, "American Medicine and the 'Organizational Synthesis,'" 655.

103. Donald Madison, "Preserving Individualism in the Organizational Society: 'Cooperation' and American Medical Practice, 1900–1920," *BHM* 70 (1996): 442–83.

104. Ibid. Starr, *The Social Transformation of American Medicine*, 198–232. Christopher Crenner, "Organizational Reform and Professional Dissent in the Careers of Richard Cabot and Ernest Amory Codman, 1900–1920," *Journal of the History of Medicine and Allied Sciences* 56 (2001): 211–37.

105. Richard Cabot, "Better Doctoring for Less Money," *American Magazine* 81 (April 1916): 7–9, 77–78; 81 (May 1916): 43–44, 76–79.

106. Crenner, "Organizational Reform and Professional Dissent," 211–37. Starr, *The Social Transformation of American Medicine*, 209–215. Quotation from article 6, sec. 2 of the AMA's "Principles of Medical Ethics" (1912), as reprinted in *The American Medical Ethics Revolution*, 353. For Philadelphia reactions to Cabot, see "Cabot's Attack on the Profession—What Will Philadelphia Physicians Do About It?" *WR* 11, no. 39 (1916): 2.

107. Donald L. Madison and Thomas R. Konrad, "Large Medical Group-Practice Organizations and Employed Physicians: A Relationship in Transition," *Milbank Quarterly* 66, no. 2 (1988): 240–82.

108. Madison, "Preserving Individualism in the Organizational Society," 480–81. Madison overlooked hospitals as sites of early corporatism in medical practice. See Edward T. Morman, introduction to *Efficiency, Scientific Management, and Hospital Standardization*, ed. Edward T. Morman (New York: Garland, 1989).

109. George Rosen, *Fees and Fee Bills: Some Economic Aspects of Medical Practice in Nineteenth Century America*, supplement no. 6 to the *BHM* (Baltimore: Johns Hopkins University Press, 1946). Burrow, *Organized Medicine in the Progressive Era*, 106–10.

110. "Physicians' Business Association Makes Headway," *WR* 12, no. 32 (1917): 6. Rosen, *Fees and Fee Bills*, 12–13.

111. "Why Join the Physicians' Business Association?" *WR* 12, no. 33 (1917): 9. See also "Philadelphia Physicians Organize for Betterment," *WR* 12, no. 31 (1917): 1; "Physicians' Business Association Makes Headway," 6; and "Physicians' Protective Association," *WR* 15, no. 12 (1919): 25.

112. David T. Beito, "The 'Lodge Practice Evil' Reconsidered: Medical Care Through Fraternal Societies, 1900–1930," *Journal of Urban History* 23, no. 5 (1997): 569–600, esp. 571–72.

113. Mabee, *The Physician's Business*, 200.

114. Starr, *The Social Transformation of American Medicine*, 200–209. Rosen, *The Structure of American Medical Practice*, 98–108.

115. "The 'Lodge Practice' Evil," *WR* 1, no. 3 (1905): 5.

116. Reilly, *Building a Profitable Practice*, 64–65.

117. "Young Men in the County Society," *WR* 9, no. 4 (1913): 2. See remarks by Dr. Gertrude A. Walker in Roberts, "The Doctor's Fee—A Plea for Honorable Dealing," 182.

118. Charles E. Rosenberg, "Social Class and Medical Care in Nineteenth-Century America: The Rise and Fall of the Dispensary," in *Sickness and Health in America*, 2nd ed. (see note 90), 273–86. "The Question of Medical Charities," *Medical News* (Nov. 28, 1903): 1041–43.

119. Rosenberg, "Social Class and Medical Care," 273–86.

120. David Rosner, *A Once Charitable Enterprise: Hospitals and Health Care in Brooklyn and New York, 1885–1915* (Cambridge: Cambridge University Press, 1982), 146–163. Gert Brieger, "The Use and Abuse of Medical Charities in Late Nineteenth-Century America," *American Journal of Public Health* 67, no. 3 (1977): 264–267. David Rosner, "Health Care for the 'Truly Needy': Nineteenth-Century Origins of the Concept," *Milbank Memorial Fund Quarterly/Health and Society* 60, no. 3 (1982): 355–85.

121. "The Question of Medical Charities," 1041–43. Leo J. O'Hara, *An Emerging Profession: Philadelphia Doctors, 1860–1900* (New York: Garland, 1989), esp. 329–31.

122. "Philadelphia Investigates Its Hospitals," *The Modern Hospital* 3 (December 1904): 388–90. For an example of one hospital's internal investigation, see "Minutes of the Hospital Committee of the Board of Managers of Jefferson Hospital," June 1, 1911, June 24, 1912, December 15, 1913, June 15, 1914, January 17, 1916, and February 14, 1916, TJU Archives. See also Thomas McCrae, "Dispensary Abuse Study at Jefferson Hospital," *WR* 11, no. 27 (1916): 5.

123. G. A. Kleene, "The Problem of Medical Charity," *Annals of the American Academy of Political and Social Science* 23 (May 1904): 1–15. Rosenberg, "Social Class and Medical Care," 273–86.

124. E. E. Montgomery, "Attend County Meeting on Doctor's Incomes," *WR* 11, no. 18 (1916): 2. See similar discussions in "How Practice Lessens Here," *WR* 6, no. 20 (1911): 9, and "Medicine's Earnings," *The Jeffersonian* 9, no. 69 (1907): 9. In actuality, the typhoid fever mortality declined dramatically at this time: Gretchen A. Condran,

Henry Williams, and Rose A. Cheney, "The Decline in Mortality in Philadelphia from 1870 to 1930: The Role of Municipal Services," in *Sickness and Health in America: Readings in the History of Medicine and Public Health*, ed. Judith W. Leavitt and Ronald Numbers, 3rd ed. (Madison: University of Wisconsin Press, 1997), 452–566.

125. "General Practitioner's Fees Small," *WR* 6, no. 9 (1910): 7.

126. "Don't Do It, Specialists," *WR* 6, no. 43 (1911): 3.

127. Reilly, *Building a Profitable Practice*, 243–45. For discussion in Philadelphia, see Boardman Reed, "Specialism—Its Evils and the Remedy," *PMJ* 8, no. 2 (1904): 755–77 and G. G. Davis, "The Study of Specialties," *WR* 10, no. 11 (1914): 19–21.

128. See, for example: E. E. Montgomery, "What Should the Young Graduate Know of Gynecology?" *The Jeffersonian* 6, no. 46 (1905): 103–5; "The General Practitioner in Emergencies," *WR* 10, no. 34 (1915): 10; and "When Shall the General Practitioner Treat the Eye or the Ear?" *WR* 10, no. 10 (1914): 17.

129. "The Question of Medical Charities," 1041–43.

130. "The General Practitioner," *PMJ* 4, no. 3 (1900): 223. This article was excerpted from *The Clinical Recorder*, but the editors of the *PMJ* digested it for the Pennsylvania readership.

131. "Medical Philadelphia," *Montgomery County Medical Bulletin* 1, no. 4 (1913): 51–53.

132. Beito, "The 'Lodge Practice Evil' Reconsidered," 593–94.

133. Harry Marks, "'Until the Sun of Science . . . The True Apollo of Medicine Has Risen': Collective Investigation in Britain and America, 1880–1910," *Medical History* 50 (2006): 147–66.

134. Roberts, "The Doctor's Fee," 177–78 for Dr. Taylor's comments.

135. Ibid., 180 for Dr. Lautenbach's comments.

136. Thomas Goebel, "The Uneven Rewards of Professional Labor," *Journal of Social History* 29, no. 4 (1996): 749–77; Madison, "Preserving Individualism in the Organizational Society," 442–83; and Crenner, "Organizational Reform and Professional Dissent," 211–07.

3. Downtown Specialists and Neighborhood GPs

1. Catharine MacFarlane, [Autobiography], 20–40, 52–59, Catherine MacFarlane Papers, Acc 195, box 1, DUCOM Archives.

2. Daniel W. Cathell, *The Physician Himself and Things That Concern His Reputation and Success*, 12th ed. (Philadelphia: F.A. Davis Company, 1913), 3–4.

3. I borrow the term "location behavior" from early studies of the distribution of doctor's offices conducted by economists in the 1930s–1950s and geographers in the 1970s. Doctors' location behavior—or the observed distribution of doctor's offices—did not necessarily conform to career and business advice.

4. Lewis Mayers and Leonard V. Harrison, *The Distribution of Physicians in the United States* (Chicago: General Education Board, 1924), 3–39. Raymond Pearl, "Distribution of Physicians in the United States," *JAMA* 84, no. 14 (1925): 1024–25. George Rosen, *The Structure of American Medical Practice, 1875–1941*, ed. Charles E. Rosenberg (Philadelphia: University of Pennsylvania Press, 1982), 25–36, 53–61. Paul Starr, *The Social Transformation of American Medicine* (New York: Basic Books, 1982), 60–78.

5. George Rosen, *The Specialization of Medicine with Particular Reference to Ophthalmology* (New York: Froben Press, 1944). Rosen, "Whither Specialization," in *Medicine and Society: Contemporary Medical Problems in Historical Perspective*, no. 4 (Philadelphia:

American Philosophical Library, 1971), 196–219. George Weisz, "Mapping Medical Specialization in Paris in the Nineteenth and Twentieth Centuries," *Social History of Medicine* 7, no. 2 (1994): 177–211. Weisz, *Divide and Conquer: A Comparative History of Medical Specialization* (New York: Oxford University Press, 2006), 63–83.

6. C. R. Mabee, *The Physician's Business and Financial Adviser*, 4th ed. (Cleveland: Continental Publishing, 1900), 93. Thomas Reilly, *Building a Profitable Practice: Being a Text-Book on Medical Economics* (Philadelphia: J. B. Lippincott, 1912), 30. Philip H. Moore, "Beginning a Medical Career," *The Jeffersonian* 9, no. 74 (1908): 2.

7. Paul L. Knox, James Bohland, and Neil Larry Shumsky, "The Urban Transition and the Evolution of the Medical Care Delivery System in America," *Social Science and Medicine* 17 (1983): 37–43.

8. David Rosner, *A Once Charitable Enterprise: Hospitals and Health Care in Brooklyn and New York, 1885–1915* (Princeton, NJ: Princeton University Press, 1982), 13–35. Rosen, *The Structure of American Medical Practice*, 25–36, 53–60. Neil Larry Shumsky, James Bohland, and Paul Knox, "Separating Doctors' Homes and Doctors' Offices: San Francisco, 1881–1941," *Social Science and Medicine* 23, no. 10 (1986): 1051–57. Paul F. Mattingly, "The Changing Location of Physician Offices in Bloomington-Normal, Illinois: 1870–1988," *Professional Geographer* 43, no. 4 (1991): 465–74. See also Anne Marie Adams and Stacie Burke, "A Doctor in the House: The Architecture of Home-Offices for Physicians in Toronto, 1885–1930," *Medical History* 52, no. 2 (2008): 163–94.

9. U.S. Bureau of the Census, *Twelfth Census of the United States, 1900* (Washington, DC: United States Census Office, 1901), vol. 1, pt. 1: *Population*, table 22, lxix. U.S. Bureau of the Census, *Thirteenth Census of the United States, 1910* (Washington, DC: U.S. G.P.O., 1913), vol. 3, *Population*, 527. U.S. Bureau of the Census, *Fourteenth Census of the United States, 1920* (Washington, DC: U.S. G.P.O., 1921), vol. 1, *Population*, table 40, 64.

10. Ibid. and Nathaniel Burt and Wallace E. Davies, "The Iron Age, 1876–1905," in *Philadelphia: A 300-Year History*, ed. Russell F. Weigley (New York: W. W. Norton, 1982), 471–523. U.S. Dept. of Commerce and Labor, Bureau of Statistics, *Statistical Abstract of the United States, 1904* (Washington, DC: U.S. G.P.O., 1905), no. 27, 427–28. U.S. Dept. of Commerce, Bureau of Foreign and Domestic Commerce, *Statistical Abstract of the United States* (Washington, DC: U.S. G.P.O., 1917), no. 39, 111. U.S. Bureau of the Census, *Thirteenth Census of the United States, 1910* (Washington, DC: U.S. G.P.O., 1913), vol. 3, *Population*, table 5, 605.

11. Allen F. Davis and Mark H. Haller, eds., *The Peoples of Philadelphia: A History of Ethnic Groups and Lower-class Life, 1790–1940* (Philadelphia: Temple University Press, 1973). William W. Cutler III and Howard Gillette Jr., eds., *The Divided Metropolis: Social and Spatial Dimensions of Philadelphia, 1800–1945* (Westport, CT: Greenwood Press, 1980). Sam Bass Warner Jr., *The Private City: Philadelphia in Three Periods of Its Growth*, 2nd ed. (Philadelphia: University of Pennsylvania Press, 1987).

12. U.S. Bureau of the Census, *Thirteenth Census of the United States, 1910* (Washington, DC: U.S. G.P.O., 1913), vol. 8, *Manufactures*, table 1, 84.

13. W.E.B. Du Bois, *The Philadelphia Negro: A Social Study* (1899; repr. Philadelphia: University of Pennsylvania Press, 1996), 97–146 (quote 111). Isabel Eaton, "Special Report on Negro Domestic Service in the Seventh Ward, Philadelphia," in *The Philadelphia Negro* (see above), 427–509. On immigrants, see Caroline Golab, "The Immigrant and the City: Poles, Italians, and Jews in Philadelphia, 1870–1920," and Maxwell Whiteman, "Philadelphia's Jewish Neighborhoods," in *The Peoples of*

Philadelphia (see note 11), 203–30, 231–54; Burt and Davies, "The Iron Age," 471–523; Lloyd Abernathy, "Progressivism," in *Philadelphia: A 300-Year History* (see note 10), 524–65; and Theodore Hershberg et al., "A Tale of Three Cities: Blacks, Immigrants, and Opportunity, 1850–1880, 1930, 1970," in *Philadelphia: Work, Space, Family, and Group Experience in the Nineteenth Century: Essays Toward an Interdisciplinary History of the City*, ed. Theodore Hershberg (New York: Oxford University Press, 1981), 461–91.

14. Warner, *The Private City.* Hershberg et al., "A Tale of Three Cities," 461–91. Janet Rothenberg Pack, "Urban Spatial Transformation: Philadelphia 1850 to 1880, Heterogeneity to Homogeneity?" *Social Science History* 8, no. 4 (1984): 435–54. Stuart Blumin, *The Emergence of the Middle Class: Social Experience in the American City, 1760–1900* (Cambridge: Cambridge University Press, 1989).

15. Lisa Rosner, "Thistle on the Delaware: Edinburgh Medical Education and Philadelphia Practice, 1800–1825," *Social History of Medicine* 5, no. 1 (1992): 31–32, 39–40.

16. Hershberg et al., "A Tale of Three Cities," 461–91. I borrow Hershberg's term "opportunity structure," which refers to the total opportunities for habitation, employment, education, and recreation at a given point in time. These opportunities are unequally distributed across space and social groups, giving the opportunity structure an "ecological" form.

17. Philip Scranton, *Figured Tapestry: Production, Markets, and Power in Philadelphia Textiles, 1885–1941* (Cambridge: Cambridge University Press, 1989). Stephanie W. Greenberg, "The Relationship between Work and Residence in an Industrializing City: Philadelphia, 1880," in *The Divided Metropolis* (see note 11), 141–68. Warner, *The Private City.*

18. Du Bois, *The Philadelphia Negro.* Warner, *The Private City.*

19. Greenberg, "The Relationship between Work and Residence," 141–68. Greenberg, "Industrial Location and Ethnic Residential Patterns in an Industrializing City: Philadelphia, 1880," in *Philadelphia: Work, Space, Family, and Group Experience* (see note 13), 204–232. Greenberg, "Neighborhood Change, Racial Transition, and Work Location: A Case Study of an Industrial City, Philadelphia, 1880–1930," *Journal of Urban History* 7, no. 3 (1981): 267–314. John H. Hepp, IV, "'Such a Well-Behaved Train Station:' Evolving Spatial Patterns at Philadelphia's Late Victorian Central Passenger Depots, 1876–1901," *Pennsylvania History* 70, no. 1 (2003): 1–27.

20. Jeffrey P. Roberts, "Railroads and the Downtown: Philadelphia, 1830–1900," and Margaret S. Marsh, "The Impact of the Market Street 'El' on Northern West Philadelphia: Environmental Change and Social Transformation, 1900–1930," in *The Divided Metropolis* (see note 11), 27–55, 169–92. Hepp, "'Such a Well-Behaved Train Station,'" 1–27.

21. Kenneth T. Jackson, *Crabgrass Frontier: The Suburbanization of the United States* (New York: Oxford University Press, 1985). Margaret S. Marsh, "Suburbanization and the Search for Community: Residential Decentralization in Philadelphia, 1800–1900," *Pennsylvania History* 44 (1977): 99–116. Gary R. Hovinen, "Suburbanization in Greater Philadelphia," *Journal of Historical Geography* 11, no. 2 (1985): 174–95. John Henry Hepp IV, *The Middle-class City: Transforming Time and Space in Philadelphia, 1876–1926* (Philadelphia: University of Pennsylvania Press, 2003).

22. DuBois, *The Philadelphia Negro.* The Octavia Hill Association, "Certain Aspects of the Housing Problem in Philadelphia," *Annals of the American Academy of Political and Social Science* 20 (1902): 111–20. Emily Wayland Dinwiddie, "Some Aspects of Italian Housing and Social Conditions in Philadelphia," *Charities (and*

the Commons) 12 (1904): 490–93. Dinwiddie, "Housing Conditions in Philadelphia," *Charities (and the Commons)* 14 (1905): 631–38. John F. Sutherland, "Housing the Poor in the City of Homes: Philadelphia at the Turn of the Century," in *The Peoples of Philadelphia* (see note 11), 175–201.

23. Colin Gordon, *Mapping Decline: St. Louis and the Fate of the American City* (Philadelphia: University of Pennsylvania Press, 2008). Michael Davis, *City of Quartz: Excavating the Future of Los Angeles* (New York: Vintage Books, 1990).

24. Warner, *The Private City*, 185–93. Roberts, "Railroads and the Downtown," 27–55. Hepp, *The Middle-class City.* Jerome P. Bjelopera, *City of Clerks: Office and Sales Workers in Philadelphia, 1870–1920* (Urbana: University of Illinois Press, 2005). On domestic service, see Du Bois, *The Philadelphia Negro*, 97–141; Eaton, "Special Report on Negro Domestic Service"; and Dennis Clark, " 'Ramcat' and Rittenhouse Square: Related Communities," in *The Divided Metropolis* (see note 11), 125–40.

25. Warner, *The Private City*, 183–185. Golab, "The Immigrant and the City," 203–30. Whiteman, "Philadelphia's Jewish Neighborhoods," 231–54. Richard N. Juliani, *The Social Organization of Immigration: The Italians in Philadelphia* (New York: Arno Press, 1980). Stefano Luconi, *From Paesani to White Ethnics: The Italian Experience in Philadelphia* (Albany: State University of New York Press, 2001), 17–38. Octavia Hill Association, "Certain Aspects of the Housing Problem in Philadelphia," 111–20. Dinwiddie, "Some Aspects of Italian Housing and Social Conditions in Philadelphia," 490–93. Dinwiddie, "Housing Conditions in Philadelphia," 631–38. Sutherland, "Housing the Poor in the City of Homes," 175–201. Jeffrey P. Brosco, "Tales of Medicine and Poverty: Child Health in South Philadelphia, 1910–1930," *Current Problems in Pediatrics* 27 (1997): 196–212.

26. Warner, *The Private City*, 178–83.

27. Ibid., 194–97. Marsh, "Suburbanization and the Search for Community," 99–116. Marsh, "The Impact of the Market Street 'El,'" 169–92. Anne E. Krulikowski, "'Farms Don't Pay': The Transformation of the Philadelphia Metropolitan Landscape, 1880–1930," *Pennsylvania History* 72, no. 2 (2005): 194–227.

28. Warner, *The Private City*, 197–200. Meredith Savery, "Instability and Uniformity: Residential Patterns in Two Philadelphia Neighborhoods, 1880–1970," in *The Divided Metropolis* (see note 11), 193–226. Robert Fishman, *Bourgeois Utopias: The Rise and Fall of Suburbia* (New York: Basic Books, 1987), 134–54. David R. Contosta, *Suburb in the City: Chestnut Hill, Philadelphia, 1850–1990* (Columbus: Ohio State University Press, 1992).

29. Warner, *The Private City*, 161–223. William W. Cutler III, "The Persistent Dualism: Centralization and Decentralization in Philadelphia, 1854–1975," in *The Divided Metropolis* (see note 11), 249–84.

30. U.S. Bureau of the Census, *Twelfth Census of the United States, 1900* (Washington, DC: U.S. G.P.O., 1904), Special Reports, *Occupations*, table 43, 672, 676; U.S. Bureau of the Census, *Thirteenth Census of the United States, 1910* (Washington, DC: U.S. G.P.O., 1914), vol. 4, *Population*, table 3, 193; and U.S. Bureau of the Census, *Fourteenth Census of the United States, 1920* (Washington, DC: U.S. G.P.O., 1923), vol. 4, *Population*, table 19, 218. See the appendix for discussion.

31. Cathell, *The Physician Himself*, 4. See also Joseph McDowell Matthews, *How to Succeed in the Practice of Medicine* (Philadelphia: W. B. Saunders, 1905), 23, and Mabee, *The Physician's Business and Financial Adviser*, 91.

32. Data based on a 20 percent skip-interval sample of all listed doctors for Philadelphia, Pennsylvania, in the *AMD* (Chicago: AMA Press, 1909). See the appendix for

details on the sample. Of the 664 Philadelphia doctors sampled, 632 were in active practice and there were 724 practice addresses (some doctors had more than one practice address). 701 of these practices were able to be ward coded. The number of practices in any given ward was extrapolated from the sample number by multiplying by five. For example, the ninth ward had 34 practices in the sample, or 170 when extrapolated. Practice concentrations were calculated using ward-level population data in the federal census. For example, the ninth was had 170 practices per 5,071 residents, or a concentration of 3,352 private practices per 100,000 residents. This does not mean that the ninth ward had 3,352 practices or 100,000 residents. Rather, the calculation of practice concentration simply permits comparison across wards of different residential sizes.

33. Cathell, *The Physician Himself*, 6–7.
34. Mabee, *The Physician's Business*, 91–93, Reilly, *Building a Profitable Practice*, 33–34.
35. "What Doctors Want," *WR* 10, no. 23 (1915): 15.
36. Shumsky et al., "Separating Doctors' Homes and Doctors' Offices," 1051–57. Adams and Burke, "A Doctor in the House," 163–94.
37. "Central Offices for Physicians," *WR* 11, no. 5 (1915): 3.
38. "All Doctors Wishing Offices," *WR* 10, no. 23 (1915): 15.
39. Du Bois, *The Philadelphia Negro*, 287–309. Octavia Hill Association, "Certain Aspects of the Housing Problem in Philadelphia," 111–20. Eaton, "Special Report on Negro Domestic Service," 444–55.
40. Data not shown. See the appendix for details on the sample.
41. See analysis by Joel D. Howell and Catherine G. McLaughlin, "Race, Income, and the Purchase of Medical Care by Selected 1917 Working Class Urban Families," *Journal of the History of Medicine and Allied Sciences* 47 (1992): 439–61.
42. See table 5. Cathell, *The Physician Himself*, 6–7.
43. Edith Flower Wheeler, "She Saunters Off into Her Past," 119–22, Edith Flower Wheeler Papers, Acc x.2002.2.1–5, box 1, DUCOM Archives.
44. Steven J. Peitzman, *A New and Untried Course. Woman's Medical College and the Medical College of Pennsylvania, 1850–1998* (New Brunswick, NJ: Rutgers University Press, 2000), 66. Christine Stansell, *City of Women: Sex and Class in New York, 1789–1860* (Chicago: University of Illinois Press, 1987).
45. Wheeler, "She Saunters Off into Her Past," 127.
46. Cathell, *The Physician Himself*, 5.
47. Mabee, *The Physician's Business and Financial Adviser*, 82.
48. Reilly, *Building a Profitable Practice*, 31–32.
49. Mabee, *The Physician's Business and Financial Adviser*, 91–92.
50. Reilly, *Building a Profitable Practice*, 139.
51. On expected fees in Manayunk versus elsewhere, see "Physicians' Business Association Makes Headway," *WR* 12, no. 32 (1917): 6 and Dr. E.J.G. Beardsley, "A Doctor of the Old School," *WR* 18, no. 41 (1923): 15, 17, 19; 18, no. 42 (1923): 9, 11, 13, 15.
52. Shumsky et al., "Separating Doctors' Homes and Doctors' Offices," 1051–57. Adams and Burke, "A Doctor in the House," 163–194. Mattingly, "The Changing Location of Physician Offices," 465–74.
53. Rosner, *A Once Charitable Enterprise*, 13–35.
54. Of the 664 Philadelphia doctors in the 20-percent sample from the *AMD* (1909), the educational history of 650 were given. Of these 650 Philadelphia doctors, 588 (or 90 percent) had earned their medical degree in Philadelphia. See the appendix for details on the sample.

55. One can see immediate evidence of this in *WR* by comparing the titles of papers given at the weekly meetings of local medical associations versus those given before the PCMS. On the community and neighborhood organization of health care in the pre-industrial city, see Rosner, *A Once Charitable Enterprise*, 13–16 and Steve Peitzman, "'The City of Medicine': Doctors and Patients in Old Philadelphia," talk at the College of Physicians of Philadelphia, September 17, 2003.

56. "Membership in the Branches," *WR* 3, no. 16 (1907): 7.

57. See the appendix for details on the *AMD* (1909) sample.

58. In 1909, Philadelphia specialists had been in practice for an average of 21.4 years, as compared to 17.7 years for GPs. Differences in the mean experience of specialists and GPs were significant when measured by Student's t-test (p < .01). Data not shown. See the appendix for details.

59. 139 of the 701 practices with determinable addresses in the *AMD* (1909) sample were located in the eighth ward or on its border streets (19.8 percent). Leo J. O'Hara suggested that Rittenhouse Square was home to Philadelphia's medical aristocracy in the late nineteenth century. See *An Emerging Profession: Philadelphia Doctors, 1860–1900* (New York: Garland, 1989), 295–327.

60. Advertisement for a "Chestnut Street" office in *WR* 10, no. 26 (1915): 15.

61. Howard A. Kelley, "Success in Life," *The Jeffersonian* 8, no. 64 (1907): 88.

62. Ella B. Everitt, "Timely Suggestions to the Recent Graduate," *The Iatrian* 3, no. 8 (1912): 3.

63. Of the 408 college fellows who resided or practiced in Philadelphia, 288 had downtown practice locations in 1910 (or 70.5 percent). Address data from the *Transactions of the College of Physicians of Philadelphia*, 3rd ser., 32 (1910): vii–xlix. In contrast, only 210 of the 664 doctors in our *AMD* (1909) sample had a practice located Downtown (31.6 percent). The College of Physicians had always been a bastion of the medical elite in Philadelphia: Whitfield J. Bell Jr., *The College of Physicians of Philadelphia: A Bicentennial History* (Canton, MA: Science History Publications, 1987), vii. See the appendix for details on the sample.

64. See "Central Offices for Physicians," 3.

65. Of 632 doctors in active practice in the *AMD* 1909 sample, 93 had two practice addresses (14.7 percent). Of these 65 had one of their two practices located Downtown (70 percent). Specialists, in particular, valued having a second address—28.2 percent of specialists, as compared to 14.7 percent of all doctors, had two practice addresses. See the appendix for details on the sample.

66. All but two of these specialists were in solo practice. See *The Professional Directory of Doctors and Druggists of Philadelphia, Including Camden and Atlantic City and Eighty Nearby Towns* (Philadelphia: Edward Trust, 1910), 151, for the names of doctors in the Professional Building. Their specializations are in the *AMD* (1909).

67. Northeast Philadelphia had the lowest rate of position-holding (23 percent). South Philadelphia had a slightly higher rate (39 percent), and the city average was 41 percent. Data not shown. See the appendix.

68. Of the 44 doctors listed in the street directory of *The Professional Directory* as having offices in the second and third wards, 33 could be found in the manuscript census for 1910. Of these, 9 were Italian-born (24.2 percent) and 10 were Russian-born Jews (30.3 percent). See the appendix for details.

69. David McBride, *Integrating the City of Medicine: Blacks in Philadelphia Health Care, 1910–1965* (Philadelphia: Temple University Press, 1989), 5–30. Of the 48 doctors listed in *The Professional Directory* as having locations in the thirtieth ward, 39

could be found in the manuscript census for 1910. Of these, 10 were listed as "black or Negro" or "mulatto" (25.6 percent). See the appendix for details.

70. Jeffrey P. Brosco, "Policy and Poverty: Child and Community Health in Philadelphia, 1910–1930," *Archives of Pediatric Medicine* 149 (1995): 1381–87. Brosco, "Tales of Medicine and Poverty," 196–212.

71. "Desirable Office and Home," *WR* 12, no. 2 (1916): 12.

72. Reilly, *Building a Profitable Practice*, 30–31.

73. Rita S. Finkler, "Good Morning Doctor!" (1967), 79, Rita S. Finkler Papers, R 154.F5, DUCOM Archives.

74. Ibid., 81–82.

75. Kelley, "Success in Life," 89.

76. Finkler, "Good Morning Doctor!" 86.

77. Mabee, *The Physician's Business and Financial Adviser*, 129.

78. MacFarlane, [Autobiography], 32–35.

79. Ibid., 52.

4. New Career Paths, New Business Methods

1. For an introduction, see Morris J. Vogel, *The Invention of the Modern Hospital, Boston, 1870–1930* (Chicago: University of Chicago Press, 1980); David Rosner, *A Once Charitable Enterprise: Hospitals and Health Care in Brooklyn and New York, 1885–1915* (Cambridge: Cambridge University Press, 1982); Charles E. Rosenberg, *The Care of Strangers: The Rise of America's Hospital System* (Baltimore: Johns Hopkins University Press, 1987); Diana E. Long and Janet Golden, eds., *The American General Hospital: Communities and Social Contexts*, (Ithaca, NY: Cornell University Press, 1989); and Rosemary Stevens, *In Sickness and in Wealth: American Hospitals in the Twentieth Century*, paperback ed. (Baltimore: Johns Hopkins University Press, 1999). For an overview of Philadelphia hospitals, see Steven J. Peitzman, "'Thoroughly Practical': America's Polyclinic Medical Schools," *BHM* 54 (1980): 166–87; Charles E. Rosenberg, "From Almshouse to Hospital: The Shaping of Philadelphia General Hospital," *Milbank Memorial Fund Quarterly / Health and Society* 60, no. 1 (1982): 108–54; Rosemary Stevens, "Sweet Charity: State Aid to Hospitals in Pennsylvania, 1870–1910," *BHM* 58 (1984): 287–314; Edward T. Morman, "Clinical Pathology in America, 1865–1915: Philadelphia as a Test Case," *BHM* 58 (1984): 198–214; David McBride, *Integrating the City of Medicine: Blacks in Philadelphia Health Care, 1910–1965* (Philadelphia: Temple University Press, 1989); and Leo J. O'Hara, *An Emerging Profession: Philadelphia Doctors, 1860–1900* (New York: Garland Publishing, 1989).

2. George Rosen, *The Structure of American Medical Practice, 1875–1941*, ed. Charles E. Rosenberg (Philadelphia: University of Pennsylvania Press, 1983), 46. Rosenberg, *Care of Strangers*, 310–52.

3. Vogel, *The Invention of the Modern Hospital*, 5–28, 97–119. Rosner, *A Once Charitable Enterprise*, 16–23, 36–61. Rosen, *The Structure of American Medical Practice*, 43–51. Rosenberg, *The Care of Strangers*, 97–121. Joan E. Lynaugh, "From Respectable Domesticity to Medical Efficiency: The Changing Kansas City Hospital, 1875–1920," and Vanessa Gamble, "The Negro Hospital Renaissance: The Black Hospital Movement, 1920–1945," in *The American General Hospital* (see note 1), 21–39, 67–81.

4. Joel D. Howell, *Technology in the Hospital: Transforming Patient Care in the Early Twentieth Century* (Baltimore: Johns Hopkins University Press, 1995). Rosenberg, *The Care of Strangers*, 142–65.

5. Stevens, *In Sickness and In Wealth*, 106, table 51. Judith Walzer Leavitt, *Brought to Bed: Childbearing in America, 1750 to 1950* (New York: Oxford University Press, 1986).

6. Vogel, *The Invention of the Modern Hospital*, 97–119. Rosner, *A Once Charitable Enterprise*, 62–93. Rosenberg, *The Care of Strangers*, 237–61. Stevens, *In Sickness and In Wealth*, 105–131.

7. Stevens, *In Sickness and In Wealth*, 142.

8. Rosen, *The Structure of American Medical Practice*, 43–51. Rosenberg, *The Care of Strangers*, 66–89. William G. Rothstein, *American Medical Schools and the Practice of Medicine, A History* (New York: Oxford University Press, 1987), 131–34.

9. Oswald Hall, "The Informal Organization of Medical Practice in an American City" (PhD diss., University of Chicago, 1944), 27–29, 85–90. Rosenberg, *The Care of Strangers*, 179–89.

10. Rosner, *A Once Charitable Enterprise*, 95–121. Rosenberg, *The Care of Strangers*, 166–211, 237–85.

11. J. A. Curran, "Internships and Residencies: Historical Backgrounds and Current Trends," *Journal of Medical Education* 34, no. 9 (1959): 873–84. Rosemary Stevens, "Graduate Medical Education: A Continuing History," *Journal of Medical Education* 53 (1978): 1–18. Rosen, *The Structure of American Medical Practice*, 78–81. Rothstein, *American Medical Schools and the Practice of Medicine*, 134–36. Kenneth M. Ludmerer, *Time to Heal: American Medical Education from the Turn of the Century to the Era of Managed Care* (New York: Oxford University Press, 1999), 79–101. "Hospital Service in the United States: Nineteenth Annual Presentation of Hospital Data by the Council on Medical Education and Hospitals of the AMA," *JAMA* 114, no. 13 (1940): 1157–1256, esp. 1157.

12. *Final Report of the Commission on Medical Education* (New York: 1932), appendix, table 80. *Graduate Medical Education: Final Report of the Commission on Graduate Medical Education* (Chicago: University of Chicago Press, 1940), 256, table 4.

13. H. G. Weiskotten and Marion E. Altenderfer, "Trends in Medical Practice," pt. 2, *Journal of Medical Education* 27, no. 5 (1952): 1–41, esp. 36, table 35.

14. George D. Wolf, *The Physician's Business: Practical and Economic Aspects of Medicine* (Philadelphia: J. B. Lippincott, 1938), 1.

15. Carl C. Fischer, "Chapter Six—'Men in White': The Interne Year, 1928–1929," and "Chapter Seven: The Private Practice of Pediatrics, 1931–1969," in Fischer Memoirs (Edited BW), 1–2, 4, Carl C. Fischer Papers, DUCOM Archives.

16. For general overviews, see: *Graduate Medical Education*, 96–103; Curran, "Internships and Residencies," 873–84; Stevens, "Graduate Medical Education," 1–18; Rosemary Stevens *American Medicine and the Public Interest: A History of Specialization*, updated ed. (Berkeley: University of California Press, 1998), 77–131, 149–266; Rosen, *The Structure of American Medical Practice*, 78–81; and George Weisz, *Divide and Conquer: A Comparative History of Specialization* (New York: Oxford University Press, 2006), 127–46.

17. Stevens, "Graduate Medical Education," 1–18. Jennifer L. Gunn, "Science and Skill: Educating the Medical Practitioner at the Graduate School of Medicine of the University of Pennsylvania" (PhD diss., University of Pennsylvania, 1997).

18. Stevens, *American Medicine and the Public Interest*, 127–31, and 542, table A1.

19. Ibid., 218, 543, table A2.

20. "Hospital Service in the United States," 1171.

21. The formalization of specialty qualifications was initially intended to check the growth of specialization in the American medical profession, but the opposite occurred. See Rosen, *The Structure of American Medical Practice*, 85–94.

22. Weiskotten and Altenderfer, "Trends in Medical Practice" (1952), 36, table 35. H. G. Weiskotten et al., "Trends in Medical Practice: An Analysis of the Distribution and Characteristics of Medical College Graduates, 1915–1950," *Journal of Medical Education* 35, no. 12 (1960): 1071–1121, esp. 1092, table 16.

23. Nathan Sinai and Alden B. Mills, *A Survey of the Medical Facilities of the City of Philadelphia, 1929*, Publications of the Committee on the Costs of Medical Care, no. 9A (Washington, DC, 1929), 4–5.

24. Weiskotten et al., "Trends in Medical Practice" (1960), 1093, table 17.

25. Harold G. Scheie, Letter to Parents, Jan. 23, 1938, Scheie Papers, UPT 50/S318, box 2, folder 5, UPA.

26. Harold G. Scheie, Letter to Parents, July 30, 1938, Scheie Papers, UPT 50/S318, box 2, folder 5, UPA.

27. Harold G. Scheie, Letter to Parents, Jan. 25, 1939, Scheie Papers, UPT 50/S318, box 2, folder 6, UPA.

28. Harold G. Scheie, Letter to Parents, Mar. 25, 1940, Scheie Papers, UPT 50/S318, box 2, folder 7, UPA.

29. Sinai and Mills, *A Survey of the Medical Facilities*. 5–6, figure 1 and 25, table 1.

30. I. S. Falk, Rufus Rorem, and Martha D. Ring, *The Costs of Medical Care: A Summary of Investigations of Economic Aspects of the Prevention and Care of Illness*, Publications of the Committee on the Costs of Medical Care, no. 27 (Chicago: University of Chicago Press, 1933), 242. Their data were adapted from R. G. Leland, "Income from Medical Practice," *JAMA* 96, no. 20 (1931): 1689, table 14.

31. Paul A. Dodd and E. F. Penrose, *Economic Aspects of Medical Services: With Special Reference to Conditions in California* (Washington, DC: Graphic Arts Press, 1939), 250.

32. Hermann C. Weiskotten, et al., "Trends in Medical Practice: An Analysis of the Distribution and Characteristics of Medical College Graduates, 1915–1950," *Journal of Medical Education* 35, no. 12 (1960): 1078.

33. See the appendix and table 19 of this book for details.

34. See the appendix of this book for details.

35. Hall, "The Informal Organization of Medical Practice," 10, 14–29, 35–39, 58–69, 125–26, 137–46, 156–65, 174–96, 241–49. Unfortunately, Hall used surnames to determine ethnic affiliation, though he had the aid of "representative members of each main group." Ibid., 14–15.

36. Campbell Gibson, "Population of the 100 Largest Cities and Other Urban Places in the United States, 1790 to 1990," U.S. Bureau of the Census, Population Division Working Paper No. 27, table 17, "Population of the 100 Largest Urban Places: 1940" (Washington, DC, 1998), http://www.census.gov/population/www/documentation/twps0027.html. *AMD* (1940): 1530–31, 1571, 1636, and 1639. In 1940, Providence had 559 doctors and 10 hospitals as compared to 4,392 doctors and 80 hospitals in Philadelphia. Note that the *AMD* (1940) included hospitals "for the care of tuberculosis, communicable diseases, and mental conditions," unlike the *Philadelphia Hospital and Health Survey, 1929* (Philadelphia: Philadelphia Health and Hospital Survey Committee, 1930), 566.

37. For an overview, see Ludmerer, *Time to Heal*, 60–65.

38. Philadelphia had slightly higher a higher representation of women in the medical profession, or 6.4 percent vs. 4.6 percent nationwide. See table 11 and Ellen S. More, *Restoring the Balance: Women Physicians and the Profession of Medicine, 1850– 1995* (Cambridge, MA: Harvard University Press, 1999), 97–99.

39. Ludmerer, *Time to Heal*, 60–65. McBride, *Integrating the City of Medicine*, 94–99.

40. Carol Lopate, *Women in Medicine* (Baltimore: Johns Hopkins University Press, 1968), 195. From 1949 to 1958, dropout rates were 15.5 percent for women and 8.3 percent for men. No data were available on the dropout rates of African American versus white medical students.

41. McBride, *Integrating the City of Medicine*, 89–90, esp. table 15. Of the 60 women in the *AMD* (1940) sample of Philadelphia doctors, 45 had attended a medical school for women. See the appendix of this book for details.

42. McBride, *Integrating the City of Medicine*, 85–122, esp. 99–106 for data cited.

43. Ibid., 31–122, esp. 31–84 on public health. For comparisons in the South, see Todd L. Savitt, "Entering a White Profession: Black Physicians in the New South, 1880– 1920," *BHM* 67, no. 4 (1987): 507–40, and Thomas J. Ward Jr., *Black Physicians in the Jim Crow South* (Fayetteville: University of Arkansas Press, 2003). See also Gamble, "The Negro Hospital Renaissance," in *The American General Hospital* (see note 1), 82–105, and James Wolfinger, *Philadelphia Divided: Race and Politics in the City of Brotherly Love* (Chapel Hill: University of North Carolina Press, 2007).

44. Mary Roth Walsh, *"Doctors Wanted: No Women Need Apply": Sexual Barriers in the Medical Profession, 1835–1975* (New Haven: Yale University Press, 1977), 219–24. More, *Restoring the Balance*, 105–12.

45. More, *Restoring the Balance*, 95–112. Lopate, *Women in Medicine*, 199.

46. Of the 879 doctors in the *AMD* (1940) sample of Philadelphia, 868 had names of discernable gender. Of these, 60 were women (or 6.9 percent, similar to federal census data in table 11). 20 women were specialists (partial or full-time), while 315 of 808 men were specialists (partial or full-time). See the appendix of this book for details.

47. More, *Restoring the Balance*, 170–81.

48. On the growth of specialization in this period, see George Rosen, "Changing Attitudes of the Medical Profession to Specialization," *BHM* 12 (1942): 343–54; Rosen, *The Specialization of Medicine with Particular Reference to Ophthalmology* (New York: Froben Press, 1944); Milton Terris and Mary Monk, "Changes in Physicians' Careers: Relation of Time after Graduation to Specialization," *JAMA* 160, no. 8 (1956): 653–55; Weiskotten et al., "Trends in Medical Practice" (1960); Stevens, *American Medicine and the Public Interest*, 75–289; and Weisz, *Divide and Conquer*, 63–83, 127–46.

49. Weiskotten and Altenderfer, "Trends in Medical Practice" (1952), 36–38. *Graduate Medical Education*, 13–23.

50. *Graduate Medical Education*, 91–92.

51. Stevens, *American Medicine and the Public Interest*, 251–57, 305–14.

52. Specialization and experience data were gathered from the *AMD* (1909) and *AMD* (1940) samples of Philadelphia doctors. See the appendix of this book for details. In 1940, GPs and full specialists had been in practice an average of 21.6 years and 24.1 years, respectively, and this difference was significant when measured by Student's t-test ($p < .05$). However, when comparing GPs to all specialists (full and partial), specialists had been in practice an average of only 22.5 years, an insignificant difference from GPs when measured by Student's t-test ($p > .05$).

53. Terris and Monk, "Changes in Physicians' Careers," 653–55. Terris and Monk only measured full specialization, lumping partial specialists in with GPs.

54. These numbers were calculated from individual data for the 1935 and 1940 classes in Weiskotten and Altenderfer, "Trends in Medical Practice" (1952), 31–34, and table 33.

55. These numbers were calculated from Leland, "Income from Medical Practice," 1689, table 14. Reliance upon salaried work varied greatly from one specialty to another, however.

56. Rosen, *The Structure of American Medical Practice*, 88. See also Leven, *The Incomes of Physicians*, 115–16, tables 11A and 12A; Leland, "Income from Medical Practice," 1687, table 9 and chart 3, Falk et al., *The Costs of Medical Care*; William Allan Richardson, "How Much the Doctor Collects," *Medical Economics* 18 (December 1940): 52–55; and Dodd and Penrose, *Economic Aspects of Medical Services*. Incomes differed considerably by specialty, though only a handful of specialties were less lucrative than general practice.

57. William Allan Richardson, "Physicians' Incomes," *Medical Economics* 17 (September 1940): 38–48. Dodd and Penrose, *Economic Aspects of Medical Services*, 208–20.

58. Rosen, *The Structure of American Medical Practice*, 88. Terris and Monk, "Changes in Physicians' Careers," 655.

59. Denise Bystryn Kandel, "The Career Decisions of Medical Students: A Study in Occupational Recruitment and Occupational Choice" (PhD diss., Columbia University, 1960), 290.

60. Ibid., 253, esp. table 82.

61. Ibid., 268, esp. table 88.

62. Ibid., 438–50, esp. table 137.

63. Leven, *The Incomes of Physicians*, 59–64

64. Leland "Income from Medical Practice," 1685, table 4. Leven *The Incomes of Physicians*, 41–49, 114, table 10A; and Richardson "Physicians' Incomes," 42, chart 4A.

65. Sinai and Mills, *A Survey of Medical Facilities of the City of Philadelphia*, 7–8, figure 2.

66. Leland, "Income from Medical Practice," 1683–91, esp. 1689, table 12. Percentages were calculated from raw data.

67. Beatrix Hoffman, *The Wages of Sickness: The Politics of Health Insurance in Progressive America* (Chapel Hill: University of North Carolina Press, 2001). Ronald L. Numbers, *Almost Persuaded: American Physicians and Compulsory Health Insurance, 1912–1920* (Baltimore: Johns Hopkins University Press, 1978). Theda Skocpol, *Protecting Soldiers and Mothers: The Political Origins of Social Policy in the United States* (Cambridge, MA: Harvard University Press, 1992). James G. Burrow, *Organized Medicine in the Progressive Era: The Move towards Monopoly* (Baltimore: Johns Hopkins University Press, 1977), 133–53.

68. *Medical Economics* 1, no. 1 (1923): 6. Circulation data were printed on the title page in the 1930s. In all likelihood, the journal was sent free of charge to AMA members and funded by advertising revenue. Nevertheless, advertisers would not have continued to pay for advertisement space unless the journal was widely read.

69. Wolf, *The Physician's Business*.

70. Ibid., 37–69.

71. Bureau of Medical Economics, *Collecting Medical Fees* (Chicago: AMA Press, 1938), 1.

72. Ibid., 2–3.

73. Leven, *The Incomes of Physicians*, 42.

74. Ibid., 41–49. Sinai and Mills, *A Survey of the Medical Facilities of Philadelphia*, 7.

75. Sinai and Mills, *A Survey of the Medical Facilities of Philadelphia*, 6–7. Altogether, expenses consumed 40 percent of the average gross income of Philadelphia doctors in 1929.

76. Dodd and Penrose, *Economic Aspects of Medical Services*, 234, table 117.

77. Hall, "The Informal Organization of Medical Practice," 151–52, 242–47.

78. Dr. M. Agnes Gowdey, "More Ramblings 2/25/02" and "Notes from conversation between M. Agnes Gowdey MD and Grace Palmer (compiler) Nov. 23, 2001," Gowdey Papers, Acc 241, new acquisitions, 2003–2004, DUCOM Archives.

79. Samuel Bernard Hadden, "First Case as a Medical Doctor, 1926," Hadden Papers, UPT 50/H126, box 1, folder 9, UPA. Hadden's office location and specialization were determined from the *AMD* (1929), 1283.

80. Rosen, *The Structure of American Medical Practice*, 40–43.

81. Jeffrey Brosco, "Policy and Poverty: Child and Community Health in Philadelphia, 1900–1930," *Archives of Pediatric Medicine* 149 (1995): 1381–87.

82. Skocpol, *Protecting Soldiers and Mothers*, 480–524.

83. George Rosen, *Preventive Medicine in the United States, 1900–1975* (New York: Science History Publications, 1975), 58–61. Mitchell H. Charap, "The Periodic Health Examination: Genesis of a Myth," *Annals of Internal Medicine* 95 (1981): 733–35. Audrey B. Davis, "Life Insurance and the Physical Examination: A Chapter in the Rise of American Medical Technology," *BHM* 55 (1981): 392–406. Francis Ashley Faught, "What the Periodic Health Examination Should Disclose," *WR* 30, no. 41 (1935): 1195. A. I. Rubenstone, "Why Periodic Health Examinations? General Considerations, Value to Laity, the Individual Patient, and the Community," *WR* 30, no. 42 (1935): 1241–44. Committee on Periodic Health Examination, "Periodic Health Examinations: Letters and Blanks Now Ready," *WR* 30, no. 40 (1935): 1165.

84. Charles Miller Scott, "Your Yearly Inventory," *WR* 24, no. 2 (1928): 17, 19. W. Burrill Odenatt, "Have You a Family Doctor?" *WR* 26, no. 17 (1930): 23, 25. F. F. Borzell, "Consult Your Physician," *WR* 26, no. 25 (1931): 25, 27, 30.

85. James M. Dodson, "The Growing Importance of Preventive Medicine to the General Practitioner," *JAMA* 81, no. 17 (1923): 1427–29.

86. "Income from Preventive Medicine in Private Practice," *PMJ* 38 (1935): 524.

87. For Philadelphia-area examples of this effort, see J. T. Ullom, "The Boundaries of General Practice," *Transactions of the College of Physicians of Philadelphia*, 3rd series, 44: 451–58; Thomas A. Miller, "Problems of Diagnosis from the Standpoint of the General Practitioner," *PMJ* 32 (1929): 562–65; J. L. Atlee, "When Should the General Practitioner Refer the Patient to a Specialists from the Cancer Viewpoint?" *WR* 26, no. 46 (1931): 21; Howard A. Kelley, "A Letter to the Doctors of Pennsylvania," *PMJ* 35 (1932): 316–17; James Ewing, "A Letter to the Doctors of Pennsylvania," *PMJ* 35 (1932): 648–49; Edwin H. McIlvain, "The General Practitioner and Industry," *PMJ* 35 (1932): 834–44; Maurice J. Karpeles, "The Modern Family Doctor in Relation to the Specialist," *WR* 28, no. 43 (1933): 21–23, 31; George C. Yeager, "The Modern Family Doctor," *WR* 28, no. 44 (1933): 13–14.

88. Francis A. Faught, "Economic Value of the Periodic Health Examination," *PMJ* 36 (1933): 261–64. Rosen, *Preventive Medicine in the United States*, 58–61.

89. Donald L. Madison and Thomas R. Konrad, "Large Medical Group-Practice Organizations and Employed Physicians: A Relationship in Transition," *Milbank Quarterly* 66, no. 2 (1988): 240–82.

90. For analysis, see Barbara B. Perkins, "Economic Organization of Medicine and the Committee on the Costs of Medical Care," *American Journal of Public Health* 88, no. 11

(1998): 1721–23, and Forrest A. Walker, "Americanism versus Sovietism: A Study of the Reaction to the Committee on the Costs of Medical Care," *BHM* 53 (1979): 489–504.

91. Madison and Konrad, "Large Medical Group Practice Organizations," 240–46.

92. For a helpful taxonomy of group practices in Providence, Rhode Island, in 1940, see Hall, "The Informal Organization of Medical Practice," 170–72.

93. Wolf, *The Physician's Business*, 34.

94. For a discussion of efficiency and early hospital standardization impulses, see Edward T. Morman, "Introduction," in *Efficiency, Scientific Management, and Hospital Standardization*, ed. Edward T. Morman (New York: Garland, 1989).

95. Weiskotten and Altenderfer, "Trends in Medical Practice" (1952), 31–33. Leland, "Income from Medical Practice," 1689, table 14.

96. Peter Buck, "Why Not the Best? Some Reasons and Examples from Child Health and Rural Hospitals," *Journal of Social History* 18 (1985): 413–31.

97. Rosner, *A Once Charitable Enterprise*, 94–121. Stevens, *American Medicine and the Public Interest*, 251–57.

98. David P. Adams, "Community and Professionalization: General Practitioners and Ear, Nose, and Throat Specialists in Cincinnati, 1945–1947," *BHM* 68 (1994): 664–84.

99. Ibid., 678–84. Stevens, *American Medicine and the Public Interest*, 293–317.

100. Margaret B. Tinkcom, "Depression and War, 1929–1946," in *Philadelphia: A 300-Year History*, ed. Russell F. Weigley (New York: W. W. Norton, 1982), 601–48, esp. 612–13. Gladys L. Palmer, "Recent Trends in Employment and Unemployment in Philadelphia," *National Research Project on Reemployment Opportunities and Recent Changes in Industrial Techniques*, report no. P-1 (Philadelphia: Philadelphia Labor Market Studies, 1937), esp. 8–9, chart 3.

101. Gladys L. Palmer, "Employment and Unemployment in Philadelphia in 1936 and 1937. Part I: May 1936," *National Research Project on Reemployment Opportunities and Recent Changes in Industrial Techniques*, report no. P-3, part I (Philadelphia: Philadelphia Labor Market Studies, 1938), esp. 15–22, tables 5 and 8.

102. Richardson, "Physicians' Incomes," 38–48, esp. chart 2A.

103. "Some Answers!" *WR* 28, no. 11 (1932): 11.

104. Fischer, "Chapter Seven: The Private Practice of Pediatrics, 1931–1969," 2–3.

105. Dodd and Penrose, *Economic Aspects of Medical Services*, 210–211 and tables 95 and 96.

106. "The Aid Association," *WR* 28, no. 12 (1932): 3, 5.

107. "Some Answers!" *WR* 28, no. 11 (1932): 11.

108. "Report of Open Meeting on Medical Economics," *WR* 28, no. 22 (1933): 15–16, 18; 28, no. 23 (1933): 24–26; 28, no. 24 (1933): 24–26.

109. Richard W. Larer, "The Economic Problems of the Physician," *WR* 28, no. 10 (1932): 19–22, 24.

110. "And Yet Another 'Clinic'!" *PMJ* 38 (1935): 533–34.

111. See, for example, "The Hospital as a Competitor of the Family Physician," *PMJ* 36 (1933): 845.

112. Summarized in a series of articles under the title "What Your Society Is Doing. Medical Economics Committee Activities," in *WR* 28, no. 40 (1933).

113. L. W. Deichler, "Report of the Section on Dispensary Abuses and Social Service Departments," *WR* 28, no. 40 (1933): 13–19.

114. L. W. Deichler, "Section on Dispensary Abuses," *WR* 29, no. 48 (1934): 1443–44.

115. "The Hospital and the Extensively-Studied Dispensary Case," *WR* 29, no. 50 (1934): 1493, 1495, 1497, 1499, 1501, 1503, 1505–13.

5. From Center City to Suburb

1. Judith Walzer Leavitt, *Brought to Bed: Childbearing in America 1750 to 1950* (New York: Oxford University Press, 1986). Joel D. Howell, *Technology in the Hospital: Transforming Patient Care in the Early Twentieth Century* (Baltimore: Johns Hopkins University Press, 1995). Rosemary Stevens, *In Sickness and in Wealth: American Hospitals in the Twentieth Century*, paperback ed. (Baltimore: Johns Hopkins University, 1999).

2. David Rosner, "Doing Well or Doing Good: The Ambivalent Focus of Hospital Administration," in *The American General Hospital: Communities and Social Contexts*, ed. Diana E. Long and Janet Golden (Ithaca, NY: Cornell University Press, 1989), 157–69. Rosner, *A Once Charitable Enterprise: Hospitals and Health Care in Brooklyn and New York, 1885–1915* (Princeton: Princeton University Press, 1982). Stevens, *In Sickness and in Wealth.*

3. Ronald L. Numbers, *Almost Persuaded: American Physicians and Compulsory Health Insurance, 1912–1920* (Baltimore: Johns Hopkins University Press, 1978). Beatrix R. Hoffman, *The Wages of Sickness: The Politics of Health Insurance in Progressive America* (Chapel Hill: University of North Carolina Press, 2001).

4. Forrest A. Walker, "Americanism versus Sovietism: A Study of the Reaction to the Committee on the Costs of Medical Care," *BHM* 53 (1979): 489–504. Barbara Bridgman Perkins, "Economic Organization of Medicine and the Committee on the Costs of Medical Care," *American Journal of Public Health* 88, no. 11 (1998): 1721–25. Committee on the Costs of Medical Care, *Medical Care for the American People: The Final Report of the Committee on the Costs of Medical Care* (Chicago: University of Chicago Press, 1932). I. S. Falk, C. Rufus Rorem, and Martha D. Ring, *The Costs of Medical Care: A Summary of Investigations on the Economic Aspects of the Prevention and Care of Illness*, Publications of the Committee on the Costs of Medical Care, no. 27 (Chicago: University of Chicago Press, 1933).

5. Lewis Mayers and Leonard V. Harrison, *The Distribution of Physicians in the United States* (New York: General Education Board, 1924), 164–66. Raymond Pearl, "Distribution of Physicians in the United States," *JAMA* 84, no .14 (1925): 1024–28. H. G. Weiskotten, "Tendencies in Medical Practice: A Study of 1925 Graduates," *Journal of the Association of American Medical Colleges* 7, no. 2 (1932): 65–85. R. G. Leland and the AMA Bureau of Medical Economic Research, *Distribution of Physicians in the United States* (Chicago: AMA Press, 1935), 35–39. H. G. Weiskotten, "Trends in Medical Practice," *Journal of the Association of American Medical Colleges* 12, no. 5 (1937): 321–56. Paul A. Dodd and E. F. Penrose, *Economic Aspects of Medical Services, with Special Reference to Conditions in California* (Washington, DC: Graphic Arts Press, 1939), 25–29. *Graduate Medical Education: Report of the Commission on Graduate Medical Education* (Chicago: University of Chicago Press, 1940), 267, table 15. Joseph W. Mountin, Elliott H. Pennell, and Virginia Nicolay, "Location and Movement of Physicians, 1923 and 1938: General Observations," *Public Health Reports* 57, no. 37 (1942): 1363–75. Mountin, Pennell, and Nicolay, "Location and Movement of Physicians, 1923 and 1938: Effect of Local Factors upon Location," *Public Health Reports* 57, no. 51 (1942): 1945–53. Mountin, Pennell, and Nicolay, "Location and Movement of Physicians, 1923 and 1938: Age Distribution in Relation to County Characteristics," *Public Health Reports* 58, no. 12 (1943): 483–90. George Rosen, *The Specialization of Medicine with Particular Reference to Ophthalmology* (New York: Froben Press, 1944). Joseph W. Mountin, Elliott H. Pennell, and Georgie S. Brockett, "Location and Movement of Physicians, 1923 and 1938: Changes in Urban and Rural Totals for Established Physicians," *Public Health Reports* 60, no. 7 (1945):

173–185. William Weinfeld, "Incomes of Physicians, 1929–1949," *Survey of Current Business* 31 (1951): 9–26.

6. R. G. Leland, "Income from Medical Practice" *JAMA* 96, no. 20 (1931): 1683–91. Maurice Leven, *The Incomes of Physicians: An Economic and Statistical Analysis*, Publications of the Committee on the Costs of Medical Care, no. 24 (Chicago: University of Chicago Press, 1932), 34–40. Dodd and Penrose, *Economic Aspects of Medical Services*, 211–12. William A. Richardson, "Physicians' Incomes," *Medical Economics* 17 (1940): 38–48. Richardson, "How Much the Doctor Collects," *Medical Economics* 18 (1940): 52–55.

7. Mountin et al., "Location and Movement of Physicians, 1923 and 1938: General Observations," 1373.

8. Earl Shepard Johnson, "A Study in the Ecology of the Physician" (master's thesis, University of Chicago, 1932), James H. S. Bossard, "A Sociologist Looks at the Doctors," in *The Medical Profession and the Public: Currents and Counter Currents* (American Academy of Political and Social Science, 1934); and Oswald Hall, "The Informal Organization of Medical Practice in an American City" (PhD diss., University of Chicago, 1944).

9. Bossard, "A Sociologist Looks at the Doctors," 9.

10. "The Medical Profession and the Public," *WR* 29, no. 25 (1934): 727, 729, 731, 733. See also PCMS, Commission on Medical Economics, "The Medical Profession and the Public: A Critical Analysis of the Argument Advanced in Support of Socialized Medicine at the Joint Meeting of the College of Physicians of Philadelphia and the American Academy of Political and Social Science, Irvine Auditorium, Philadelphia, February 7, 1934," *WR* 29, no. 31 (1934): 922–27, 929, 931.

11. Walker, "Americanism versus Sovietism."

12. Campbell Gibson, "Population of the 100 Largest Cities and Other Urban Places in the United States: 1790 to 1990," U.S. Bureau of the Census, Population Division Working Paper no. 27 (Washington, DC, 1998), http://www.census.gov/population/www/documentation/twps0027.html. U.S. Bureau of the Census, *Sixteenth Census of the United States* (Washington, DC: U.S. G.P.O., 1942), *Population*, vol. 1, "Number of Inhabitants" 912, table 3.

13. Philip Scranton, "Large Firms and Industrial Restructuring: The Philadelphia Region, 1900–1980," *Pennsylvania Magazine of History and Biography* 116, no. 4 (1992): 419–65. Jerome P. Bjelopera, *City of Clerks: Office and Sales Workers in Philadelphia, 1870–1920* (Urbana: University of Illinois Press, 2005), 9–31.

14. U.S. Bureau of the Census, *Sixteenth Census of the United States, 1940* (Washington, DC: U.S. G.P.O., 1943) *Population*, vol. 2, "Characteristics of the Population," 210, table B-35.

15. Richard A. Varbero, "Philadelphia's South Italians in the 1920s," in *The Peoples of Philadelphia: A History of Ethnic Groups and Lower-Class Life, 1790–1940*, ed. Allen F. Davis and Mark H. Haller (Philadelphia: Temple University Press, 1973), 255–75. Stefano Luconi, "Bringing Out the Italian-American Vote in Philadelphia," *Pennsylvania Magazine of History and Biography* 117, no. 4 (1993): 251–85.

16. Eugene P. Ericksen and William L. Yancey, "Work and Residence in Industrial Philadelphia," *Journal of Urban History* 5, no. 2 (1979): 147–82. Stephanie W. Greenberg, "Neighborhood Change, Racial Transition, and Work Location: A Case Study of an Industrial City, Philadelphia, 1880–1930," *Journal of Urban History* 7, no. 3 (1981): 267–314.

17. Frederick Miller, "The Black Migration to Philadelphia: A 1924 Profile," *Pennsylvania Magazine of History and Biography* 108 (1984): 315–50.
18. U.S. Bureau of the Census, *Thirteenth Census of the United States, 1910* (Washington, DC: U.S. G.P.O., 1913), vol. 3, *Population*, table v, 605. U.S. Bureau of the Census, *Sixteenth Census of the United States, 1940* (Washington, DC: U.S. G.P.O., 1943) *Population*, vol. 2, "Characteristics of the Population," 210, table B-35.
19. Miller, "The Black Migration to Philadelphia," 329–33.
20. John F. Bauman, "Public Housing in the Depression: Slum Reform in Philadelphia Neighborhoods in the 1930s," in *The Divided Metropolis: Social and Spatial Dimensions of Philadelphia, 180–1975*, ed. William W. Cutler III and Howard Gillette Jr. (Westport, CT: Greenwood Press, 1980), 227–48. Amy E. Hillier, "Redlining and the Home Owners' Loan Corporation," *Journal of Urban History* 29, no. 4 (2003): 394–420. Hillier, "Who Received Loans? Home Owners' Loan Corporation Lending and Discrimination in Philadelphia in the 1930s," *Journal of Planning History* 2, no. 1 (2003): 3–24. Hillier, "Searching for Red Lines: Spatial Analysis of Lending Patterns in Philadelphia, 1940–1960," *Pennsylvania History* 71, no. 1 (2005): 25–47. Hillier, "Residential Security Maps and Neighborhood Appraisals: The Home Owners' Loan Corporation and the Case of Philadelphia," *Social Science History* 29, no. 2 (2005): 207–33. Russell A. Kazal, "The Interwar Origins of the White Ethnic," *Journal of American Ethnic History* 23, no. 4 (2004): 78–131, esp. 98–108. James Wolfinger, *Philadelphia Divided: Race and Politics in the City of Brotherly Love* (Chapel Hill: University of North Carolina Press, 2007).
21. Ericksen and Yancey, "Work and Residence in Industrial Philadelphia," 147–82, and Greenberg, "Neighborhood Change, Racial Transition, and Work Location," 267–314. Miller "The Black Migration to Philadelphia," 334–37. U.S. Bureau of the Census, *Sixteenth Census of the United States, 1940* (Washington, DC: U.S. G.P.O., 1943), vol. 3, *Population*, 48–53, table 13. Wolfinger, *Philadelphia Divided*, 1–33.
22. Miller, "The Black Migration to Philadelphia," 347–49.
23. Theodore Hershberg et al., "A Tale of Three Cities: Blacks, Immigrants, and Opportunity in Philadelphia, 1840–1880, 1930, 1970," in *Philadelphia: Work, Space, Family, and Group Experience in the Nineteenth Century*, ed. Theodore Hershberg (New York: Oxford University Press, 1981), 461–91. Greenberg, "Neighborhood Change, Racial Transition, and Work Location," 267–314. Even when controlling for the effects of occupational status, African-Americans earned less than their white counterparts in the 1930s. See Clara Hardin, *The Negroes of Philadelphia: The Cultural Adjustment of a Minority Group* (Bryn Mawr, Pa.: Craft Press, 1945), 77–79, 166. Some of Hardin's data were extracted from Alice C. Hanson, U.S. Dept. of Labor, Bureau of Labor Statistics, Cost of Living Division, *Bulletin No. R. 556*.
24. Elizabeth Fones-Wolf, "Industrial Unionism and Labor Movement Culture in Depression-Era Philadelphia," *Pennsylvania Magazine of History and Biography* 109 (1985): 3–26. Jerome P. Bjelopera, "White Collars and Blackface: Race and Leisure among Clerical and Sales Workers in Early Twentieth Century Philadelphia," *Pennsylvania Magazine of History and Biography* 126, no. 3 (2002): 471–90. John Henry Hepp IV, *The Middle-Class City: Transforming Space and Time in Philadelphia, 1876–1926* (Philadelphia: University of Pennsylvania Press, 2003).
25. For comparisons, see James Borchert and Susan Borchert, "Downtown, Uptown, Out of Town: Diverging Patterns of Upper Class Residential Landscapes in Buffalo, Pittsburgh, and Cleveland, 1885–1935," *Social Science History* 26, no. 2 (2002): 311–46.

26. Hepp, *The Middle-Class City*. Gary R. Hovinen, "Suburbanization in Greater Phila-delphia," *Journal of Historical Geography* 11, no. 2 (1985): 174–95. Hillier, "Search-ing for Red Lines," 25–47.

27. Scranton, "Large Firms and Industrial Restructuring," 419–65. Greenberg, "Neigh-borhood Change, Racial Transition, and Work Location," 267–314. Hillier, "Resi-dential Security Maps and Neighborhood Appraisals," 207–33. For comparisons, see Colin Gordon, *Mapping Decline: St. Louis and the Fate of the American City* (Philadelphia: University of Pennsylvania Press, 2008).

28. Ericksen and Yancey, "Work and Residence in Industrial Philadelphia," 168–70. Stephanie Dyer, "'Holding the Line Against Philadelphia': Business, Suburban Change, and the Main Line's Suburban Square, 1926–1950," *Business and Economic History* 27, no. 2 (1998): 279–91.

29. Sam Bass Warner Jr., *The Private City: Philadelphia in Three Periods of Its Growth*, 2nd ed. (Philadelphia: University of Pennsylvania Press, 1987), 169–77.

30. U.S. Bureau of the Census, *Census of Business: 1935*, "Intra-City Business Census Sta-tistics for Philadelphia, Pennsylvania" (Washington, DC: U.S. G.P.O., 1937), 15, fig. 2.

31. Ibid., 25–27.

32. Warner, *The Private City*, 185–94. As acknowledged elsewhere, I borrow Warner's district divisions in my analysis. See also Hepp, *The Middle-Class City*.

33. *The WPA Guide to Philadelphia*, comp. by the Federal Writers' Project of the Works Progress Administration for the Commonwealth of Pennsylvania (1937; repr. Phila-delphia: University of Pennsylvania Press, 1988), 443.

34. Margaret S. Marsh, "The Impact of the Market Street 'El' on Northern West Phil-adelphia: Environmental Change and Social Transformation, 1900–1930," in *The Divided Metropolis* (see note 20), 169–92.

35. Kazal, "The Interwar Origins of the White Ethnic," 86–107. Wolfinger, *Philadelphia Divided*, 11–82.

36. U.S. Bureau of the Census, *Sixteenth Census of the United States* (Washington DC: U.S. G.P.O., 1943), *Population*, vol. 3, "The Labor Force," 30, table 11, and *Sixteenth Census of the United States* (Washington DC: U.S. G.P.O., 1942), *Population*, vol. 1, "Number of Inhabitants" 912, table 3. See the appendix of this book for details. For national trends, see William G. Rothstein, *American Medical Schools and the Practice of Medicine: A History* (New York: Oxford University Press, 1987), esp. 120, table 6.1 and 143, table 7.2.

37. David McBride, *Integrating the City of Medicine: Blacks in Philadelphia Health Care, 1910–1965* (Philadelphia: Temple University Press, 1989).

38. The median net income of Philadelphia doctors in 1929 was $4,207: Nathan Sinai and Alden B. Mills, *A Survey of the Medical Facilities of the City of Philadelphia: 1929*, Publications of the Committee on the Costs of Medical Care, no. 9A (Chicago: University of Chicago Press, 1931), 4–8. There were no other systematic studies of the income of Philadelphia doctors in this period.

39. For a discussion of sources and methods, see the appendix of this book.

40. George D. Wolf, *The Physician's Business: Practical and Economic Aspects of Medi-cine* (Philadelphia: J. B. Lippincott, 1938), 31.

41. Neil Larry Shumsky, James Bohland, and Paul Knox, "Separating Doctors' Homes and Doctors' Offices: San Francisco, 1881–1941," *Social Science and Medicine* 23, no. 10 (1986): 1051–57.

42. *The WPA Guide*, 145. Warner, *The Private City*, 191–94. Hepp, *The Middle-Class City*, 168–207.

43. There were 155,000 business and 191,000 residential telephones in Philadelphia by 1937 (about one for every ten residents, or one for every three households): *The WPA Guide*, 140–41. See also Claude S. Fischer, *America Calling: A Social History of the Telephone to 1940* (Berkeley: University of California Press, 1992), 181, 287–91.

44. Daniel Cathell, *Book on the Physician Himself and Things That Concern His Reputation and Success*, 12th ed. (Philadelphia: F. A. Davis Company, 1913). "Passing of the Country Doctor?" *Bucks County Medical Monthly* 16, no. 11 (1925): 82. "The Doctor's Telephone," *WR* 30, no. 47 (1935): 1369.

45. On office-building construction in Chicago (1871–1930), see: R. D. McKenzie, "The Rise of Metropolitan Communities," in *Recent Social Trends in the United States*, ed. President's Research Committee on Social Trends (New York: McGraw-Hill, 1933), 477. I discovered this source in George Rosen, *The Structure of American Medical Practice, 1875–1941*, ed. Charles E. Rosenberg (Philadelphia: University of Pennsylvania Press, 1983), 54n53.

46. For examples, see: "Proposed Central Doctor's Building," *WR* 5, no. 16 (1909): 1, and "Central Medical Building," *WR* 20 (May 16, 1925): 27.

47. See office rental prices in the following: "Proposed Central Doctor's Building," 1; "Advertisement for Office Space," in *WR* 12, no. 26 (1917) and *WR* 12, no. 32 (1917); "Offices in Professional Center," *WR* 24, no. 40 (1929): 25–26.

48. Sinai and Mills, *A Survey of the Medical Facilities of the City of Philadelphia*, 4–8. In 1929, the median net income of Philadelphia doctors ($4,250) was well above the national median net incomes for doctors ($3,705), as measured in Leven, *The Incomes of Physicians*, 20.

49. "Central Medical Building," *WR* 20 (May 16, 1925): 23–30.

50. "The Baker Biochemical Laboratories," *WR* 25, no. 43 (1930): 16. "Central Medical Building," 30. Ads for private laboratories had become common in Northeast cities by the 1910s to 1920s: Christopher Crenner, "Private Laboratories and Medical Expertise in Boston circa 1900," in *Devices and Designs: Medical Technologies in Historical Perspective*, ed. Carsten Timmermann and Julie Anderson (New York: Palgrave Macmillan, 2006), 61–73.

51. For examples of advertisements targeted to group practices, see: "Central Medical Building," 23–30, and "Two-Physician Suites," *WR* 25, no. 43 (1930): 16.

52. Shumsky et al., "Separating Doctors' Homes and Doctors' Offices," 1054, only briefly mention this important factor.

53. "Central Medical Building," 30.

54. Hepp, *The Middle-Class City*, 3–12.

55. Shumsky et al., "Separating Doctors' Homes and Doctors' Offices," 1056–57. See also Paul Starr, *The Social Transformation of American Medicine* (New York: Basic Books, 1982).

56. "Advertisement for Office Space."

57. For example, see Samuel Hopkins Adams, "The Vanishing Country Doctor," *Ladies' Home Journal* 40, no. 10 (1923): 23, 178, 180; Adams, "Why the Doctor Left," *Ladies' Home Journal* 40, no. 11 (1923): 26, 218–19; "Passing of the Country Doctor," *Bucks County Medical Monthly* 16, no. 11 (1925): 82; and "The Old-Fashioned 'Country Doctor' Disappearing," *WR* 20 (1925): 21, 23. For Philadelphia examples, see Edgar A. Guest, "The Family Doctor," *Bucks County Medical Journal* 13, no. 4 (1922): 40; "Hospital Faddism," *Bucks County Medical Journal* 15, no. 4 (1924): 33; "Editorial Department," *WR* 23, no. 16 (1927): 9, 20; "Concerning Specialism," *PMJ* 34 (1930): 45; Jay Frank Schamberg, "The Salvage of the Family Physician," *WR* 27, no. 15

(1931): 21–22, 25; and "Family Physician Stages a Comeback," *Montgomery County Medical Bulletin* 19, no. 8 (1932): 73–84. For critiques of the "old-time doctor," see: Charles Falkowsky, "The Individual Practitioner," *WR* 22, no. 28 (1927): 21.

58. "Advertisement for Office Space."

59. Paul Starr argued that automobiles increased the incomes of doctors in general: *The Social Transformation of American Medicine*, 70–71. Other historians have showed that the automobile transformed rural medical practice: Michael Berger, "The Influence of the Automobile on Rural Health Care, 1900–1929," *Journal of the History of Medicine and Allied Sciences* 28 (1973): 319–35, and Guenter B. Risse, "From Horse and Buggy to Automobile and Telephone: Medical Practice in Wisconsin, 1848–1930," in *Wisconsin Medicine: Historical Perspectives*, ed. Ronald L. Numbers and Judith W. Leavitt (Madison: University of Wisconsin Press, 1981), 25–45. The influence of automobiles on urban practice, however, remains poorly understood. I thank Christopher Crenner for calling to my attention this historiographical point.

60. "Why Join the Physicians' Motor Club?" *WR* 12, no. 30 (1917): 11. "Physicians' Motor Club Run," *WR* 8, no. 40 (1913): 2.

61. Of the 497 elected college fellows who resided and had a private medical practice in Philadelphia, 371 had a downtown office in 1939 (75 percent). Analysis was based on membership lists: *Transactions of the College of Physicians of Philadelphia*, 4th ser., 8, no. 1 (1940): 67–90. Office addresses were confirmed using the *AMD* (1940). In contrast, from our twenty percent sample of Philadelphia doctors in the *AMD* 1940, only 220 of the 695 doctors (in active practice with a determinable address) had a downtown office (or 32 percent). See the appendix of this book for details.

62. Wolf, *The Physician's Business*, 31.

63. In Philadelphia in 1940, 11 percent of employed African American men worked as janitors, and 23 percent in all nondomestic service jobs combined. Another 29 percent worked as nonfarm and nonmine laborers. 60 percent of employed African American women still worked as domestic servants. By comparison, of employed white men, only 1 percent worked as janitors, only 5 percent worked in all service nondomestic service jobs combined, and only 6 percent worked as nonfarm and nonmine laborers; of employed white women, only 5 percent worked as domestic servants. Data from U.S. Bureau of the Census, *Sixteenth Census of the United States, 1940* (Washington, DC: U.S. G.P.O., 1943), vol. 3, *Population*, 48–53, table 13.

64. Hardin, *The Negroes of Philadelphia*. Miller, "The Black Migration to Philadelphia," 315–50. Charles Pete Banner-Haley, "*The Philadelphia Tribune* and the Persistence of Black Republicanism during the Great Depression," *Pennsylvania History* 65 (1998): 190–99.

65. Hardin, *The Negroes of Philadelphia*, 77–79, 166.

66. Ericksen and Yancey, "Work and Residence in Industrial Philadelphia," 147–82. Marsh, "The Impact of the Market Street 'El,'" 169–92. Greenberg, "Neighborhood Change, Racial Transition, and Work Location," 267–314. Hershberg et al., "A Tale of Three Cities," 461–91.

67. For ward level data on race, see U.S. Bureau of the Census, *Thirteenth Census of the United States, 1910* (Washington, DC: U.S. G.P.O., 1913), vol. 3, *Population*, table 5, 605–8, and U.S. Bureau of the Census, *Sixteenth Census of the United States, 1940* (Washington, DC: U.S. G.P.O., 1942), *Population and Housing: Statistics for Census Tracts*, "Philadelphia, Pa." table 1, 4–5 and table 5, 140–63.

68. McBride, *Integrating the City of Medicine*, 1–122. Of the 632 doctors in active practice in the *AMD* (1909) sample, 40 had offices in the forty-seventh ward, and 36

could be found in the manuscript census for 1910. Of these 1 was listed as "black or Negro" or "mulatto" in 1910; the remainder (35) were white. By comparison, of the 695 doctors in active practice in the *AMD* (1940) sample, only 19 had offices in the forty-seventh ward, and 19 could be found in the manuscript census for 1940. Of these, 4 were listed as "black or Negro," and 15 were white. See table 7 for percentage comparisons and the appendix of this book for details on sources and methods.

69. "Central Offices for Physicians," *WR* 11, no. 15 (1915): 3.

70. For example, see add listed under "For Rent" in *WR* 24, no. 40 (1929): 25–26.

71. Wolf, *The Physician's Business*, 30.

72. For ward-level data on population, see U.S. Bureau of the Census, *Thirteenth Census of the United States, 1910* (Washington, DC: U.S. G.P.O, 1913), vol. 3, *Population*, 549, table 1, and U.S. Bureau of the Census, *Sixteenth Census of the United States, 1940* (Washington DC: U.S. G.P.O., 1942), *Population*, vol. 1, "Number of Inhabitants," 931, table 6. Data on the number of private practices per ward were extrapolated from the *AMD* (1940) sample. See the appendix and table 20 of this book.

73. Bossard, "A Sociologist Looks at the Doctors," 7–8.

74. Sinai and Mills, *A Survey of the Medical Facilities of the City of Philadelphia*, 4–8. See also Leven, *The Incomes of Physicians*, 54–60, and Richardson, "Physicians' Incomes," 38–48.

75. Sinai and Mills, *A Survey of the Medical Facilities of the City of Philadelphia*, 7. R. G. Leland, "Income from Medical Practice," 1684–1685. Leven, *The Incomes of Physicians*, 44–49. Richardson, "Physicians' Incomes," 42.

76. U.S. Bureau of the Census, *Sixteenth Census of the United States, 1940* (Washington, DC: U.S. G.P.O., 1942), *Population and Housing*, "Statistics for Census Tracts: Philadelphia, Pa.," table 1, 4–6, table 2, 25, and table 5, 149. The number of residents per doctor was extrapolated from the *AMD* (1940) sample. See the appendix of this book for details.

77. Harold G. Scheie, Letter to Parents, October 26, 1935 and Thanksgiving Day, 1935, Scheie Papers, UPT 50/S318, Box 2, Folder 2, UPA.

78. "For Rent: Physician's Office," in *WR* 28, no. 40 (1933): 35. "Physician's Office and Residence, S.E. Phila.," in *WR* 20 (June 13, 1925): 29.

79. Dr. Lee Winston Silver, "Summary for 50th Reunion" (1983), Silver Papers, Acc 1995.x.15, Box 1, DUCOM Archives. *AMD* (1940), 1602.

80. "Physician's Office and Residence, S.E. Phila.," 29.

81. "For Sale—Suburban Office and Home Ideally Combined," in *WR* 32, no. 52 (1937): 1535. For discussion, see George Wolf, *The Physician's Business*, 32–33.

82. "For Sale—Suburban Office and Home Ideally Combined," 1535.

83. On the growing commerce of Philadelphia suburbs in this period, see Dyer, "'Holding the Line against Philadelphia," 279–91.

84. U.S. Bureau of the Census, *Census of Business: 1935*, "Intra-City Business Census Statistics for Philadelphia, Pennsylvania" (Washington, DC: U.S. G.P.O., 1937), 26, 30.

85. In an example to be discussed shortly, pediatric specialist Dr. Carl Fischer located his office in the Germantown Professional Building in the late 1930s.

86. Wolf, *The Physician's Business*, 34–35.

87. For examples, see: "For Sale—Physician's Office and Residence, S.E. Philadelphia," 29; "For Sale," *WR* 28, no. 40 (1933): 35; "Opportunity for Physician to Acquire Office and Residence" and "Physicians Home and Office, Together with Practice," in

WR 24, no. 40 (1929): 25–26; and "Unusual Opportunity for Quick Buyer," *WR* 33, no. 48 (1938): 1479.

88. Carl C. Fischer, "Chapter Seven: The Private Practice of Pediatrics, 1931–1969," 1, Carl C. Fischer Papers, uncatalogued collection, Fischer Memoirs, chapter 7 (edited BW), DUCOM Archives.

89. Ibid., 1–2.

90. Ibid., 2.

91. John Modell, "An Ecology of Family Decisions: Suburbanization, Schooling, and Fertility in Philadelphia, 1880–1920," *Journal of Urban History* 6, no. 4 (1980): 397–417.

92. Carl C. Fischer, "Chapter Seven," 9.

93. Ibid., 4.

94. Ibid., 15.

95. For example, see N. D. Jewson, "The Disappearance of the Sick-Man from Medical Cosmology, 1770–1870," *Sociology* 10 (1976): 225–44; Mary E. Fissell, "The Disappearance of the Patient's Narrative and the Invention of Hospital Medicine," in *British Medicine in an Age of Reform*, ed. Roger French and Andrew Wear (London: Routledge, 1991), 92–109; and Stephen Jacyna, "Construing Silence: Narratives of Language Loss in Early Nineteenth-Century France," *Journal of the History of Medicine and Allied Sciences* 49 (1994): 333–61. On the United States, see Steven M. Stowe, "Seeing Themselves at Work: Physicians and the Case Narrative in the Mid-Nineteenth Century American South," *American Historical Review* 101 (1996): 41–79; John Harley Warner, *The Therapeutic Perspective: Medical Practice, Knowledge, and Identity in America, 1820–1885* (Princeton: Princeton University Press, 1997); Warner, *Against the Spirit of the System: The French Impulse in Nineteenth-Century American Medicine* (Baltimore: Johns Hopkins University Press, 1998); and David J Rothman, *Strangers at the Bedside: A History of How Law and Bioethics Transformed Medical Decision-Making* (New York: Basic Books, 1991), 127–47.

96. Charles E. Rosenberg, *The Care of Strangers: The Rise of America's Hospital System* (Baltimore: Johns Hopkins University Press, 1987), esp. 97–121. "The Education of the Interne," *JAMA* 43, no. 7 (1904): 469–470. "The Hospital Intern Year," *JAMA* 60, no. 25 (1913): 2017.

97. Warner, *Against the Spirit of the System*. Russell M. Jones "American Doctors in Paris, 1820–1861: A Statistical Profile," *Journal of the History of Medicine and Allied Sciences* 25 (April 1970), 143–57. Steven M. Stowe, *Doctoring the South: Southern Physicians and Everyday Medicine in the Mid-Nineteenth Century* (Chapel Hill: University of North Carolina Press, 2004), esp. 27–39.

98. At one point during, after his selection as the assistant chief medical officer for an optional second year of internship, Dr. Scheie noted that "I see anywhere from 70 to 100 patients a day including all the emergencies so I learn plenty." See Harold Scheie to Parents, July 12, 1936, Scheie Papers, UPT 50/S318, box 2, folder 3, UPA.

99. Harold Scheie to Parents, October 16, 1935, Scheie Papers, UPT 50/S318, box 2, folder 2, UPA.

100. Ibid.

101. Harold Scheie to Parents, July 3, 1935, Scheie Papers, UPT 50/S318, box 2, folder 2, UPA.

102. Harold Scheie to Parents, August 4, 1935, Scheie Papers, UPT 50/S318, box 2, folder 2, UPA.

103. Ibid. Scheie noted later in the same letter that he hoped next to go to see places such as "Valley Forge, Independence Hall, Liberty Bell, and what not."
104. Harold Scheie to Parents, Oct. 16, 1935, Scheie Papers, UPT 50/S318, box 2, folder 2, UPA.
105. Harold Scheie to Parents, 1935 [date unknown], Scheie Papers, UPT 50/S318, box 2, folder 2, UPA.
106. Ibid.
107. Ibid.
108. Harold Scheie to Parents, Oct. 26, 1935, Scheie Papers, UPT 50/S318, box 2, folder 2, UPA.
109. Harold Scheie to Parents, Thanksgiving Day, 1935, Scheie Papers, UPT 50/S318, box 2, folder 2, UPA.
110. Harold Scheie to Parents, April 28, 1937 and July 30, 1938, Scheie Papers, UPT 50/S318, box 2, folders 4 and 5, UPA.
111. For description of his office and living arrangements, see Harold Scheie to Parents, March 20, 1939, April 10, 1939, and January 27, 1940, Scheie Papers, UPT 50/S318, box 2, folders 6 and 7, UPA.
112. Harold Scheie to Parents, 1935 [date unknown], Scheie Papers, UPT 50/S318, box 2, folder 2, UPA.
113. Harold Scheie to Parents, March 20, 1939, Scheie Papers, UPT 50/S318, box 2, folder 6, UPA.
114. Harold Scheie to Parents, March 5, 1939, Scheie Papers, UPT 50/S318, box 2, folder 6, UPA.

Conclusion

1. Paul Knox, James Bohland, and Neil Larry Shumsky first made this point in "The Urban Transition and the Evolution of the Medical Care Delivery System in America," *Social Science and Medicine* 17 (1983): 37–43.
2. Neil Larry Shumsky, James Bohland, and Paul Knox, "Separating Doctors' Homes and Doctors' Offices: San Francisco, 1881–1941," *Social Science and Medicine* 23, no. 10 (1986): 1051–57. Anne-Marie Adams and Stacie Burke, "A Doctor in the House: The Architecture of Home-Offices for Physicians in Toronto, 1885–1930," *Medical History* 52, no. 2 (2008): 163–94. David Rosner, *A Once Charitable Enterprise: Hospitals and Health Care in Brooklyn and New York, 1885–1915* (Princeton: Princeton University Press, 1982). Paul F. Mattingly, "The Changing Location of Physician Offices in Bloomington-Normal, Illinois: 1870–1988," *Professional Geographer* 43, no. 4 (1991): 465–74.
3. See, for example, Richard Harris and Robert Lewis, "The Geography of North American Cities and Suburbs, 1900–1950: A New Synthesis," *Journal of Urban History* 27, no. 3 (2001): 263–92.
4. Carolyn Adams et al., eds., with Joshua Freely and Michelle Schmitt, *Restructuring the Philadelphia Region: Metropolitan Divisions and Inequality* (Philadelphia: Temple University Press, 2008).
5. See, for example, Thomas Goebel, "American Medicine and the 'Organizational Synthesis': Chicago Physicians and the Business of Medicine, 1900–1920," *BHM* 68 (1994): 639–63; Goebel, "The Uneven Rewards of Professional Labor: Wealth and Income in the Chicago Professions, 1870–1920," *Journal of Social History* 29, no. 4 (1996): 749–77; Donald L. Madison, "Preserving Individualism in the Organizational Society: 'Cooperation' and American Medical Practice, 1900–1920," *BHM* 70 (1996): 442–83; Christopher Crenner, "Organizational Reform and Professional Dissent in

the Careers of Richard Cabot and Ernest Amory Codman, 1900–1920," *Journal of the History of Medicine and Allied Sciences* 56 (2001): 211–37; John Harley Warner, "Grand Narrative and Its Discontents: Medical History and the Social Transformation of American Medicine," and Michael S. Goldstein, "The Persistence and Resurgence of Medical Pluralism," in "Transforming American Medicine: A Twenty-Year Retrospective on The Social Transformation of American Medicine," special issue of *Journal of Health Politics, Policy, and Law* 29, no. 4–5 (2004): 757–80, 925–45.

6. I thank Christopher Crenner for bringing this important point to my attention. Any error in my articulation of this point rests solely with me.

7. For reviews of intra-urban studies, see: John W. Hambleton, "Main Currents in the Analysis of Physician Location" (Madison: Health Economics Research Center at the University of Wisconsin, 1971); Pierre de Vise, *Misused and Misplaced Hospitals and Doctors: A Locational Analysis of the Urban Health Care Crisis* (Washington, DC: Association of American Geographers, Commission on College Geography, 1973); Gary William Shannon and G. E. Alan Dever, *Health Care Delivery: Spatial Perspectives* (New York: McGraw-Hill, 1974); William A. Rushing, *Community, Physicians, and Inequality: A Sociological Study of the Maldistribution of Physicians* (Lexington, MA: Lexington Books, 1975); Barry S. Eisenberg and James R. Cantwell, "Policies to Influence the Spatial Distribution of Physicians: A Conceptual Review of Selected Programs and Empirical Evidence," *Medical Care* 14, no. 6 (1976): 455–68; Health Resources Administration, Office of Graduate Medical Education, "Literature Review of Selected Factors Affecting the Location Decisions of Physicians" (Washington, DC, 1980); Richard L. Ernst and Donald E. Yett, *Physician Location and Specialty Choice* (Ann Arbor, MI: Health Administration Press, 1985); Council on Graduate Medical Education, "Physician Distribution and Health Care Challenges in Rural and Inner-City Areas," ed. U.S. Department of Health and Human Services, Public Health Service, Health Resources and Services Administration, (Washington, DC, 1998).

8. See, for example, Joseph L. Dorsey, "Physician Distribution in Boston and Brookline, 1940 and 1961," *Medical Care* 7, no. 6 (1969): 429–40; Donald Dewey, *Where the Doctors Have Gone: The Changing Distribution of Private Practice Physicians in the Chicago Metropolitan Area, 1950–1970*, Chicago Regional Hospital Study (Chicago: Illinois Regional Medical Program, 1973); David S. Guzick and Rene I. Jahiel, "Distribution of Private Practice Offices of Physicians with Specified Characteristics among Urban Neighborhoods," *Medical Care* 14, no. 6 (1976): 469–88; Patricia Gober and Rena J. Gordon, "Intraurban Physician Location: A Case Study of Phoenix," *Social Science and Medicine* 14D (1980): 407–17; Gerald F. Pyle, "Physician Office Locations within Charlotte, North Carolina," *Southeastern Geographer* 29, no. 2 (1989): 118–35; Gerrit J. Knaap and Diane Blohowiak, "Intraurban Physician Location: New Empirical Evidence," *Medical Care* 27, no. 12 (1989): 1109–16; Mattingly, "The Changing Location of Physician Offices," 465–74; and Donald P. Albert, "Physician Office Locations and Land Use Planning: Asheville, North Carolina, 1948–1993," *North Carolina Geographer* 3 (1994): 31–46.

9. See, for example, Paul J. Jehlik and Robert L. McNamara, "The Relation of Distance to the Differential Use of Certain Health Personnel and Facilities and to the Extent of Bed Illness," *Rural Sociology* 17, no. 3 (1952): 261–65, and Richard L. Morrill, Robert J. Earickson, and Philip Rees, "Factors Influencing Distances Traveled to Hospitals," *Economic Geography* 46, no. 2 (1970): 161–71.

10. Guzick and Jahiel, "Distribution of Private Practice Offices," 469–88. Beatrix Hoffman, "Emergency Rooms: The Reluctant Safety Net," in *History and Health Policy in the United States: Putting the Past Back In*, ed. Rosemary A. Stevens,

Charles E. Rosenberg, and Lawton R. Burns (New Brunswick; NJ: Rutgers University Press, 2006), 250–72. Bonnie Lefkowitz, *Community Health Centers: A Movement and the People Who Made It Happen* (New Brunswick, NJ: Rutgers University Press, 2007). Alondra Nelson, *Body and Soul: The Black Panther Party and the Fight Against Medical Discrimination* (Minneapolis: University of Minnesota Press, 2011). On health policy arguments for using community health centers to address doctor shortages, see: Ralph C. Parker, Richard A. Rix, and Thomas G. Tuxill, "Social, Economic, and Demographic Factors Affecting Physician Population in Upstate New York," *New York State Journal of Medicine* 69 (1969): 706–12; Pierre de Vise, ed., *Slum Medicine: Chicago's Apartheid Health System* (Chicago: Community and Family Study Center, University of Chicago, 1969); David L. Brown, "The Redistribution of Physicians and Dentists in Incorporated Places of the Upper Midwest, 1950–1970," *Rural Sociology* 39, no. 2 (1974): 205–23.

11. For example, see: John C. Norman and Beverly Bennett, eds., *Medicine in the Ghetto* (New York: Appleton-Century-Crofts, 1969); de Vise, ed., *Slum Medicine;* and Jonathan P. Weiner, "A Shortage of Physicians or a Surplus of Assumptions?" *Health Affairs* 21, no. 1 (2002): 160–62.

12. Martin Powell, "Coasts and Coalfields: The Geographical Distribution of Doctors in England and Wales in the 1930s," *Social History of Medicine* 18, no. 2 (2005): 245–63. For critical discussion, see Martin Gorsky, "Local Government Health Services in Interwar England: Problems of Quantification and Interpretation," *BHM* 85, no. 3 (2011): 384–412.

13. For British examples, see Paul L. Knox, "The Intraurban Ecology of Primary Medical Care: Patterns of Accessibility and Their Policy Implications," *Environment and Planning* A10 (1978): 415–35; Knox, "Medical Deprivation, Area Deprivation, and Public Policy," *Social Science and Medicine* 13D, no. 2 (1979): 111–21; D. R. Phillips, "Spatial Variations in Attendance at General Practitioner Services," *Social Science and Medicine* 13D, no. 3 (1979): 169–81; Paul L. Knox, "The Accessibility of Primary Care to Urban Patients: A Geographical Analysis," *Journal of the Royal College of General Practitioners* 29, no. 3 (1979): 160–68; Paul L. Knox and Michael Pacione, "Locational Behaviour, Place Preferences, and the Inverse Care Law in the Distribution of Primary Medical Care," *Geoforum* 11, no. 1 (1980): 43–55; Paul L. Knox, "Measures of Accessibility as Social Indicators: A Note," *Social Indicators Research* 7, no. 4 (1980): 367–77; Knox, "Regional Inequality and the Welfare State: Convergence and Divergence in Levels of Living in the United Kingdom, 1951–1971," *Social Indicators Research* 10, no. 3 (1982): 319–35.

14. William B. Schwartz et al., "The Changing Geographic Distribution of Board-Certified Physicians," *New England Journal of Medicine* 303, no. 18 (1980): 1032–38. Joseph P. Newhouse et al., "Does the Geographical Distribution of Physicians Reflect Market Failure?" *Bell Journal of Economics* 13, no. 2 (1982): 493–505. Joseph P. Newhouse et al., "Where Have All the Doctors Gone?" *JAMA* 247, no. 17 (1982): 2392–96. Joseph P. Newhouse et al., "The Geographic Distribution of Physicians: Is Conventional Wisdom Correct?" (Santa Monica, CA: RAND Corporation, 1982). Albert P. Williams et al., "How Many Miles to the Doctor?" *New England Journal of Medicine* 309, no. 16 (1983): 958–63. Meredith B. Rosenthal, Alan Zaslavsky, and Joseph P. Newhouse, "The Geographic Distribution of Physicians Revisited," *Health Services Research* 40, no. 6, pt. 1 (2005): 1931–52. Michael L. Chernew et al., "Would Having More Primary Care Doctors Cut Health Spending Growth?" *Health Affairs* 28, no. 5 (2009): 1327–35. For a critique of the Newhouse-RAND studies, see Beatrix Hoffman, "Restraining the

Health Care Consumer: The History of Deductibles and Co-Payments in U.S. Health Insurance," *Social Science History* 30, no. 4 (2006): 501–28.

15. Newhouse et al., "The Geographic Distribution of Physicians." Barry S. Eisenberg and James R. Cantwell, "Policies to Influence the Spatial Distribution of Physicians: A Conceptual Review of Selected Programs and Empirical Evidence," *Medical Care* 14, no. 6 (1976): 455–68. Donald E. Pathman, Thomas R. Konrad, and Thomas C. Ricketts, "The Comparative Retention of National Health Service Corps and Other Rural Physicians: Results of a Nine-Year Follow-up Study," *JAMA* 268, no. 12 (1992): 1552–58. George M. Holmes, "Does the National Health Service Corps Improve Physician Supply in Underserved Locations?" *Eastern Economic Journal* 30, no. 4 (2004): 563–81.

16. See Julian Tudor Hart's classic polemic, "The Inverse Care Law," *Lancet* 297, no. 7696 (1971): 405–12. For perspective on Hart's germinal work, and subsequent revisions and rejections thereof among English health care policy scholars, see Graham Watt, "The Inverse Care Law Today," *Lancet* 360, no. 9328 (2002): 252–54.

17. Philip M. Lankford, "Physician Location Factors and Public Policy," *Economic Geography* 50, no. 3 (1974): 244–55.

18. For theories of incremental reform, see: Rosemary A. Stevens, "History and Health Policy in the United States: The Making of a Health Care Industry, 1948–2008," *Social History of Medicine* 21, no. 3 (2008): 461–83; Sven Steinmo and Jon Watts, "It's the Institutions, Stupid! Why Comprehensive National Health Insurance Always Fails in America," *Journal of Health Politics, Policy, and Law* 20, no. 2 (1995): 329–72; Jill Quadagno, "Why the United States Has No Health Insurance: Stakeholder Mobilization against the Welfare State, 1945–1996," in "Health and Health Care in the United States: Origins and Dynamics," ed. Donald W. Light and Ivy Bourgeault, extra issue, *Journal of Health and Social Behavior* 45 (2004): 25–44; Beatrix Hoffman, "Health Care Reform and Social Movements in the United States," *American Journal Public Health* 93, no. 1 (2003): 75–85; and Colin Gordon, *Dead on Arrival: The Politics of Health Care in Twentieth-Century America* (Princeton, NJ: Princeton University Press, 2003).

19. Classic studies of doctor supply include: Rashi Fein, *The Doctor Shortage: An Economic Diagnosis*, Studies in Social Economics (Washington, DC: Brookings Institution, 1967); Martha Katz, David C. Warner, and Dale Whittington, "The Supply of Physicians and Physicians' Incomes: Some Projections," *Journal of Health Politics Policy and Law* 2, no. 2 (1977): 227–56; and Richard Cooper et al., "Economic and Demographic Trends Signal an Impending Physician Shortage," *Health Affairs* 21, no. 1 (2002): 140–54. For excellent reviews, see Jonathan P. Weiner, "A Shortage of Physicians or a Surplus of Assumptions?" 160–62, and David Blumenthal, "New Steam from an Old Cauldron—the Physician-Supply Debate," *New England Journal of Medicine* 350, no. 17 (2004): 1780–87.

20. Summary adapted from Blumenthal, "New Steam from an Old Cauldron."

21. Ibid.

22. See, for example, Steven A. Schroeder and Lewis G. Sandy, "Specialty Distribution of U.S. Physicians—the Invisible Driver of Health Care Costs?" *New England Journal of Medicine* 328, no. 13 (1993): 961–63, and David H. Mark et al., "Medicare Costs in Urban Areas and the Supply of Primary Care Physicians," *Journal of Family Practice* 42, no. 1 (1996): 33–39. For dissenting views, see Michael L. Chernew et al., "Would Having More Primary Care Doctors Cut Health Spending Growth?" 1327–35.

23. See Weiner's summary of these arguments in "A Shortage of Doctors or a Surplus of Assumptions?"

24. For a summary of the debate, see David Hemenway, "The Optimal Location of Doctors," *New England Journal of Medicine* 306, no. 7 (1982): 397–401.

Appendix

1. George Weisz, "Medical Directories and Medical Specialization in France, Britain, and the United States," *BHM* 71 (1997): 23–68.
2. Ibid. Frank V. Cargill, "The American Medical Directory," in *A History of the American Medical Association, 1847–1947*, ed. Morris Fishbein (Philadelphia: W. B. Saunders Company, 1947), 1170–79.
3. The following were used: George W. Bromley and Walter S. Bromley, *Atlas of the City of Philadelphia, Complete in One Volume* (Philadelphia: G. W. Bromley and Co., 1895, 1899, and 1910 editions); *A New Map of the City of Philadelphia for C.E. Howe Co.* (1908), *Philadelphia Street Name Changes*, rev. ed. with reverse directory, prep. Jefferson M. Moak (Philadelphia: Chestnut Hill Almanac, 2001); and *Ward Genealogy of the City and County of Philadelphia*, comp. Allen Weinburg and Dale Fields, with Charles E. Hughes Jr. (Philadelphia: Department of Public Records, 1958).
4. *AMD* (1909), advt. 3.
5. *AMD* (1929), 1273–1301. Nathan Sinai and Alden B. Mills, *A Survey of the Medical Facilities of the City of Philadelphia, 1929*, Publications of the Committee on the Costs of Medical Care, no. 9A (Washington, DC, 1929), 5. See also: Maurice Leven, *The Incomes of Physicians: An Economic and Statistical Analysis*, Publications of the Committee on the Costs of Medical Care, no. 24 (Chicago: University of Chicago Press, 1932), 50–51; R. G. Leland, *Distribution of Physicians in the United States* (Chicago: AMA Press, 1935), 39–44; and Weisz, "Medical Directories and Medical Specialization."
6. *The Professional Directory of Doctors and Druggists of Philadelphia, Including Camden and Atlantic City and Eighty Nearby Towns* (Philadelphia: Edward Trust, 1910), 163–75.
7. Ibid., 209–66.
8. For discussion, see R. Darcy and Richard Rohrs, *A Guide to Quantitative History* (Westport, CT: Praeger, 1995).
9. Groups of sample doctors that were being compared varied in size. For example, the number of specialists was different from the number of GPs in the 1909 sample. There was no reason to assume a similar distribution of experience values among specialists and GPs, so we used an algorithm that did not assume equal variances in this and all Student's t-tests performed.
10. Neil Larry Shumsky, James Bohland, and Paul Knox, "Separating Doctors' Homes and Doctors' Offices: San Francisco, 1881–1941," *Social Science and Medicine* 23, no. 10 (1986): 1051–57, esp. 1053, table 1.
11. "Biographical Card Index and Directory," *JAMA* 45 (1905): 1574–75. I thank George Weisz for calling my attention to this source, and for his helpful discussion of the meaning of addresses in the *AMD* when we met at the 2004 AAHM meeting in Madison, Wisconsin.
12. *AMD* (1940), esp. "Data Following Names" description found on a pullout key entitled "How to Use the American Medical Directory."
13. Ibid.
14. *AMD* (1909), 970–72. U.S. Bureau of the Census, "Benevolent Institutions, 1910" (Washington, DC: U.S. G.P.O., 1913), 346–49, 390–93. *Philadelphia City Register* (Philadelphia: C. E. Howe Co., 1910).
15. *AMD* (1940), 1530–31.

Index

Page numbers followed by the letter *f* indicate figures; those by *m*, maps; those by *t*, tables.

About the Author

James A. Schafer Jr. is an assistant professor in the Department of History at the University of Houston. His work examines the social, political, and economic history of American medicine and health care. He began his career as a cellular and molecular biologist before earning his Ph.D. from the Institute of the History of Medicine at the Johns Hopkins School of Medicine.

Available titles in the Critical Issues in Health and Medicine series:

Alyssa Picard, *Making the American Mouth: Dentists and Public Health in the Twentieth Century*

Heather Munro Prescott, *The Morning After: A History of Emergency Contraception in the United States*

David G. Schuster, *Neurasthenic Nation: America's Search for Health, Happiness, and Comfort, 1869–1920*

Karen Seccombe and Kim A. Hoffman, *Just Don't Get Sick: Access to Health Care in the Aftermath of Welfare Reform*

Leo B. Slater, *War and Disease: Biomedical Research on Malaria in the Twentieth Century*

Paige Hall Smith, Bernice L. Hausman, and Miriam Labbok, *Beyond Health, Beyond Choice: Breastfeeding Constraints and Realities*

Matthew Smith, *An Alternative History of Hyperactivity: Food Additives and the Feingold Diet*

Rosemary A. Stevens, Charles E. Rosenberg, and Lawton R. Burns, eds., *History and Health Policy in the United States: Putting the Past Back In*

Barbra Mann Wall, *American Catholic Hospitals: A Century of Changing Markets and Missions*

Frances Ward, *The Door of Last Resort: Memoirs of a Nurse Practitioner*

CPSIA information can be obtained at www.ICGtesting.com
Printed in the USA
BVOW08s1233071113

335679BV00003B/10/P